"I find your bo⟨...⟩ ⟨...⟩n that you have proba⟨...⟩ including myse⟨...⟩ ⟨...⟩mately involved in the⟨...⟩

    Dr. J. ⟨...⟩e Witwatersrand and Johannesburg Hospital, Johannesburg, South Africa.

"This is indeed a revealing exposé of an often misunderstood syndrome depicted in detail with passion and deep personal concern. It is a factual, hardhitting, informational book, verbally illustrating the pitfalls of commission and/or omission in the diagnosis of mitral valve prolapse. The author is to be complimented in converting personal experience, backed with sound scientific knowledge, into a book of this nature. It is hoped that the publication of this book will have a profound bearing on the prevention of the complications associated with heart disease."

    Barry S. Krasner, M.D., Former Director of Cardiopulmonary Medicine, Memorial Hospital of Green County, N.Y.
    Assistant Clinical Professor, Department of Anesthesiology, Albert Einstein College of Medicine/Montefiore Medical Center, N.Y.
    Director, Ambulatory Infusion and Pain Clinic, Valatie, N.Y.

"Sharon Anderson is an exceptional and truly extraordinary cardiac patient. She has a brilliantly logical and inquisitive mind. She has written a fascinating, compelling and informative book . . . a beautifully written book which is difficult to put down . . . She has demonstrated an admirable courage and persistence in collecting information, studying the basic cardiac principles and writing this book . . . which she initially undertook to help her own situation but, in the end, realized it could benefit all MVP patients. I highly recommend that this book be read not only by cardiac patients but also by physicians, technologists and biomedically interested persons."

    Dr. Benedict Kingsley, former Adjunct Professor of Medicine (Cardiology) and former Assistant Professor of Diagnostic Radiology, Hahnemann Medical University.
    Trustee and Program Director National Foundation for Non-Invasive Diagnostics, Princeton, N.J.

MITRAL VALVE PROLAPSE

BENIGN SYNDROME?

Second Edition

Sharon Anderson

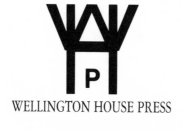

WELLINGTON HOUSE PRESS

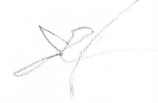

Canadian Cataloguing in Publication Data

Anderson, Sharon (Sharon Rose)
  Mitral valve prolapse : benign syndrome?

2nd ed.
Includes bibliographical references and index.
ISBN 0-9694302-1-3

1. Anderson, Sharon (Sharon Rose)
2. Mitral valve - Displacement - Patients - Biography.
3. Infective endocarditis.   4. Therapeutics, Dental.
5. Diagnostic errors.   I. Title.

RC685.V2A5 1994   362.1'96125'0092   C94-932356-X

The names of all dentists, doctors and hospitals which I refer to in my treatment, with the exception of Dr. John B. Barlow and the Mayo Clinic, are fictitious.

Wellington House Press
24 Wellington Street West
Barrie, Ontario, Canada L4N 1K2
Telephone: (705) 737-1458

Typeset by Video Text Inc., Barrie, Ontario.

In Loving Memory of Margo

FOREWORD

Drawing on her craft as a novelist, Sharon Anderson weaves the story of her personal experience with Mitral Valve Prolapse (MVP) and one of its complications (infective endocarditis) into an exciting tale which holds the attention of the reader from chapter to chapter. Some physicians would have us believe mitral valve prolapse is overdiagnosed while others believe it is underdiagnosed. This book carries a strong message, a lesson to be remembered by physicians, that, if a patient has a condition or disease, no matter how common or uncommon it is, it may markedly alter their health status and qualify of life.

In her book, Sharon provides us with some unique insights into this oft misunderstood and even maligned malady. Her personal experience with this common and usually benign condition reminds us there is a spectrum of severity with all conditions and illnesses. That there is sex bias within the medical profession and that women's complaints are often viewed as psychiatric in origin are frequent complaints of the female patient. Some physicians may well view Sharon's odyssey to find answers as neurotic doctor shopping. However, reading this book will reveal such is far from the case, that it, in fact, became necessary for her to pursue the medical care she instinctively knew was necessary for her survival. Close scrutiny of her frightening observations and experience helps us to understand the multi-faceted nature of the patient-doctor relationship and why it is that women make these complaints. Sometimes directly and sometimes by intimation, she reveals those less than admirable traits of some whose names are followed by "M.D.", such as the reluctance to accept data, information or observations from patients or others (nurses or techs). The noted Canadian physician, Sir William Osler reminded physicians nearly a century ago that we should "Listen to the patient. He's giving you the diagnosis."

With passion and deep commitment to sharing her experience and knowledge with the public and professionals alike, Sharon takes us on a journey where we become witnesses to the metamorphosis of a frightened, bewildered patient into the author who chronicles her illness in a well-documented fashion. She articulately describes the natural history of her own experience with the mitral valve prolapse syndrome and her development of infectious endocarditis even while under medical (albeit blunted) scrutiny. She discovers other less virtuous traits in some of her physician encounters when her questions and concerns were met with disinterest, lack of compassion and even hostility and termination of caregiving on the part of her physicians. Apart from these disturbing insights into the patient/physician relationship, altered by an obscure and difficult diagnostic problem, she describes the fascinating journey through the circulatory system from a patient's viewpoint. To describe her as a layperson would not be appropriate since her thirst to define her own illness extended to include a bibliography of over 500 articles and books.

From the perspective of one not associated with the medical profession, Sharon offers us valuable insights about ourselves as physicians, our relationships with our support people (nurses, technologists, aides, secretaries, etc.) and the interaction of this total medical complex with that necessary component which drives it, namely, the *patient*. In this time of increased awareness of the cardiovascular health problems of women, hers is yet another female cry in the wilderness that must be heard. She movingly contrasts the plight of the female patient, wanting to participate in her care, with that of a male patient, another layperson, Norman Cousins, whose input was welcomed by medical professionals, and who was, in his own words, in "Anatomy of an Illness", a "respected partner" in his care.

Physicians who observe multiple patients with a disease process are often able to document and describe the illness, do statistical research and educate other professionals. However, frequently, the psychosocial impact on patients and their perceptions and understanding regarding the disease are minimized or not addressed at all. Sharon points to a new kind of relationship, a sharing one, between the patient and the physician. A sharing of wisdom that is necessary to the healing process. If the patient is perceptive, some of his/her wisdom and knowledge of a given illness or condition can become a window that fully rounds out our understanding of a disease process.

This book is important to the public and professionals alike. Physicians who are in primary care medicine would be well advised to read it to better understand the often bizarre and unusual, but real, symptoms which are experienced by the large number of patients who have this condition and whom they may unknowingly encounter daily in their practice.

Some patients with mitral valve prolapse may be further frightened by her story and will require a compassionate physician to put it into proper perspective. Conversely, those who are not intimidated and those who have faced an illness will find many descriptions which often fit their own symptoms or experiences and thus this book will serve a very therapeutic, supportive and reassuring purpose.

In conclusion, it is hoped Sharon's book will have a significant impact on the understanding and prevention of complications related to heart disease and, in particular, to MVP. It is also hoped that its insights, not only into the disease process and its testing procedures but into the patient-physician relationship, will have a substantial effect on the reduction of healthcare costs.

Dr. Walt Weaver,
Cardiologist and
Clinical Professor of Medicine,
University of Nebraska.

Table of Contents

Introduction:
Flies to the Gods

A woman, 31 years of age, while playing tennis with her husband suddenly stopped the game, walked in a natural manner to the side of the court and sat down. She fumbled at her shoelacing and then called to her husband, "Come over here." To her husband's question, "What is the matter?" she replied, "I don't know; I feel sick." With these words her body relaxed, and she sank slowly to the left side, became unconscious and could not be aroused . . . the physician who was summoned arrived quickly and found her cyanotic, pulseless, but still breathing. She was taken without delay to a hospital . . . but was dead on arrival. Investigation disclosed the facts that the woman was an athletic instructor, that she was an expert swimmer and had lately been sought as a swimming instructor, for a large educational institution. She played tennis and rode horseback regularly. Her husband never knew of his wife's being ill or making any complaint . . . on the day of her death, she was in her usual health, had eaten a hearty dinner and riden in an automobile about five miles to reach the tennis court. The game had just begun as she showed her first sign of distress . . . at the bifurcation of the left coronary artery was found the cause of death, an embolus . . .[1]

The reader, in all probability, will imagine that the young woman, described in the above passage, died from a sudden heart attack. Everyone, at some time or other, has known or heard of a person, in excellent health like this tennis player, who drops dead unexpectedly. Unfortunately, many doctors would likely agree that the cause of death of this athletic, young woman was a heart attack, especially in the absence of a careful autopsy. In most cases, this is certainly all the doctor would feel is necessary to tell the grief stricken family. And certainly family and friends are likely to demand little more information. Everyone knows what a heart attack is and everyone dreads it like the sword of Damocles. The medical profession is largely responsible for the creation of this fearful bogeyman. It is doctors who have given us the term "heart attack" which conjures up the image of some dark monster hiding, waiting to spring upon us without warning. And our sins are decried: our smoking, our diets, our Type "A" personalities. In general, doctors have made it their business to simplify illness and death for the public, and few people question. But no term is more all inclusive, more sweeping, than the term, "heart attack", which the media has transformed into a household word. For the doctor it is both a convenient label to make the job easier and a cudgel, so familiar, so threatening, that the very word alone pumps adrenalin into the bloodstream in classic Pavlovian response and suppresses further investigation or any challenge of medical opinion. The heart attack is tinged with the miraculous, beyond even the power of the gods to prevent.

This athletic, young woman did not, however, die of a heart attack. Her death was caused by an infection which is called Bacterial Endocarditis (BE) or, more correctly, Infective Endocarditis (IE), a common and very serious complication for those with the heart condition called Mitral Valve Prolapse (MVP) that is the subject of this book. IE can produce the classic symptoms of a heart attack. Today, this disease is totally preventable and, in the words of one British physician, Dr. Joan Weyman, "should never happen at all."[2]

The majority of doctors believe IE is rare and rarer still in the MVP syndrome. Its rarity, however, is a myth nurtured by errors in diagnosis. IE is a disease that, for an unprepared doctor, is very difficult to diagnose and is easily mistaken for other less serious illnesses, in particular viral infections, flu, tonsillitis or even the common sore throat and cold. Another myth is that IE is an acute, fulminant infection which is immediately fatal, and that no one recovers from it without massive doses of IV antibiotics for lengthy periods of time. However, even with treatment, if it is delayed, IE can result in death, and, in virtually all cases, this common bacterial infection will cause a deformed or leaky valve in the heart to deteriorate in function. Unless the valve is repaired or replaced with an artificial device, heart failure will occur sooner or later and, when all else fails, heart transplant must inevitably be the last desperate resort. But the public rarely sees the medical or autopsy report on the cause of death, or challenges it, and, in cases similar to that of this young woman, shocked friends and relatives would never question the doctor's verdict of "heart attack", the silent kind, happening suddenly out of the blue.

The bacterial infection from which this young woman died is one to which many people with certain heart problems are susceptible. Individuals with the thickened, ballooning or bulging valves, the valvular abnormality which gives rise to the name Mitral Valve Prolapse (MVP), are particularly vulnerable to IE. In fact, their risk is 8.2 times greater than that for people with normal hearts.[3] Because this young woman had, at autopsy, no evidence of any deformity of the heart or its valves, in particular any signs of rheumatic heart disease, which the majority of doctors still incorrectly think underlies most cases of IE, she likely had MVP. But, at the time of her death in 1931, MVP and its pathological signs, that can range from the microscopic to the overt, had not been identified, and the clinical findings and patient symptoms associated with this condition most physicians of the day would have considered totally insignificant. The attitude of many of today's physicians towards MVP is, however, depressingly identical, despite voluminous research over many years on MVP. Many doctors, even currently, believe MVP is an entirely benign condition and the set of symptoms related to the heart neurotic in origin.

MVP is the "most common" of all heart diseases[4], yet ironically it remains almost unknown to the public. Even those individuals who have the condition may be unaware. And there are still a great many doctors who are unable to identify it. It is my hope that, with this book, MVP, like cancer, arthritis or heart attack, will become a household word. Most people who know they have MVP, likely came to this knowledge casually or accidentally and, for all too many, tragically, with IE and the replacement of the mitral valve in their hearts. The major reason for the lack of information about MVP is the long established opposition of the medical profession to public education in general and to granting the patient access to his or her own personal medical information, specifically when MVP is part of the medical picture.

How would you know you have MVP? There are many common and not so common symptoms: palpitations which make you more aware of the beating of your heart, various cardiac arrhythmias such as extra beats, episodes of extremely rapid and/or irregular heart beat, frequently when falling to sleep or waking, dizziness, often brief, non-disabling black-outs, especially on standing up, fatigue, which may be particularly noticeable upon waking in the morning, shortness of breath (SOB) on exertion, chest pain that is generally left sided, episodes of partial or complete fainting, myopia and migraine. In males, other clues to MVP may be narrow chest dimensions and underdeveloped physique or asthenic build, that is, tall, slender and angular with poor muscular development. Women with MVP are also frequently underdeveloped and have boyish, athletic figures with flat-chest and narrow hips. The tennis player referred to was said to have these skeletal characteristics. But most important of all, you may be entirely asymptomatic and have **none** of these physical signs nor any symptoms. It has been suggested that, "for every patient with symptomatic MVP, there are hundreds of asymptomatic persons."[5]

However, if you report these symptoms to your doctor, it is likely that he will attribute them to anxiety or a lack of physical fitness, rather than to MVP, especially if you are a woman. In fact, many doctors like to call MVP "the disease of anxious women". Doctors hold this opinion because they believe MVP is found in more women than men, in a ratio of about four to one. However, there is evidence that MVP is found equally in men and women and, over 100 years ago, was found first exclusively in men. What caused doctors to promote MVP as a disease of women? This is one of the many questions I will address in this book.

If your doctor says he has heard something unimportant in your heart, and if you have any of the aforementioned symptoms, in all likelihood you have MVP. In using this non-descriptive word, "something", I am being deliberately vague. "Something" is a word which doctors favour if they decide to tell the patient of the presence of MVP. A general physician or, perhaps a specialist — rarely does an MVP patient actually get to see a heart specialist — may have said he has heard a "funny noise', a "queer sound" or a "click" in your heart. Or your doctor might be more generous in his description and tell you that he has heard a "harmless", "functional" or "innocent" murmur. Doctors will rarely, if ever, tell you that these sounds, in particular the sound of a murmur, mean that your heart is less than perfect. Frequently, your doctor will decide not to tell you what he has found, and there is much evidence that this is a growing trend within the medical profession. But you protest, you do not want to hear that your heart is in any way imperfect, especially if you feel well. However, to keep this pump-engine running smoothly, to prevent deterioration that can halt its function altogether, you must possess this knowledge because, more often than not, your doctor will fail to protect you from IE and thus from further damage to your heart valves and the greater increase in complications that follow.

Extraordinary numbers of people in the United States, Canada and the rest of the world have MVP. Six to twenty percent of the adult population, not to mention children, have MVP according to the American Heart Association.[6] Some American researchers have attempted to estimate the actual number of people with this condition. They say it is in the range between 13 and 21.6 million people in the United States.[7] Other American researchers have reported a 21 percent incidence in healthy, young women[8], a 4 percent incidence in healthy, young men,[9] though other researchers have found MVP equally in men and women[10], and a 5 percent incidence in the general pediatric population.[11] Another study found that 7 percent of new-born baby girls have MVP.[12] If we take the number to be in the 5-10 percent range for the general population, a figure most researchers agree upon[13], 1.3 to 2.5 million Canadians would have MVP.

There are about 12,500 cases of IE that are reported annually in the US. Mandatory reporting is not required in either Canada or the United States. This means, therefore, that the actual number of cases per year is unknown. A study of four large series of IE patients admitted consecutively to American hospitals shows an incidence of 13 — 15 percent, or about 1,625 of the 12,500 cases, of patients with this disease would have underlying MVP.[14] In Canada, where our population is ten percent of that in the US, these figures might translate into approximately 1,250 cases per annum with 160 to 170 of these in association with MVP. In fact, the figure for those cases involving MVP is nearer to that of all the reported cases of the disease in association with all heart conditions that pose a risk or even the total number of recorded deaths. For example, in 1986 in Canada, there were 187 deaths from IE.[15] This is a very small number which does not reflect accurately the actual number of cases according to research I will bring forward in this book. There is convincing evidence that the incidence of IE and the mortality are greatly underestimated in both Canada and the US.

According to an important study in the American Heart Journal in 1987 individuals with MVP and a significant heart murmur are thirteen times more likely to contract IE than those with MVP without a murmur, and people over the age of forty-five are four times more likely to get IE than younger people with prolapse.[16] The benefits of keeping the condition stable are obvious, and there is information in the medical literature, as I will demonstrate, to strongly suggest that IE causes mitral valve prolapse and that IE or prolapse begets further prolapse or increased deterioration in the valves. The significance of this is underlined by the fact that two of three patients with a severe MVP murmur, or a pansystolic murmur, PSM, develop heart failure and that progression from a late systolic murmur, LSM, to a PSM is "frequently associated with clinical deterioration."[17] Yet, the patient may not know this. He or she may have noticed an increase in breathlessness with activities once performed easily or an increase in fatigue and still not know there has been any valvular deterioration.

Though many doctors still continue to think that MVP is a benign, unimportant condition, researchers have long ago proven otherwise. In addition to the bacterial infection which killed the young athlete, MVP is known to cause myocardial or cerebral infarction, that is pure heart attack, unassociated with IE, and stroke, two of the most important causes of mortality. It is not likely that your doctor will tell you MVP is a disease, one that should be taken seriously. And he will not tell you that there are these four major complications: infective endocarditis, progression to severe regurgitation and cardiac failure from a leaky mitral valve, thromboembolism and sudden death from cardiac arrhythmias. In Canada, cardiovascular disease claims over 75,000 lives each year.[18] 400,000 Americans succumb to sudden death from heart disease each year, and it is believed that, among the MVP population, individuals with MVP and mitral regurgitation have a fifty to one hundred fold greater risk of sudden death.[19] How many of these cardiovascular deaths in either country are caused from MVP?

Because MVP is so poorly understood and often not even recognized by the doctor in his day to day practice, patients, and the public in general, know even less about this condition. Many doctors claim there's not much to tell their patients because MVP has only recently been identified. However, this is incorrect, and doctors are misleading their patients. MVP, christened with at least a dozen different names, has been recognized for over a century. Its history is not only long and startling but has also included the phenomenon of war. Older doctors, who may have been aware of the characteristics of the abnormal heart sounds for years, choose to ignore them as unimportant. Such doctors do not know that the opinions of medical scientists towards this cardiac condition have changed dramatically a long time ago.

However, despite the fact that MVP is one of the most talked about topics in the medical literature, apart from a few pathological observations, very little is known of the cause of the prolapsed valves and, while researchers have observed the mechanisms of deterioration, they have made surprisingly few conclusions. There is no known "cure", so to speak, but there are reliable methods of preventing deterioration of the mitral valve. It is crucial, therefore, that doctors search diligently for MVP in all their patients.

Individuals with MVP are often said to have a totally different body chemistry, lean toward cerebral pursuits and artistic endeavors but possess a nervous or neurasthenic disposition, what doctors refer to as "anxious personalities". Some famous artists may have suffered from this common heart conditon. Maria Callas, for instance, was said to possess an unusually high palate shaped like a Gothic arch[20], and the Canadian pianist, Glen Gould, had long, spindly fingers and an asthenic body build. These physical characteristics are often associated with MVP and, in these cases, may have paradoxically contributed to the great talents of these artists as well as to their untimely deaths. Genius, Freud said, bordered on neurosis. A case might even be made for linking MVP with an impressive list of famous individuals of unique intellectual and artistic gifts whom doctors would likely call "neurotic" or "anxious". To name a few, Florence Nightingale, Elizabeth Barrett Browning and, especially, Virginia Woolf who had the distinctly angular and asthenic build found in MVP patients. All of these women had histories of "mysterious" cardiovascular disorders with symptoms similar to those found in MVP. What is only highly suspected in Maria Callas and Glenn Gould, pathologist, Dr. Frederick Zugibe, has acknowledged as virtually conclusive in Abraham Lincoln.[21]

Unfortunately, it is precisely the neurotic fog clouding the understanding of MVP that has led doctors to make diagnostic errors, which can result in tragedy, in the handling of patients who report symptoms of this disease. And it is this neurotic fog that has encouraged the study of females rather than males with this disorder. The stress doctors place on neurosis is also another reason why the public knows so little about MVP. When I was first told that I had this condition in 1976, I had never heard of MVP though extensive research had been reported in many of the medical journals for over ten years. Most readers will likely begin this book with little or no knowledge about MVP. Out of respect for the dignity and intelligence of the lay person I will not use the "ticker-belly-bum talk-down" language doctors reserve specifically for patients. There is no medical expression that cannot be dissected and rendered intelligible with the aid of a medical dictionary and an illustrated anatomy atlas. It is time that medical terminology was purged of its mystery. If we think of our high school studies of Greek mythology and of Apollo, who was both the sun god and the god of healing, we will have no trouble realizing why most medical terms come from Greek. For example, the Greek word, "haima" or "hema", for blood is the root of many medical words such as hematuria, blood in the urine, or hematology, the study of the blood and its diseases. Many other medical terms come from Latin, such as the verb, "infarcire", meaning to stuff, which is the source of the word, infarction, which means the blocking of an artery, cerebral in the brain, myocardial in the heart or, in common parlance, heart attack and stroke.

Democratic nations cherish, even revere, freedom of information, and ours is a time that demands honesty, accountability, full disclosure. Who among us does not believe it is our right to have the full truth about the military and political intrigues, the patronage scandals of our governments or the greed of industrial forces that are depleting our natural resources or polluting and ultimately destroying our environment, our very habitat? Why then are we not clamouring for the truth, for complete disclosure of personal health information? It is my hope that this book will enable the reader to appreciate the full horror of that ironic couplet from the pen of the 18th century poet, Alexander Pope, "A little Learning is a dang'rous Thing." It was this famous quotation which a specialist tossed out at me when he was greatly angered by my reading the medical literature to understand MVP. All doctors I encountered, with the exception of Dr. John Barlow of South Africa, who eventually agreed with the conclusion I drew from my medical data, as I laboriously pieced my history together, convinced me that they are the elite who conceive that only they are entitled to know what is truly in the patient's personal medical record and that they have the exclusive right to guard this information from the patient. When you turn the last page of this book, you will have drunk deep of the Pierian Spring as the wise poet cautioned us to do. And, thus, fully informed about MVP and its risks you will be able to assume a responsible role in your own health care. You will be able to benefit from years of research on MVP, as is your right, and avoid the unhappy events that overwhelmed myself and others. And, for those who do not have MVP, this is a story of one person's efforts to obtain personal health information from a very powerful group about a condition that has confused the medical establishment for over a hundred years.

Mitral Valve Prolapse: Benign Syndrome? is not a book whose sole purpose is to alarm. Its underlying objective is to inform people in order to keep them healthy. It must, therefore, be a book about oppression, not just of the sick, that long neglected minority group, but of all consumers of health care services. However, to become responsible, knowledgeable health care consumers might well be the most difficult challenge of our lives, one with seemingly insurmountable obstacles. It is that challenge which is the substance of this story of a struggle for human rights. The right to health is the inalienable right of every person but it cannot be had without the concomitant right of access to personal health information which, as Ontario Supreme Court judge, the Hon. Justice Horace Krever, said, is "a measure of human dignity".[22] We are also entitled to benefit from medical knowledge that has accumulated over the decades and to which everyone has contributed in tax dollars and in personal suffering.

The right to personal health information is being violated daily by those who do not possess but only defend medical knowledge from public acquisition. We live, in a sense, in the Dark Ages, vis-à-vis the medical profession which is one of the rare groups unwilling to share its knowledge, especially when the patient's health changes adversely. Ironically, those dedicated to relieving the oppression of illness are, in fact, often the oppressors. The only road to freedom from that oppression lies, therefore, in being fully informed and, therefore, fully armed with all the medical knowledge that has accumulated on our bodies from the first second we enter a doctor's office or a hospital and become a patient. Access to that knowledge means access to health and, to assure ourselves of this right to health, we will have to wage a formidable battle against the medical profession, its doctors, the hospitals, local medical societies, the governing colleges and all health care workers to whom we are obliged to submit, like children, for their assistance.

Recently, when I was hospitalized and was waiting impotently in a wheelchair for an echocardiogram, I chanced to look at the book containing my medical observations, tests etc., which I had been asked to carry. A technician instantly rushed toward me and slapped the book shut. "This is not for you to see," she pronounced with great anxiety. This happening confirms that, we, the patients, are the hewers of wood and drawers of water; we serve as the laboratory animals who are ultimately sacrificed so that our bodies may be studied in order to provide the medical profession with knowledge that it may or may not use. The actions of this technician, who will plead, like any good soldier, that she is only doing her duty in carrying out the orders of her superior, can only be felt as an enormous insult, a blow to the human dignity of the patient. Such orders that reflect the attitudes of the entire medical profession have no place in the enlightened societies of the world which publicly commit themselves to the protection of human rights and are praised for doing so. You may believe that your doctor is always open and frank with you, but, when questioned or challenged, when the medical record is asked for, doctors will prove themselves members of a secretive, elitist group that exercises an uncontested monopoly over personal health information which they guard from patient view at the expense of the sick entrusted to their care. It is only because of our own uncritical, unassailable faith in doctors, tantamount to that which we have given throughout the history of civilization to a god or gods, that these privileged groups continue to be permitted to hoard and defend this knowledge. It is time for the wellbeing of the patient to be put above the private interests of the doctor.

A totally preventable illness struck me, which took me many years to understand, one which I will show was the same which killed the young woman described in my opening paragraphs. When I sought an explanation for the deterioration in my health, the machinery of an army ground into place, and crucial medical records mysteriously vanished. This illness left me with symptoms that were gradually revealed as those of heart failure with two leaky valves and cardiac enlargement, but, although my doctor has prescribed drugs, diuretics and digitalis, specific for heart failure, he has continued to question its existence and deny the cause.

My experience is not unique. It is something that has happened to many people who have attempted to oppose the control of the medical profession over health information. Such a struggle, to be fully appreciated, could be compared to the struggle against a powerful dictatorship. My search for information and the disappearance of my medical history is an event equivalent, in some respects, to an event which the Czechoslovakian author, Milan Kundera, relates in his novel, *The Book of Laughter and Forgetting*. Kundera begins his tale with an impressive happening that interweaves truth and fiction. It is 1948 in Prague, a time when the fateful romance with Communism was in flower. Klement Gottwald, party co-founder and eventual President of Czechoslovakia, is addressing millions of countrymen from the balcony of the Baroque Palace in Prague. Close to Gottwald, participating in his glory, are the current political darlings of this new regime. It is a bitterly cold, wintry day. Gottwald shivers, and one, Clementis, responding with a burst of compassion, removes his fur cap and places it on the bare head of the trembling Gottwald.

This is a moment in time of vast social, political and historical significance. The flashbulbs snap; party propaganda circulates hundreds of thousands of photographs commemorating Clementis' model act of generosity towards the regime. Newspapers, magazines, posters, books, school texts, museums — all implant this fragment of history in the hearts of the Czech people. Four years later, Kundera tells us, Clementis fell from favour and was hanged for treason in one of Gottwald's great purges. It was not, however, the execution of Clementis but the events which followed in the wake of terror that accurately translate the meaning of tyranny, of the seizure of power. For Czechoslovakia, this was the wholesale slaughter of its culture, the obliteration of its history and past, that which assures the continuity and thus the significance of humanity. The completeness of the act of violence was symbolized in the Party orders to airbrush Clementis out of the photographs and re-issue new pictures showing only Gottwald alone on the balcony, a fur cap on his head, pathetic testimony that Clementis had once been favoured, had once even existed.

The fur cap tells it all. Only the traces of the truth remain while the real evidence has vanished. But, the reader will protest, Czechoslovakia is not Canada. Our people with power do not, like the oppressive nations of the world, destroy evidence, wipe out history. We do not live in the kind of meaningless world that Kundera has described. Although the events I describe in this book are on a tiny scale in comparison to those in Kundera's novel and, although the subtle replaces the obvious, the insidious the overt, the destruction of my medical history is no less an act of aggression, a violation of the rights of the patient. When all the facts are exposed, the actions of the entrusted bodies, invested with powers and privileges denied ordinary citizens, cannot possibly even faintly resemble the activities of responsible, democratic, caring citizens.

Our rights are supposedly enshrined in The Canadian Charter of Rights and Freedoms. This document represents the definitive expression of an advanced, highly moral society. But the disappearance of my medical records — and that action can only be viewed as intentional in the light of the highly suspicious circumstances surrounding their disappearance — and other coercive efforts to silence me make a mockery of the principle of justice contained in our Constitution that "Everyone has the right to life, liberty and security of the person and the right not to be deprived thereof."[23] My x-rays, print-outs of echocardiograms and other documents constituted the only evidence of my illness and of the cause of a serious deterioration in my health. Their unaccountable loss deprived me of the "right to security of person". Without them, my future health is jeopardized, the nature of my past illness and its connection with my present condition remains unclear and the contribution of my experience to the understanding of MVP will go unappreciated.

Acting like "the Party" in Czechoslovakia, my cardiologist and others who protected him by being silent "airbrushed" me out of medical history as if I had never been ill, improperly diagnosed and incorrectly treated. Without my medical records I am a person without a complete past. In Canada, with the exception of a few provinces, there is no law that allows the patient to have copies of personal medical information kept by a health care provider and, therefore, no remedy to protect injured patients from the syndrome of the vanishing medical record. My questioning of the care given by my doctors and dentists culminated in a conspiracy of silence on the part of other doctors and dentists in the city of Toronto and denials that I had even suffered a febrile illness. Subsequent attempts at providing an oral summary of my history to assure that I received the necessary care were disbelieved, and I encountered resistance in obtaining proper follow-up health care.

Medical records are part of the continuity of human experience, of memory, of consciousness, of integrity of the individual, just as the past history and the culture of a nation shapes the consciousness of its people. The suffering, anxiety and deprivation of freedom that accompanies illness is real. No individual or group has the right to annihilate that history because it may represent a threat to the powerful. Ask any former prisoner of conscience, rescued through the efforts of Amnesty International, if he or she would like to forget the mental and physical torture. The answer will be yes, but deny that he or she had ever suffered those same cruelties and there will be vigorous protest. And to any survivor of the Nazi concentration camps, deny that the holocaust ever existed and observe the fury of the response. Then you will have some idea of the despair, anxiety, depression and justifiable anger that patients feel who are victims of medical or dental incompetence and then find themselves impotent before these powerful, privileged groups that can simply airbrush mistakes out of the medical records.

The significance of our lives is intimately bound up with our past. The existentialists have cautioned us to appreciate the "now", and no one, conscious of the transitory quality of life, would deny the wisdom of such an injunction. But our continuity with the past, whether it be a past of suffering or joy, is an integral dimension of the meaningfulness of life. Medical records are a measure of that meaningfulness, and control over them affects our freedom, our self-determination and our ability to heal. Therefore, this book is also directed to the entire medical profession, not just those doctors and dentists who were involved in my care. All health care workers must ultimately accept the patient's need for truth, for access to complete personal medical information and they must understand how the fulfillment of that need is intimately related to recovery from illness.

Anger is not an emotion with which well-adjusted, responsible citizens are comfortable. In fact, anger is often only tolerated, viewed as natural, in the malajusted or the criminal. And, sometimes, anger in these people is even elevated to the status of art. Thus, the Roger Carons and the Jack Henry Abbots of the world are awarded prestigious literary prizes, hailed as "heroic" and lavishly praised for writing books "hurling with anger"[24] against what they conceive as social injustice, and the literati of the western world even help them toward freedom from their oppressors.

Yet, anger from the responsible, the well-adjusted, the sick is rarely heard. But the sick must be angry; their justifiable rage can be turned to the good of all. We must be angry because our constitutions and civil rights codes do not protect us. They contain only ineffective, flowery rhetoric that has no more credibility or force than fiction, and we are left repressing our rage and swallowing Shakespeare's bitter maxim: "As flies to wanton boys are we to the gods; they kill us for their sport."

PART ONE:

A LITTLE LEARNING IS A
DANGEROUS THING

The Personal Story of a Woman with Mitral Valve Prolapse

1

Citadel of the Gods

There is an intensive wave of enthusiasm throughout the country for athletics, both in the young and in the old. There is simultaneously a nation-wide interest in the great prevalence of cardiovascular disease. I have felt for a long time that the beneficial effects of athletics upon the circulation is very meagre . . . Certain muscles in the body may be strengthened by exercise, but I find no proof that the strength or health of the circulation is similarly improved.

Samuel A. Levine. "Some Unproved Impressions Concerning
The Subject of Heart Disease" (June 14, 1928) *The New England
Journal of Medicine* 198 (17): 885-887.

Exercise will not make you healthy. It will not make you live longer. Fitness and health are not the same thing . . . Fitness refers to the body's capacity to do physical work and to engage in physical activity. Health refers to the presence or absence of disease.

Dr. Henry A. Solomon, *The Globe and Mail*, Toronto,
May 18, 1985.

Shortly after our marriage, like many young couples, my husband and I purchased an old house and sacrificed ourselves to its restoration. But this was an old rooming house, and many months soon became years of grinding toil. While my husband went to work as a pharmacist, I scraped mummified layers of paper from the twelve foot walls. This meant standing on the top step of a ladder with a thirty pound steamer tray full of boiling water in one hand and a scraper in the other. On my husband's free evenings and weekends, we worked together, sanding floors clogged with years of dirt and motorcycle grease, scraping off paint and varnish, ripping up mouldy, rubber tile, linoleum and rotting particle board with chisel and crowbar and demolishing or erecting walls. We were caught up in the craze of reviving the ghostly beauty of the old, the neglected or abused, restoring wood to its natural beauty and hanging jungles of green plants in big bay windows, tiny symbols of survival in an age bent on destruction of the natural environment or even the whole universe.

The reader may wonder what the restoration of an old house has to do with my story of Mitral Valve Prolapse and the medical profession. My aim is to stress the kind of work I was doing at the time my heart began to show the first signs of rebelling. In the beginning, we had no reason to believe that I would be unable, physically, to perform these Herculean tasks. Even after an eight or nine hour gruelling day, I was able to drum up the energy to cycle three miles, all uphill, back to the place we had rented until our new home was liveable.

One day when we had moved into our old house and I was heaving the steamer against the wall, I felt extraordinary fatigue even though it was only mid morning. My legs began to feel wobbly, and I found myself taking longer rests. Usually, when I was mechanically steaming and scraping, I was embellishing some scene or other in a novel I was working on, creating poetry, which I would rush to write down in the midst of my labours, or rehearsing some music I was practicing as part of my repertoire for my piano degree towards which I was working while I waited to find a teaching position in my new home town.

However, this particular day, my mind was too tired to compose, and the steamer tray leapt perversely from my exhausted grip and plunged noisily to the floor where it lay hissing at me. I had simply pushed myself beyond the limits of human endurance. Though I took a longer rest than usual, I did not quit, and, in the evening, I staggered up to bed and flopped down fully clothed. I immediately drifted off into sleep but was awakened by a burst of sustained rapid heart beat like rain drumming. As my consciousness dimmed, I called to my husband on the other side of the room. My voice seemed far away. My whole body felt numb, and there was a cold, prickly sensation in my hands and feet. My husband tried to take my pulse but it was so rapid that separate beats were indistinguishable. This episode lasted long enough for my husband to cross the room and attempt, several times, to record my pulse.

This was an entirely unexpected experience for me. All my husband and I could think of was heart attack, the doctor's buzz word, like "inferiority complex" of the shrink and "head space" of the druggie, to cover most heart problems and simple enough for the lay person to comprehend. On my father's side, there had been three victims of sudden cardiac deaths, a grandfather at 47, an aunt at 35 and an uncle at 26. When I questioned my mother about these deaths, she would say, "I don't know anything about them. The doctors said they died of heart attacks." When I pressed for more information, she added, "Well, your uncle was a blue baby. He had a hole in his heart and he had a heart attack."

This brief episode certainly did not send me scurrying to my doctor. Instead, I attributed this bizarre event to exhaustion and immediately plunged back into the inhuman labour. Occasionally, at night, a burst of rapid heart beat would wake me but it was so brief that I ignored it. It was only after a second episode, identical to the first, which occurred again just as I was falling asleep, that I even thought of consulting a doctor. But, still, I allowed several months to elapse before I made an appointment with my GP. Our desire to have a child was an important factor in our decision to seek a cardiac assessment.

Since the rapid heart beat had taken place a long time ago, I felt silly about having a check-up. However, my GP said he heard a murmur and decided to send me to an internist. He, too, heard the murmur but said he heard, "something else" as well which he could not identify.

At first I was a little shocked to hear that I had a murmur since I had never paid any attention to my heart, and murmurs, in my mind, were synonymous with pale, sickly individuals with little stamina who were warned to avoid sports or heavy work, neither of which I had ever avoided. And I did not want to believe that the rapid heart beat or the murmur were, in any way, related to the hard work since I wanted to continue just as I was doing.

Although I told both my GP and the internist that I was unaware of a murmur, I recalled later that, a few years ago, when I was living in Toronto, my doctor had said that he had heard a murmur on one of my rare check-ups about a year after my tonsils had been removed. He too had sent me on to a specialist who x-rayed my heart and reported that I had an enlarged aorta, the great vessel that transports the blood away from the heart to all parts of the body. In explaining the findings, this Toronto specialist had declared that the minor alteration in my aorta caused turbulence of the blood flow, but the sound was not really that of a murmur, and his advice to me was to ignore this new finding. This is, of course, exactly what I had done.

A second heart x-ray revealed no abnormality, not even the supposedly enlarged aorta. However, the internist referred me to a cardiologist, whom I will call Dr. G. N. Austin, who would be able to explain the "something else" heard in my heart. The internist considered him "one of the best cardiologists" in Toronto. In fact, this man was the Chief of the Department of Cardiology at a hospital which I will call The Toronto Medical Science Centre, TMSC.

Recently, I glanced at a little book for beginning readers in our school system. Pictures with appropriate words teach the young child whom to idolize, respect and trust: father, minister and doctor, the trinity of paternalism: God the Father, God the Son and God the Holy Spirit who literally breathes life into our ailing bodies. I, too, had been nourished on similar fairy tales and, as an adult, retained the child's trust, respect and awe for these worthies encountered in the first marvellous act of reading. I did not suspect that my relationship with this cardiologist would precipitate a disastrous chain of events, riddled with danger, medical incompetence, dishonesty and insensitivity and, although I would come out alive, my health would be as compromised as my blind, unquestioning faith in doctors.

My reluctance to consult a doctor can only be attributed to the subtle conditioning of poverty. When I was a child, there was no government supported medical insurance plan assuring universal access. Doctors were unaffordable luxuries for a father who was an unskilled labourer, often unemployed. From my earliest years into adulthood, I suffered two and three episodes of severe tonsillitis each year with fever and swollen lymph glands.

On only one occasion, when I was particularly ill, did I see a doctor who gave me a shot of some drug or other in the buttocks.

Poverty and illness are inevitable though unwilling bedfellows. Medical care, beyond the wildest dreams of the poor, becomes magical care and the doctor a miracle worker. The child of poverty stricken parents learns to live with irremediable illness. Tonsillitis became a normal state of affairs, as dependable as summer and Christmas holidays. Needless to say, no friendly authority ever whispered in my ear that severe upper respiratory infections could damage my heart. All through high school and university, I didn't have a doctor and I avoided the infirmary at the university out of the persistent belief that any illness, if ignored, would go away. Only when I became a teacher and could pay the insurance premiums for medical care did I visit a doctor on an annual basis. But, by then, it was too late; I had already become one of poverty's victims.

Such educational and social conditioning made it difficult for me to shed my awe of the doctor who could dissolve pain, if only my parents had enough money to pay for his medical magic. And, when I finally saw Dr. Austin in the summer of 1976, I regarded him as one of those near divinities who could transplant human hearts in God-like defiance of death. The media constantly pumped out stories of mysterious, dazzling feats that only confirmed my childhood fantasies about these miracle workers. In comparison, a few flutters of the heart seemed as insignificant as a birthmark. It did not occur to me that the medical profession's obligation was to prevent me from becoming the victim of such acts of heroism.

At last, the day of my appointment arrived, and the cardiologist's secretary ushered me into the examining room. An uneasy glance at my husband and I was alone. This woman's impersonal efficiency and immensely dignified air advertised the importance of the personage who was about to probe the secrets of my fragile flesh. And the whispering, tip-toeing technician, who tried to silence the indecent clatter of a complicated looking machine she was wheeling into the room, only magnified the notion that I was soon to be thrust into the presence of a deity. The machine, of course, was an electrocardiograph. I had never seen one before. My knowledge of the doctor's tools extended to the stethoscope and the black bag, the symbols of the medicine man I had learned about as a child in the little readers like the one I just described. I had no idea what this queer machine did and little interest in its erratic scrawls on the graph paper. Besides, I couldn't imagine my heart being anything but normal.

As I lay on the examining table, waiting for Dr. Austin, I felt embarrassed for seeking attention for symptoms that had almost disappeared. Dr. Austin glided calmly into the room. He was an older man who exuded an aura of well-being and prosperity and, when he spoke in distant, imperious tones, it was to direct me through a series of postures: sit up, lie down, lie on my left side, squat, stand, lie down. Towards the end of his examination, a flock of his brothers materialized as if Dr. Austin were a genie who had rubbed a magic lamp. Having rarely used the health care system, I was completely unfamiliar with the procedure at a large, teaching hospital. I was surprised and apprehensive at the thought of more portentous souls examining my naked flesh, and doubt, the cardinal sin in the lay person, made me wonder if Dr. Austin was no more skillful in identifying the "noises" than the lowly GP or even the internist. Or were the noises so unusual he wanted others to have a crack at hearing them? Naturally, it was lost on me that these other doctors represented the hierarchy of a training institution, frequently the undergraduate working for the summer, the recent graduate doing his internship, the internist or resident in cardiology and usually another specialist, equal to the chief, to confirm his opinion.

Dr. Austin stepped back from the examining table and, with a puzzling look that had to me something of scorn in it, said, "Come and see what we've got here!" All the others crowded around the examining table as though I were a controversial insect that had defied identification by the entomologist and, when labelled at last, would be hugely disappointing. My composure disintegrated, and I responded in my most polished teacher voice, "I don't care to be a guinea pig." It was my only defense against an increasing feeling of dehumanization. "This is a teaching hospital. We all have to examine," Dr. Austin scolded. There was a certain self-righteousness in that remark which acted as a warning not to meddle in affairs that didn't concern me. "You can't expect these doctors to get any practice if you refuse them the opportunity."

What he said sounded reasonable, and, so, I swallowed my pride as the first of these doctors, the most experienced and obviously the equal of Dr. Austin, began examining me. My objection had not in the least disturbed his impregnable armour of professionalism. Like a drill sargeant, he fired out identical postural orders as he passed his stethoscope over different areas of my chest. When he was finished, he and Dr. Austin exchanged conspiratorial grins. "Mitral Valve Prolapse," Dr. Austin announced with established authority. "Yup," the other nodded in agreement.

I heard some bizarre Latin terms. Pectus excavatum. Hypomastia. Then the flurry of listeners, each putting me through the same routines. A kind of cockiness prevailed, a bit of private joking about this cryptic entity and an unmistakeable haste to get the business over with. As if to speed up the fumblings of the more lowly, perhaps the undergraduate or the intern, Dr. Austin offered crisp advice. "In these Mitral Valve Prolapsers, the murmur is quite erratic, can even disappear altogether. It helps to have them squat or try the left lateral decubitus."

Though I had always loved Latin in school, it had by now completely deserted me, and, besides, I was no longer feeling like a human being but like an insect that had been identified. I was just a Mitral Valve Prolapser. My passivity was consumate. I scrunched up in my worn carapace like a wounded turtle escaping the vindictive jabs of cruel boys with sticks. The neck, hands, fingers, toes, legs were examined, and, then, the ten minute lesson on Mitral Valve Prolapse was over. The doctors hurried out discussing the more glamorous heart attack, and the heroic by-pass. The silliness of MVP dissipated quickly and gratefully.

After dressing, I waited with my husband outside Dr. Austin's office, occasionally glancing expectantly at his door. "Well?" my husband asked. "Mitral Valve Prolapse," I whispered timidly, perplexed that, though a big long name seemed to mean nothing, I felt as if some unknown assailant had taken a swipe at me. When my husband asked what that was I could only reply that I hadn't the foggiest idea.

At last the door opened, and Dr. Austin crooked his finger to summon me. I meekly obeyed, and it occurred to me that he had not used this gesture with his colleagues to draw them around the examining table. There was in that crooking finger something of the outraged parent who silently orders a disobedient child to stop kicking the neighbour's garbage can and proceed to the place of punishment. It was a style seemingly cultivated for patients, evidently only female, for, later he would introduce himself to my husband, shaking hands and chatting politely.

"Sit down," he commanded icily. I took the chair opposite his huge, shiny desk that stretched intimidatingly between us. A multitude of questions tumbled in my mind, but his opening remark, designed to overshadow everything else he might say, silenced me. It was unforgettable. "Mitral Valve Prolapse is an entirely insignificant condition." He paused and looked directly at me as if waiting for that to sink in. "It is totally benign. It does not get worse."

"Was I born with it?" I asked timidly, unable to suppress my curiosity.

A smile hovered about his mouth. "Possibly." Head bowed, pen scratching, he asked, "Did you ever have swollen, inflamed joints?"

"Not that I recall, just a general achiness with the tonsillitis which I had two and three times a year until my tonsils were removed when I was . . ."

"No inflamed joints. No rheumatic fever," his voice marched on. He was decidedly not interested in my tonsils. "Any heart problems in your family?"

I told him about my relatives, their stories seeming so dramatic as to barely relate to what I had. However, his interest perked up. "Well, you're not going to drop dead!" he uttered sternly. "People with Mitral Valve Prolapse do not drop dead suddenly!" He seemed to grit his teeth, and what I earlier had thought was scorn became more obvious as if he were determined to squash a fear that he imagined might eat away at my reason.

As the interview continued, my need to question such an unimportant condition seemed frankly silly. Dr. Austin then described MVP. If any lecture was intended to encourage trust in him and dispel fear and curiosity, this was it. His words sedated me like a powerful tranquilizer. "What you have is a valve — the one on the left side of your heart — that bulges just a little." He leaned back in his chair and pyramided his fingers to demonstrate this bulge. "When it does this, it causes a little noise in your heart which we can hear with the stethoscope."

Again I felt like a child in grade school. From what he said I could not tell whether the valve bulged continuously or just at certain times or how that bulging related to the episodes of rapid heart beat and semi-fainting.

"For some reason, more women than men have MVP, one in five to one in twenty. It's extremely common. There's nothing wrong with the valve. In fact, it's normal, just shaped a bit differently, like a bugging eyeball." A sneer seemed to creep into his voice. "The sound we hear is just part of its normal function. The best thing for you to do is go home and forget about it. I understand you expressed some concern over having children. MVP poses absolutely no problem at all. It's a completely benign condition."

This was the second time I had been told to ignore my symptoms, to regard them as nothing more than a curiosity, but somehow it wasn't as easy to do. I was on the verge of asking about the rapid heart beat which he appeared to have forgotten was my main reason for coming when his next question cut me off. "Are you planning a family immediately?"

"Well, not quite. Next fall."

"Are you on any birth control pills?"

"Yes."

"I'd like you to come off them immediately. Our opinion is that contraceptives are not good for women in general."

"What about the rapid heart beat?" I finally got out. "Could that affect the baby?" I described the episodes, not leaving out any detail.

"A few little palpitations do bother MVP patients. But they're nothing to worry about and they certainly can't harm the baby. Nor do they cause heart attack." He levelled his gaze at me. "You have to learn to live with this nuisance. We had one woman with MVP who died unexpectedly while she was nursing her six month old baby. But our feeling is that MVP had nothing to do with her death."

Why did you mention that I wanted to ask, but, already, he was on to something else. "Women with MVP live long, healthy, normal lives. As a rule, the hearts of these patients beat a little faster than normal. If this nuisance of palpitations is causing you anxiety, we'll give you something for that." He wrote out a prescription and handed it to me.

"It was more than a nuisance," I ventured a little impatiently. "My heart beat seemed a lot faster than what you describe. My husband couldn't take my pulse. I felt as if I were about to faint. It happened when I was lying down." I then described the type of labour in which I was involved.

"The work you were doing didn't cause the palpitations," he said flatly, not looking up. "The majority of MVP patients have palpitations. You just have to live with them. It's not necessary to change your activities at all!"

I had the feeling he was totally unable to appreciate the kind of work I was doing. "But what did cause them then?"

"MVP patients are a whole lot more anxious and nervous than most people and, so, they get a few palpitations. Doctors really don't know why. But these pills will help. You'll live to a ripe old age," he said, chuckling softly. If anxiety was causing these "palpitations", why wasn't I getting them now I reasoned or whenever I was anxious about something? But this was not the case. Dr.

Austin sprung up then with the energy of a thirty year old and hustled me toward the door. "If it makes you feel better," he threw out, "you can come back in a year or two for a reassessment and some fancy tests."

The sound of his door banging behind me might as well have been the loud clanking of iron bars. I felt incarcerated in my own ignorance and timidity. His advice was to change what I felt, not what I did, and the rapid heart beat would disappear. My interview had taught me nothing about the heart or the mitral valve. And, amidst all his reassurances, the story of the woman dying shortly after childbirth bothered me. Was this a Freudian slip? And, if MVP was so common, so insignificant, why couldn't the internist, if not the GP, have told me just as much as Dr. Austin.

Although Dr. Austin succeeded in stifling my questions, he had not, somehow, suppressed my curiosity about MVP. And, although uppermost in my mind was a distinctly guilty feeling, fired in the crucible of my childhood, that I had wasted this important man's time, his overbearing, patriarchal attitude kindled in me a tiny spark of indignation. He seemed to be treating my head, not my heart. I felt short changed, cheated out of a more satisfying explanation, one more appropriate to an intelligent, educated person, to any human being with sensitivity and curiosity.

2

The Second Opinion

A Little Learning is a dang'rous Thing;
Drink deep, or taste not the Pierian Spring;
There shallow Draughts intoxicate the Brain,
And drinking largely sobers us again.

Alexander Pope: *An Essay on Criticism*: Lines 215-218

If you ask if I sit down and I take this out and I say, "Now I want you to know you may die of blood clotting or you may get hepatitis or you may get this, that or the other thing . . . then I would say 'no'. I don't believe it is good practice with any medication to go through the list of complications.

Dr. Robert Kistner, Harvard Medical School, in Corea, Gena.
The Hidden Malpractice (New York: Harper & Row Publishers,
Inc., 1977), p. 155.

The drug which Dr. Austin had prescribed to stop my anxiety or my rapid heart beat — I couldn't tell which — was propranolol, known to the public under its trade name, Inderal. For a description of this drug I consulted the *Compendium of Pharmaceuticals*, or CPS, which lists all drugs alphabetically by trade and generic or family name. It is a book found in every pharmacist's dispensary. Propranolol is a beta-adrenergic receptor blocking agent. This means it prevents certain chemicals, called epinephrine and norepinephrine, from reaching the heart by occupying the specific receptors intended for them.[1] These substances are naturally produced in the body at the terminals of nerve fibres in the sympathetic nervous system. Adrenalin is the drug industry's trade name for epinephrine which can overstimulate the heart. We all know what adrenalin does: increases blood pressure and heart rate, causes dry mouth, sweating, dizziness, all the physical signs of anxiety or fear.

Any drug will produce side effects, ranging from minor to major, but we were concerned only with those relating to pregnancy. The CPS warned that propranolol's safety during pregnancy had not yet been established. Researchers had observed several side effects such as small placenta and intrauterine growth retardation which raised the spectre of a complicated pregnancy and thus mental retardation of the unborn child. Infants born to mothers who had taken propranolol could have hypoglycemia and/or bradycardia, that is, excessively low pulse usually below sixty. Hypoglycemia is a condition involving the pancreas with symptoms of sweating, trembling, palpitations, weakness and lightheadedness. Despite the fact that this information came from the highest authority on drugs, the *Canadian Pharmaceutical Association*, which publishes the compendium, we, in good faith, accepted the judgement of Dr. G. N. Austin. We reasoned that my dosage was very small, 40 mgm. at night, presumably because my rapid heart beat occurred just as I was falling asleep, and 20 mgm. in the morning. And, how, we asked ourselves, could "one of the best cardiologists in the city" prescribe a potentially dangerous drug during pregnancy for a symptom he considered nothing more than a "nuisance" and totally harmless to the fetus! We, therefore, decided not to seek a second opinion.

Because Dr. Austin had described MVP and its symptoms as so insignificant, I considered returning to him only in the event of pregnancy when I might legitimately require a reassessment. However, a fertility problem arose which complicated matters. Although we intended ruling out all causes, we naturally wondered whether MVP or propranolol might be contributing factors. There was some basis for our suspicions of propranolol. In *The Pharmacological Basis of Therapeutics*, the bible of the pharmaceutical profession, edited by two professors of pharmacy, propranolol is said to increase "the activity of the human uterus, more in the non-pregnant than in the pregnant state."[2] We, therefore, wondered if this drug could prevent conception. The pharmaceutical association forwarded further information to my husband which linked propranolol with premature labour, a factor which only seemed to compound the problem of intrauterine growth retardation.[3]

We, therefore, felt a second opinion, especially with regard to the use of this drug, was warranted. However, we were busy people, and it was not until a year and a half later, early in 1978, that we arranged an appointment with an obstetrician-gynecologist, Dr. Grady, at a second Toronto hospital which I will call the Toronto Cardiology Institute (TCI). While this doctor did not believe propranolol was responsible for the infertility, he opposed its use during pregnancy and added that, in view of a cardiac arrhythmia, I would be, in his opinion, a "high risk" patient and should be prepared for hospitalization at any time during my pregnancy even for as long as nine months. This opinion conflicted dramatically with that of Dr. Austin. Dr. Grady was kind and concerned and did not ridicule my fears. He recommended that my care during pregnancy should be shared with a heart specialist and arranged for me to see Dr. Neville Rhodes at the same hospital in early April of 1978.

Like Dr. Austin, Rhodes was an elderly doctor and Chief of the Cardiology section. I relayed my complete history to him and the fact that I had seen Dr. Austin at TMSC. It did not occur to me that I would in any way prejudice the independence of this second opinion. Dr. Rhodes informed me he was both a friend and colleague of Dr. Austin's. After an electrocardiogram which he conducted himself, Dr. Rhodes affirmed the presence of MVP and gave me an identical but even briefer description of this condition than Dr. Austin had, saying that it was totally benign, that more women than men had it and that, while there was no risk in having children, he agreed propranolol should not be used.

Dr. Rhodes refused to answer any other questions until after I had an echocardiogram which he vowed was the gold standard for identifying MVP. The "echo", he said, was a non-invasive, completely harmless procedure using sound waves that allowed him to see how the heart and its valves functioned. The need for this test left us with the feeling that Dr. Rhodes was not entirely certain I had MVP and my hopes revived that I did not.

During the long wait of two and a half months for this test, we realized that, if we were truly to address our uneasiness, we would have to be able to formulate the relevant questions to ask Dr. Rhodes. We thus set about reviewing our sketchy high school knowledge of the heart. At first, the task of gathering medical information was a frustrating, haphazard and superficial effort beginning with the most unsatisfactory place, the public library in our city.

We managed to put together a picture of how the heart and its valves worked. The heart is a four-chambered hollow organ with a tough, muscular wall, called the myocardium, the Greek root, "kardia", meaning heart. The myocardium is surrounded by a thin, membranous sac, the pericardium. The Greek prefix, "peri", means around. This sac contains about five to twenty gms. of clear liquid, resembling amber coloured serum, which acts as a shock absorber. The myocardium is lined with a thin, strong membrane, the endocardium, "endo" for inner.

A wall or septum, from the Latin word,"sepire", to enclose, divides the heart cavity down the middle into "right" and "left" hearts which are really two pumps. Each pump is in turn divided into an upper chamber (atrium, pl. atria), which is a thin-walled storage tank that receives the blood, and a lower, thicker-walled chamber (ventricle) which is the heart's pump. The openings between the atrium and ventricle on either side are controlled by valves. The mitral valve on the left has two leaflets and is so called because it is shaped like a bishop's mitre. It opens to allow fresh, oxygenated blood from the lungs to enter the left ventricle and the aortic valve allows this blood to pass out of the left ventricle into the aorta and, so, to all parts of the body.

In the right heart, there are the tricuspid (tri for three leaflets) and pulmonic valves which function like the valves in the left heart. Two large veins transport the blood to the heart. Blood goes to the right heart from the upper part of the body via the superior vena cava and from the lower body via the inferior vena cava. This deoxygenated blood, which is dark-bluish red in colour because it has delivered its oxygen and nutrients to body tissues, enters the right atrium and passes through the tricuspid valve into the right ventricle from where it is pumped out by the right ventricle through the pulmonic valve and pulmonary artery to the right and left lungs. There it releases waste gas, carbon dioxide, and picks up oxygen which turns it bright red again. The oxygenated blood then re-enters the left atrium through the pulmonary vein and the circulation starts all over again. The cardiac cycle consists of the contraction and relaxation phases. The relaxation phase or diastole is the period when the blood fills the heart. Diastole is a Greek word meaning to stretch apart and implies the heart expands as it is filled with blood. Systole, likewise a Greek word meaning to collect, is the contraction phase, literally when all the blood has been collected from the atria and then is pumped out of the ventricles.

We could find nothing in our public library about MVP but, then, we were not yet aware that this common cardiac disorder had not reached the public conscience like hypertension, heart attack, arthritis or cancer. But, at least, we knew the location of the mitral valve in the heart, what it looked like and how the heart worked. Our next stop was the medical bookstore at the University of Toronto from which we had both graduated. To see this obscure term, MVP, in the index of a heart textbook surprised and delighted us. Our hopes rose that we would learn more than Dr. Austin or Dr. Rhodes had told us. However, our enthusiasm soon dissipated. In the particular textbook we glanced at there was only one brief paragraph on MVP describing its history, prevalence in the general population and preference for women, symptoms of fatigue, dizziness, lightheadedness and palpitations. Another complication was mentioned but, because of its long, difficult name and the author's opinion of its uncommonness, it didn't stick in our minds as relevant to us. Two Chiefs of Cardiology had stressed the complete harmlessness of the condition as well and, so, in effect, we were brainwashed early in our search. Besides, we were only interested in propranolol and pregnancy, but on this there was nothing.

Several weeks later, my husband suggested we see if either Rhodes or Austin had written anything on MVP. Our next stop was, therefore, the medical library at the University of Toronto which contains about 2000 medical journals from around the world. In finding information, we were complete novices. Knowledge begets knowledge, but we had very little base from which to begin. We had looked up Austin and Rhodes on the Video Index under periodicals. Each doctor had written an article. After some searching, we found the relevant journals on the shelves. We also came across a book on MVP, the result of a symposium. But, since neither pregnancy nor propranolol showed up in its index, we set it aside for the time being. The lack of information on the subject of MVP and pregnancy encouraged us to believe that Austin was, perhaps, right about the lack of problems in pregnancy.

I concentrated on deciphering the papers of Austin and Rhodes with the help of a medical dictionary. Both their articles mentioned sudden death as a complication. This came as a great shock to us since Dr. Austin had so vigorously denied this in spite of my family history. Austin's paper seemed unrelated to me because it dealt with chest pain which I had never experienced other than indigestion. Both papers indicated that there were degrees of prolapse, ranging from very mild to severe. This confused us because both Rhodes and Austin had laid great stress on the benign, unchanging nature of MVP. Some patients had what was called "clicks" and others clicks and murmurs. There appeared to be two parts to the mitral valve, an anterior and a posterior portion called leaflets, which closed the valve. More than one part of the valve could be prolapsed. Some patients had regurgitation. We were uncertain of the meaning of this word but guessed that it might refer to a leaky valve. Though this sounded ominous, we had no idea of its significance. And, certainly, from what we had been told, we did not think it applied to us.

A list of questions formulated quickly. Was the echocardiogram able to determine which leaflets were involved and the extent of the prolapse? What was the cause of this condition? Did I have mitral regurgitation? If so, we wondered if this would become a problem in pregnancy. Since Dr. Austin had told me that heavy labour had not caused the arrhythmia, could the prolapse itself or the regurgitation have caused it? If I discontinued the propranolol would rapid heart beat deprive the fetus of oxygen? Would the strain of pregnancy increase the prolapse or the regurgitation if there was any? And, with respect to sudden death, what was the significance of Dr. Austin's story of the young mother dying shortly after childbirth? These were some of our questions which we compiled for our second meeting with Dr. Rhodes. Answers to them would dispel our vague fears. And we hoped that Rhodes would be more prepared to explain MVP to us than Austin had been. Since I felt so well, he would surely also confirm that my prolapse was mild. As responsible future parents, we wanted reassurance that I would be a healthy and, therefore, happy mother who could look forward to the prospect of raising a child.

It had never occurred to me to establish ahead of time how the technician would operate the equipment for the echocardiogram test, no more than I would have learned the technical aspects of the apparatus the optometrist uses to examine my eyes. On the day of the test, the technician gave me the two line description, as Dr. Rhodes had, on how ultrasound picked up valve activity and translated it into an image on the screen of a closed circuit television. A printed computer read-out provides a permanent record.

What took place in the examining room helped shape my unfortunate decision not to return to the TCI. After the technician had the examination under way, a Dr. Croft entered the room presumably in accordance with a prior arrangement. From their few words, his purpose appeared to be to learn how to do an echocardiogram, though this was never clarified for me. Apart from applying a lubricant to prevent friction between the skin and the transducer which picks up the sound waves, the technician did not touch me. Dr. Croft watched a few minutes, then asked to take over. The technician sat on a stool with her back to us, her attention turned to the video screen. At the time, I was lying on my left side. I first became uneasy when Dr. Croft pressed my left breast repeatedly with lingering gestures. I felt anxious and uncomfortable but was afraid to say anything that made me appear unduly suspicious since I didn't know if his behaviour were part of his inexperience, that he, in fact, was simply trying to find the appropriate spot with his fingers for placing the transducer. However, it seemed that Dr.Croft was not placing the transducer on the areas he had touched. My suspicions were increased when he began methodically pressing the right breast. My discomfort was by then acute but I was paralyzed as to how to protest for fear that my suspicions were incorrect. In fact, I had difficulty believing that sexual harassment could actually be taking place in such a situation. Out of conditioned respect for authority, I doubted my own senses. When I at last became bold enough to speak, I asked Dr. Croft, as nicely as I could, what he was doing. He replied that he was trying to locate the aorta and quickly placed the transducer on the sternum. But, at that moment, the technician intruded abruptly, taking the transducer from him, indicating she would show him. She guided his hand for the rest of the examination.

The technician then turned on the light and instructed me to dress. Dr. Croft, however, insisted on listening to my heart. The technician busied herself with other matters at a desk behind a portable screen. After his cursory examination, which did not appear improper, Croft remained, arms crossed, rudely staring at me, at a distance of two to three feet, while I prepared to dress in the tiny room. As a hint to leave, I asked if he wished to speak further with me. Since he responded negatively, I was forced to turn my back to him and dress in his presence. He had no apparent reason for being in the room except to speak to the technician after I had gone. Afterwards, I realized he likely remained because he did not want to give me an opportunity to speak with her about his behaviour.

In subconscious obeisance to the paternalism of the medical profession, I wrote to Dr. Rhodes asking for his opinion rather than to some "impartial governing body" which, of course, I did not know existed at the time. I described Dr. Croft's behaviour in detail and asked if it were in any way improper under the circumstances. My letter resulted in a long distance telephone call from Dr. Croft who made no attempt to defend his behaviour or to convince me that I had misinterpreted actions that were perfectly appropriate for a person learning how to operate an echocardiogram. Instead, he apologized contritely and promised that "it" would never happen again, presumably with other women. Of course, Dr. Rhodes would have spoken to the technician to verify my story. Her hasty intrusion suggested she had noted improper conduct. If she hadn't, Dr. Croft would not have called me. Either she or Dr. Rhodes would have written to explain that Dr. Croft's behaviour was perfectly compatible with the procedure. I have now had conversations with several technicians and many echocardiograms, done by both experienced and inexperienced technicians, and no one has ever remotely behaved like Dr. Croft.

In itself, this sexual assault may not have persuaded me to choose Dr. Austin over Dr. Rhodes. Even though Croft appeared to be a regular staff member at the TCI, I was not likely to encounter him again. This hospital had maternity facilities with co-ordinated care which TMSC did not have. However, after my second meeting with Dr. Rhodes the decision became unfortunately inevitable. This time I asked if my husband could be present.

Dr. Rhodes protested vigorously that this was not customary, but, over his objections, my husband followed me into the office.

Dr. Rhodes' unpleasantness was foreboding and made me all the more timid. I tremulously plunged into my questions, prefacing them with the remark that we hoped he did not mind if we read his article which helped clarify MVP. "You what!" he exclaimed in astonishment. I literally froze. He regained his composure after passing a hand over his face in a gesture of extreme abhorrence at this unpardonable transgression. We could only conclude that we had trespassed on forbidden territory in reading his material which was meant only for the eyes of doctors.

I continued with the questions, beginning with those on the extent of my valve prolapse. Again, he intruded impatiently, "Why are you going into all this! What you have is nothing more than a curiosity, like a hangnail, a completely benign condition. I don't have time to answer all these questions."

With a mixture of guilt, anger and frustration, I jumped to the questions on pregnancy, believing that he might consider them more relevant.

"Look," he articulated sternly, "you're wasting my time. I'm not going to answer any questions about this unimportant condition!" He rose, proof of his opposition. I hastily folded my question paper and tucked it into my handbag. Embarrassment and total bewilderment swept over me; it was as if my questions constituted an outrageously indecent act. "A little learning is a dangerous thing you know," he warned, his manner suddenly jovial in an effort to smooth over his outburst.

I had a Masters degree in English literature and, naturally, was very familiar with Pope's *Essay on Criticism*, but, only much later, would I appreciate the full irony of those next lines, "Drink deep or taste not the Pierian Spring/ There shallow Draughts intoxicate the Brain/And drinking largely sobers us again." Flinging Pope at me was an insult. Rhodes had interpreted my deep sincerity about the responsibility of childbirth as a puerile undergraduate's attempt to impress the professor with clever questions. He regarded himself as entitled to extract wisdom from the vast corpus of English literature, in which he had no training, and use "a little bit of learning" to discourage me from claiming a similar right to even a small part of his exclusive knowledge, even though I had far more than an academic interest. The injustice of such a situation should have aroused my angry opposition, but I only retreated cowardly. Dr. Rhodes, seeing the opportunity my weakness afforded, parried with a final blow. "Did you know that she was like this when you married her?" he asked my husband. The meaning was clear. Any man in his right mind should be outraged by such forward, unbecoming behaviour in a female and a wife. Women, like children, should be seen and not heard. "Oh she must have been!" he concluded as he slapped my husband on the back in an attempt at camaraderie. The implication seemed to be that my husband obviously knew this before marriage or he would have divorced me once he found out.

"What does this mean?" my husband asked as he picked up the echocardiogram report which lay on Dr. Rhodes' desk. "It says there's no indication of mitral prolapse. Is Dr. Austin wrong then?"

"Let me see," I said excitedly, but Dr. Rhodes snatched the report out of my husband's hand.

"It may say that," he countered defensively, "but you do have prolapse. Our machine is old."

I dissolved into renewed uncertainty. I wanted to believe I did not have MVP partly because there was no possibility of getting answers. Surely, Croft's attempts, if included in the report, were bound to be inaccurate. "I have another patient now," Rhodes announced hastily as he clearly prepared to show us out. But, as we were about to leave, he said, as if in afterthought, "There's one more thing you should know before you leave. It's our policy here at this hospital to give our patients antibiotics during childbirth in case of infection. We also give them for dental work. I'll give you a prescription now for the dental visits," he said cheerfully.

Since I was still recovering from the shock of this interview, his instruction was anti-climactic and made no impression on me. If anything, I was now totally confused. Dr. Grady had stressed the danger of drugs during pregnancy and Rhodes had agreed. Now he was advising antibiotics at delivery and with dental work which I was likely to have during my pregnancy. Questions were unthinkable. I had been crushed into submission. Dr. Rhodes escorted us out of his office.

Afterwards, rage smouldered within me, but all that came out was a series of ejaculations of astonishment. "How could he behave this way!" was the topic of our conversation for the entire evening, during shopping, dinner and, later, as we prepared for bed. We both agreed I would return to Austin. At least he hadn't expressed such disapproval and had not insulted me, but we knew that was probably because I had not read any of the medical literature and asked few questions.

My fate was sealed. At the termination of our meeting, Rhodes had casually tacked on the most crucial information for a MVP patient, the use of antibiotics. From my perspective at that time, a safe pregnancy was all that interested me. As for antibiotics, I had rarely used them and didn't even understand how they worked. When you are poor, illness, like tonsillitis in my childhood, was something you waited out. Not something you cured. The habit continued on into adulthood. Rhodes' precious bit of information was then and later to become even more insignificant. But we could not know this. How could we know that a vague word, like "infection", had anything to do with the heart? He had not taken the time to explain the serious purpose for which these antibiotics were used and clearly implied that it was a policy only at "their" hospital, not all hospitals. There was no hard and fast rule about their usage. This meeting with Rhodes had thoroughly convinced me that I was being unnecessarily cautious, even neurotic in expressing concern, in asking questions about a condition equated with a hangnail, a bugging eyeball or a "nuisance"! His advice delivered so casually and so incompletely in such a stressful atmosphere was lost upon us. Dr. Rhodes' attitude had destroyed even the tiniest dimension of seriousness attached to MVP. So ended the "democratic" second opinion.

After the interview, I concentrated on having the necessary tests to rule out an infertility problem, and, in late November of 1978, I saw Dr. Austin a second time since, in spite of the propranolol, I frequently experienced little bursts of rapid heart beat in the night, usually just as I was falling asleep. Dr. Austin arranged a series of tests, echocardiogram, treadmill exercise stress test, the name of which describes the routine activity, a second chest x-ray, electrocardiogram and a Holter monitor, a device the size of a small portable tape recorder, that is strapped to the body and records the heart's electrical activity over a 24 hour period. All these tests, Austin said, were normal. He repeated his initial description that this was a benign, unimportant condition that did not require regular checking or any treatment other than propranolol for the "nuisance" of palpitations.

However, my husband, remembering Dr. Rhodes's last minute advice, asked Dr. Austin if I should have antibiotics at delivery or with dental work. Dr. Austin replied that there was no risk and antibiotics were not necessary for MVP patients. He then dismissed me with four-plus reassurance of a long, normal life.

I did not ask Dr. Austin any questions. Rhodes' brief, unexplained reference to "infection", as we were leaving, had made little impression on me of the gravity of the risk if I did not take them. I, therefore, put this out of my mind once Dr. Austin said antibiotics were entirely unnecessary. To us, that seemed wiser, too, during pregnancy and delivery. Furthermore, Rhodes' behaviour had effectively silenced me. Asking questions only aroused a doctor's anger and even the possibility of being denied care. By returning to Austin, I had committed myself totally to his judgement. If any problem should arise during my pregnancy, I would have to consult him. Though I saw the obstetrician-gynecologist at the TMSC, there was no possibility of co-ordinated care since this hospital did not have a maternity ward. Unlike Dr. Grady, this doctor believed I didn't require this kind of comprehensive care. In his opinion, neither propranolol nor MVP created any problem during pregnancy.

My brief encounter with the apostles of Aesculapius had ended in increased confusion, ignorance and unknown danger. The only practical response, on my part, was to repress both the natural desire for answers and the anxiety that came of not getting them. It was clear to me that silence was the price a woman had to pay for medical services rendered. Doctors were still the same lofty, inscrutable magic workers of my childhood who would not bother to help the poor if they couldn't pay and to whom I had many times prayed, as to some "deus ex machina", to deliver me out of the misery of tonsillitis. My earlier reluctance to go to a doctor now seemed instinctively correct. The two episodes of rapid heart beat with the sensation of a precipitous decline in consciousness we now regarded as normal just as I had once thought of tonsillitis. To express concern, as I had done for the "nuisance" of MVP was, in these doctors' eyes, to behave neurotically. I had learned a lesson that would cost me my health.

3

The Turning Point

I am the sun in my white coat,
Grey faces, shuttered by drugs, follow me like flowers.

Sylvia Plath: "The Surgeon at 2 a.m." from *Crossing The Water.*

In late April of 1979, a minor, forgettable episode in the lives of individuals without a heart murmur triggered a whole series of unhappy events in my life. A sudden toothache, a rare occurrence, became within hours a full blown pulp infection in a lower left second molar. The stage for this problem had been set much earlier in a childhood of extreme poverty. Teeth are the most expendable item in the budget of poor families. If medical doctors were a luxury in my childhood, dentists were practically unheard of. There was no such thing as regular dental check-ups to prevent tooth decay or periodontal problems. Nothing was done about a tooth unless there was pain which, if it became intolerable, was relieved expediently and inexpensively by pulling the tooth.

I did not see a dentist until I was fourteen when I had begun to work at a part-time job after school. Though I might occasionally experience a mild stinging if I ate a sweet, I had never had a toothache, and no black caries or other visible marks could be found on my teeth. We had moved from the country to the city, and my new friends all went to dentists regularly. I felt different and thought I should have a check-up like everyone else.

Consistent with my upbringing, I was alone on this visit. My father was dead, and my mother was working and thus unable to accompany me to the dentist's office. Innocent, totally uninformed and scared, I swallowed every word of the white-coated luminary from another planet. He told me that I had seventeen or more cavities which must be drilled and filled or I would lose all my teeth before I was out of my teens. I gulped and fought back my tears at this terrible sentence. Three of my cousins had lost their teeth before they had reached the drinking age. Their favorite game was "pass the dentures". They would remove their teeth and giggle ecstatically at their lisping speech. Afterwards, they passed the teeth around, crowing delightedly at their artificial beauty that beat, they said, the beauty of even a movie star's teeth. But I never saw anything funny or glamorous in having false teeth.

Knowing nothing and having been weaned on unquestioning obedience to authority, I easily fell prey to this horrible malediction. There was only enough breath in my body to squeak out that I would have to pay the staggering sum of $300.00 on time, a phrase I loathed from my early childhood. I committed my salary from the Towers Food store and promised eagerly to pay the whole debt off in the summer when my income would be greater. The dentist smiled in a fatherly way and patted me on the back in acknowledgement of my deprivation, and I stumbled out of his office. My mother, needless to say, did not challenge the wisdom of this educated person.

This dentist left only four teeth unfilled, the front teeth, top and bottom and two other teeth. After this shocking experience, I did not return to a dentist until my first year of university when an infected wisdom tooth had to be extracted and someone recommended a Dr. Mary Slapek who sent me to an oral surgeon. In the meantime I practiced good dental hygiene in accordance with what I knew. However, I never doubted that this first dentist had been right; I didn't have enough knowledge to doubt. It was only fear that something else would be found to be wrong that had kept me out of the dentist's office. My life experiences certainly had not taught me independence of thought nor the art of shopping around for a doctor or a dentist. For the next twelve years, I was Dr. Slapek's devoted patient, never questioning her work. I held the mistaken belief that anyone who offered a health care service did so out of a love of humanity and, therefore, did everything right.

Once I was earning money as a teacher, I continued to see Dr. Slapek regularly even when I moved away from Toronto. Hence when my toothache began on a Friday night, I had no dentist to call upon and had to wait until Monday morning to contact her. The pain became so severe that I was taking two extra strength Tylenol tablets every two to three hours with little effect. But I had learned in childhood to accept pain stoically and without complaining to a doctor. My temperature rose steadily, and, by late Saturday night, it was 105° F and I was almost delirious with pain and a raging fever. All night long, I shook with chills, sweats and fever.

I did not go to the hospital because my childhood conditioning had taught me that teeth were treated by dentists, not doctors. My husband had frequently talked with patients who had experienced severe pain and facial swelling from a root canal infection and, so, we assumed correctly, it would turn out, that this must be the source of the pain and fever. But two cardiologists I had seen had in no way connected the teeth and the heart for us. That was a leap that lay people simply could not make on their own. By Sunday afternoon, the pain and fever began to subside. I continued with the Tylenol, but mild fever, sweats and chills persisted.

At some point during this extremely high fever, I feared that the infection would cause grotesque facial swelling. Both my husband and I were under enormous pressure because of the unrelievable pain I was suffering. I simply assumed that on the Monday Slapek would extract the tooth. That there was any other remedy did not occur to me. My husband and I discussed whether I should take the penicillin Rhodes had prescribed. His prescription was for penicillin to be taken after a dental procedure, and his instructions to us were "in case of infection". Thus we had never once imagined that this drug was for anything other than a local infection in the mouth that might arise after dental work. Dr. Rhodes had not explained that the penicillin was to protect my heart valves from a potentially lethal infection. My husband had filled this prescription so that I would have it on hand in our medicine cabinet. Since I had seen Rhodes just under a year ago, I had visited Slapek only twice. In a casual conversation about pregnancy back in 1976, I had told Dr. Slapek of my MVP murmur, and she had recorded this information in her records. The subject, however, never arose again. She had never discussed the use of antibiotics with me, and subsequent investigation would show her records contained no reference to the use of antibiotics. No infection had ever developed from her interventions, and, therefore, I had never had a reason to take the antibiotics or to remember Rhodes' prescription until that night of the very high fever. To this day, because of the severe pain and near delirium, neither my husband nor I can recall exactly whether I took any of the penicillin. I have a vague memory of having swallowed "some" of the antibiotic tablets in the hope of preventing an infection in my face.

The only thing we could infer from Rhodes' instructions was that MVP patients must be more inclined to get local infections, such as of the gums or bone, in association with dental work. He had stressed that the use of antibiotics with childbirth and dental work was a policy unique to his hospital and not specifically for MVP patients. My husband was aware that some rheumatic heart disease (RHD) patients might take penicillin daily or before dental work, but, given his knowledge at that time, he was unable to make a comparison with MVP and, certainly, the stress that had been laid on the insignificance of that condition would not have inspired him to do so. MVP had never been a topic in pharmacy school, and timing and dosage, not reasons, are what appear on prescriptions. Thus, he could not make the mental leap to connect the teeth and MVP any more than I could, particularly as two specialists had done everything in their power to convince us that I had a normal heart. Furthermore, it is not surprising that lay people would think that penicillin taken prior to or after dental work was to prevent local infection in the mouth since, for many years after the introduction of antibiotics, dentists, themselves, held the mistaken opinion that the aim of such antibiotic therapy was to sterilize the mouth and any foci of infection,[1] not to prevent infection of the heart valves.

On Monday, Dr. Slapek took an x-ray which showed a pulp abscess. She refused to extract the tooth herself and arranged for me to see an endodontist who could, she said, remove the infected nerves and save the tooth. About a week later, I saw Dr. Marvin Cohen. Even though I believed MVP was an entirely benign condition, I still noted it on Dr. Cohen's brief history questionnaire in the space which solicited such information and specifically mentioned that I was taking propranolol for the rapid heart beat. But, Cohen, like Slapek, would never look at my history and never ask me any questions about my heart.

If I had taken any of the penicillin on the night of my fever and pain or what remained of it on my first endodontal visit, it was only from fear that my face would swell up, not because I knew my heart was in danger. Ironically, my heart was the furthest thing from my mind. The entire endodontal treatment was to consist of three visits. Dr. Cohen emphasized that the first visit was the most difficult and risky. Naturally I feared the pain would recur and that I would have swelling, but Dr. Cohen reassured me that this was not likely to happen and that, if I got through the first visit without any problem, I should have no further difficulties. I did not bring up the subject of the penicillin because it never occurred to me that a dentist as well as a doctor could prescribe these drugs. Dr. Austin had insisted that I did not need antibiotics and had not given me a prescription.

Like Dr. Slapek, Dr. Cohen took an x-ray before beginning. "I'll do everything I can to save that tooth," he declared heroically, "but it's not an easy tooth to work on. It's got three roots." His vigorous commitment made me confident in his work. But, after my second visit, I was forced to return on an emergency basis. A sensation of pressure within the tooth, aching and soreness in the jaw and a stinging sensation on chewing even the soft foods Dr. Cohen recommended made me fear that the dreaded infection had set into my face. After this first visit I, of course, had no more penicillin. I was now Dr. Austin's patient and I knew I could not get any more since he opposed its use.

My recollection of the situation that day has always remained very clear, in fact, unforgettable. I blurted out my fears and my confusion to Dr. Cohen, relating that one cardiologist I had seen some time ago had mentioned antibiotics for dental work, but that my present cardiologist, Dr. Austin, had said I did not need them. I then timidly asked his opinion. His reply, "Oh, it might be a good idea," was vague and not reassuring. "But, after I open the tooth and clean out more debris," he promised, "you'll be all right. This'll clear up the problem." Much later, I would realize that the fact that I was seeing a cardiologist did not make any impression whatsoever on Dr. Cohen, though it should have.

However, no amount of reassurance was sufficient, and I asked Dr. Cohen if he had any antibiotics on hand, not realizing, of course, the completely improper nature of my request, let alone the importance of correct dosage, drug and timing. To me, at that time, an antibiotic taken improperly was no more dangerous than an aspirin. Dr. Cohen rummaged in his drawer and gave me one orange and yellow capsule which, when I asked, he said was tetracycline. My husband afterwards verified this. Much later, I would realize that Dr. Cohen had made no more connection between the endodontal work and my MVP than I, the patient, had done.

The root canal therapy was completed at the end of June 1979. Since the temporary white filling was not strong, Dr. Cohen cautioned me not to chew any hard substances until after I had the permanent crown affixed some time in October. It was not difficult to comply since chewing even soft substances during the treatment caused pain and made my face break out in a sweat and, for some time afterwards, I felt hot and feverish. When I told Dr. Cohen this on the second visit, he said there was considerable inflammation of the jaw bone from the original pulp abscess that would linger. On a final follow-up visit in August, he made the same response to the same complaints, adding that it would take up to a year for the inflammation to heal and that evidence of the infection would remain on the x-ray for as long.

Since Dr. Cohen said nothing more could be done, I simply avoided chewing on that tooth. But my problems were hardly over. The fixation of the crown was an agonizing experience. Dr. Slapek began by grinding the tooth down to prepare for the porcelain crown. After taking an impression she then affixed what she called a temporary crown. This covering resembled a bottle cap and was the width of a dime. It had straight edges which she trimmed unevenly with an instrument that resembled pliers in order to get the proper height. The jagged edges lacerated the tissues so that chewing was unbearable, and gobs of rough, irritating adhesive clung to the edges of the tin. In effect this covering did not cleave to the tooth but sat on top of the gum, actually glued to the tissues. I, of course, had absolutely no knowledge of the crowning procedure, any more than I had of the endodontal process, and, so, once again could not protest.

When I left Dr. Slapek's office, I felt extremely uncomfortable with this hemp-like bulk in my mouth. Two days later, again on a weekend, this "crown" fell off. I was very alarmed when I saw the inflamed and bleeding tissue around the tooth. I had no idea what to do. I called a dentist, Dr. Blair, whom my husband had occasionally visited, though he was not a regular patient. This doctor was not available on a weekend. The switchboard service suggested hospital emergency. Since there was no dentist on duty there either, a nurse contacted a Dr. Lowry who lived just outside of our city. He was angry because he had to drive thirty miles to the hospital on his weekend and, from his experience, he knew that the local hospital was not equipped to handle dental emergencies. This confirmed, of course, my initial impression that tooth problems belonged in the dentist's office. Lowry refused to affix the "tin can", the term he used for Slapek's crown, and gave, as his reasons, that it was injurious to the tissues and did nothing to prevent them from readhering to the tooth. After a prolonged search he located a box of stainless steel crowns shaped like teeth. Scissors and glue sent him on another search. Because the fixing compound had long passed the expiry date, he explained that he had to press the crown hard and for several minutes to assure retention. I had to ask him to stop because of the pain and, for several hours afterward, my jaw ached.

When Dr. Slapek finally affixed the porcelain crown, it was hopelessly bulky. Over the next couple of months, she tried, several times, to correct the occlusal problem by grinding down the top tooth. This way of addressing the problem seemed to me would unnecessarily weaken that tooth and, therefore, only increased my anxiety. It was impossible to chew on this new crown because of the malocclusion and the stinging pain that did not cease. The sweats, chills and low grade fever continued as before. My complaints angered Dr. Slapek, and she refused to do anything further, saying the problem was peculiarly mine. I was just one of those people who could not adjust to a crown.

By this time I was not thinking too much about pregnancy. I was feeling so unwell. My right jaw and facial muscle ached from having chewed for seven months on the one side. Effort exhausted me, and a half hour of practicing the piano made my clothing wet with sweat. My annual appointment with Dr. Austin on November 27, 1979 arrived. This was some consolation because I had suddenly developed chest pain, a dull ache in the central and left side of my chest that went into my shoulder. Also, my sleep was fitful because the rapid heart beat had returned almost nightly now, and propranolol seemed ineffective. By the time I saw Dr. Austin, I had all but abandoned the idea of conceiving. This whole experience, which would drag on for several years, was, for many reasons, a factor in my not having children. All I could think of at that time was the day when I would feel better and be able to chew on both sides of my mouth.

Dr. Austin first addressed me with the well-worn question, polite and conventional, "Well, how are you today?"

"Miserable,"I responded truthfully and poured out all the problems of my tooth, the endodontal work, crowning, continuous stinging pain, sweats and fever, never once imagining that the sweats and fever were related to anything but the tooth. But, at that time, I thought dental problems were not the concern of a cardiologist and I felt guilty for having dumped them on him and for wasting his time. I turned quickly to the heart problems, expressing my bewilderment at the unaccustomed chest pain and the now excessive fluttering of my heart. Dr. Austin listened quietly to my complaints, then said, "Well, MVP patients do get sticky chest pains. We don't know why. It's a common symptom, but it's nothing to worry about."

"But I've never had chest pain before," I remonstrated.

"Look at it this way. Some people have headaches. You have chest aches." He took my blood pressure but not my temperature. After an electrocardiogram, he listened to my heart while he put me through the same postures as he had on previous occasions. "Mmmm," he said, shaking his head, "I can't hear the click today."

"What's that?" I asked.

"Oh, it's just a noise I've always heard in your heart. It means nothing. It comes and it goes. The murmur is likely just covering it today. Nothing to worry about," he said smiling reassuringly.

"The rapid heart beat is worse," I stressed, thinking it might relate to what he said. "A half dozen times every night short bursts wake me from my sleep. They're not as long as the first two episodes I described to you in 1976 but they seem to be as fast. And I'm so tired because I don't sleep well."

"Propranolol won't control the palpitations completely. You'll always have them. We can increase the dosage if you like. More in the daytime to maintain a higher blood level at all times."

"I don't really want to increase the drug," I responded dully. The much wanted pregnancy flitted through my mind. "In case of pregnancy."

"The propranolol is harmless," he repeated. "You've already been reassured on that point. You can see the obstetrician again if you like once you get the tooth problem sorted out."

After a chest x-ray and an echocardiogram, we returned home. A couple of days later, I received a brief letter from Dr. Austin stating that my chest x-ray showed "a minor but significant change in the configuration of the heart as compared to previous films." A follow-up appointment was set for Tuesday, January 29, 1980 at 2 p.m. for a "fluoroscopy with barium of the heart". This news was an enormous shock to both of us, especially in view of the fact that I was feeling so unwell. Even with our limited knowledge, an increase in the size of my heart sounded ominous. But we still could not make any connection between teeth and heart. They were just too remote, and no doctor I had seen had ever established the connection.

For the first time in my life, my health caused me psychological anguish. All through the month of December, including the busy Christmas season, I never felt quite well though not sick enough to take to my bed. The chills, sweats and decrease in appetite continued, and being able to chew on only one side increased my distaste for food. I began documenting my temperature which varied between 37.8°C and 38.5°C. Any kind of exertion fatigued me greatly, and the rapid heart beat grew more terrifying. Many nights I sat up, dozing in a chair until morning because as soon as I lay flat on my back, my heart fluttered so rapidly that I began to get shortness of breath.

I called Dr. Slapek in desperation and told her the tooth situation was unbearable and that the gum was now increasingly inflamed. She was unfriendly, distant, and wanted to wash her hands of the whole matter though she never suggested I see someone else. She blamed the problem on me and refused to give me an appointment until after Christmas. "I'm booked solid," she said. "Really, I don't know what else I can do. I always told you some people can't adjust to crowns. I've filed down the top tooth. There's nothing else I can do. You have to live with it."

Though Dr. Slapek had succeeded in convincing me it was my fault, her attitude was difficult to accept. Long afterwards, I would talk with people who had crowns that they could not distinguish from their natural teeth. Deeply depressed, I called Dr. Austin about my heart symptoms. Not once did I imagine that Slapek and Austin should have, all along, been in communication about the changes in my health. Dr. Austin was equally indifferent. Exhaustion had got the better of me and I was crying when I talked to him. I managed a thin veneer of self-control as I told him of the excessive, rapid heart beat that occurred when I lay flat on my back and the accompanying shortness of breath. He told me that I was being neurotic, over-reacting, and that neurosis was part of the syndrome of MVP. "Have you increased the propranolol?" he replied. I answered that I had but that I was getting headaches. "Well, it shouldn't do that. You're getting too upset about this drug. MVP patients get palpitations and shortness of breath. That's perfectly normal. Shortness of breath is a subjective sensation. You're just more aware of your heart now that you know you have MVP. Increase the propranolol a little and your heart will settle down."

When I asked if the very rapid heart beat was related to my new x-ray findings, he said it wasn't and I would have to wait until he saw me in January to know the cause. I went to see Dr. Cory, my family physician, and related everything to him. I wanted a clarification of Dr. Austin's brief, evasive letter. His letter to Dr. Cory was more detailed; my heart had enlarged by 2.5 cm. or one inch in the transverse diameter. Dr. Cory didn't know what that meant. He asked if the chest pain went into my arms. When I said no, he reassured me I was too young for angina anyway and that I was not having a heart attack. I must be patient and wait for my January appointment. He was pleased to be able to tell me that the fluoroscopy was harmless, non-invasive, that is, that nothing would enter my body and, therefore, I should be relieved. I went home confused, desperate and profoundly depressed.

4

The Teeth and the Heart

A little science is a dangerous thing, and
science in science-tight compartments is worse.
Bring to bear on every department the
co-ordinated science of all the other
departments, and the doctors will be promptly
driven beyond their crudities and follies . . . into
as sound positions . . . as humanity is capable of.

George Bernard Shaw: *Doctors' Delusions.*

The next four months were chaotic. By the time Christmas was over, a
large periodontal abscess had formed, ironic proof that what I had been suffering
for eight months was not due to my imagination nor my inability to tolerate
a crown.

Once again, I called Slapek who suggested I contact Dr. Cohen. He
reminded me that he had warned me that second molars were extremely
difficult, almost impossible, to treat. Endodontists, he stressed, had very little
success with molars but he believed he had done his work well and was quite
proud of it. I felt a subtle shift in blame to myself for having consented to
the endodontal treatment.

An x-ray confirmed an aveolar abscess. Dr. Cohen suspected the cause
was a cracked root which, he emphasized, would not show up on x-ray. There
was nothing in my arsenal of knowledge to refute this. Cohen then went to
consult a periodontist, Dr. Mentlik, who had an office in the same building.
Mentlik took several x-rays but, likewise, insisted the illusive cracked root was
invisible on the films. That a patient has a right to view the x-rays simply
didn't occur to me and, if it had, I was conditioned to believe I would be unable
to appreciate their content.

"There's only one way to be certain," Dr. Mentlik vowed, "and that's with
exploratory surgery to cut away the gum tissue so I can have a look at the
exposed root. I won't know if the tooth can be saved without doing this."

"What would be the consequences of extraction?" I asked rather regretfully
since I had put out $600.00 so far on a tooth I had not been able to use.

Dr. Mentlik rhymed off the unpleasant results. The two top teeth would descend unless wired to their neighbour. There could be periodontal problems because these teeth would have nothing to bite on. Eventually they would have to be extracted. Then the bottom lower first molar would begin to shift a little, and chewing would not be as easy on that side because of the absence of two teeth, this one and the wisdom tooth. I had visions of either a lot of hardware or a gaping hole. At that time, I did not have the influencing factor of knowing what damage this tooth had done and could still do to my heart, and Dr. Austin had rejected my new cardiac symptoms as common and unimportant in MVP. Therefore, I consented to the surgery. The decision was not one of an informed patient, who was aware of all the risks, but of a fearing patient caught between two unsatisfactory ultimatums.

In the day or two before the surgery that was to take place on January 7, 1980, my husband and I tried to find out if or how MVP related to the sudden, inexplicable cardiac enlargement. We returned to the medical library at the University and re-examined the symposium book on MVP that we had found by chance on our first visit. Although we were unable to find anything on cardiac enlargement in association with MVP, we noted some articles on the relationship between cardiac arrhythmia and sudden death in the bibliography. This was of interest to us because of the irregularities in my heart beat. Our readings led us to believe that my two earlier isolated episodes of very rapid heart beat with near fainting seemed to resemble, not the innocent "palpitations" of Dr. Austin, but what was called "paroxysmal atrial tachycardia" or PAT. Such an arrhythmia meant the heart was beating at 150-250 beats per minute. If the heart rate were 250-350 beats per minute, the arrhythmia was called atrial "flutter".[1] Curiously, "flutter" was the word I myself had chosen to describe these episodes of rapid heart beat to Austin on my first visit.

Certain case studies stuck in our minds, such as that of a 27 year old woman who had collapsed at a picnic during the normal excitement and exertion of an egg rolling contest and who later suffered a fatal cardiac arrest while engaged in an argument at a furniture store.[2] Both these events seemed less arduous and stressful than heaving a thirty pound steamer up to twelve foot walls eight hours a day six days a week. Somehow, the ongoing rapid heart beat I was experiencing over the past few months seemed more ominous. Was cardiac enlargement related to this rapid heart beat or was it a prelude to sudden death?

In our reading, we frequently came across the name of Dr. John Barlow. We located several of his articles in which he warned that MVP patients require prophylaxis against bacterial endocarditis (BE).[3] Neither this strange sounding entity nor its cause were explained in the articles. BE led to deterioration of the condition of MVP. For some reason, this one-line warning caught our attention amidst masses of detail, but, of course, we could not know whether this disease would explain my symptoms or enlarged heart. We knew "prophylaxis" signified prevention but we didn't know what measures were to be taken nor the nature of the disease to be prevented. Ironically, it never occurred to us that the "infection" that Rhodes had spoken of was identical with BE. We naturally wondered if the cardiac enlargement was a sign of a change for the worse in my condition. An article by doctors Devereux and Perloff et al, 1976, stated that "The cardiac silhouette (silhouette and config-uration, the word Austin had used, seemed to us to be identical) is normal in patients with uncomplicated mitral prolapse. Enlargement of left ventricle or left atrium awaits serious mitral regurgitation."[4] Was my cardiac enlargement causing serious regurgitation and, therefore, the symptoms I was experiencing? But we were not certain what regurgitation meant and whether or not I even had it.

This information gave us some kind of focus. Just before my periodontal surgery, we accidentally came upon a 1974 edition of *The Heart*, edited by Willus Hurst et al, on the clear-out table in Coles Book Store. Somewhere in this gargantuan work of 2,000 pages, we stumbled upon the disease of bacterial endocarditis.[5] The words leapt off the page: the teeth could cause an infection of the heart and its valves. That these two remote parts of the anatomy were connected profoundly shocked us. My heart had suddenly enlarged while I had a root abscess that progressively worsened. But was there the same danger from a root abscess as from the ordinary dental manipulations listed? The disease could be prevented, the authors said, with the use of penicillin with dental procedures in susceptible patients with rheumatic heart disease or congenital abnormalities. I supposed I had not had rheumatic fever in childhood but was MVP included in the cardiac abnormalities? We had no way of knowing the answers to these questions. Austin had said MVP was "probably" congenital. It would be some time before we understood the instructions regarding the use of penicillin or how it prevented this disease.

But at least we had learned something about this "infection" of the heart. Endocarditis is caused by bacteria (microorganisms) that enter the blood stream which transports them to the heart. The word, "itis", always means inflam-mation and thus "endocarditis" signifies an inflammation of the smooth endothelial tissue that lines the myocardium and covers the valves. The microscopic invaders are ingenious in defending themselves against destruction by human immunological forces. The bacteria become deeply embedded inside layers of necrotic, cellular debris cast off by the body: platelets, fibrin, white and red blood cells and strands of collagen. The resultant sandwich-like formation is called a vegetation, a word that implies the presence of life. It is also called simply an endocarditic lesion, a word that signifies an alteration in the tissues from disease or injury. The vegetations are engrafted to sites in the heart and on the valves. These microorganisms could enter the body in a number of ways, but we were, at this time, only interested in the teeth as the causal factor.

Though we were unable to fully understand this infection, we realized that Dr. Rhodes must have given me the penicillin to prevent this disease, even though he had used the vague term, "infection", and had not connected the teeth with the heart. Some of the classic symptoms of BE were given, such as fever, in a patient with a new organic murmur of aortic or mitral regurgitation. However, we were still confused about the meaning of regurgitation and whether or not I had it. Dr. Rhodes had refused to answer that question. If I did not have it, had I developed it thus explaining the new symptoms? I had certainly had fever every step of the way.

A detail which Austin had casually related to me on November 27, 1979 now begged interpretation. He had said he could not hear the click that day. When I asked what this click was, he had said it was an unimportant noise in the hearts of MVP patients and that the murmur was likely covering it. There had obviously been some change in the sound he had heard in my heart, but we had no idea of the significance. A murmur, from his explanation, meant simply an additional "noise" in the heart. And, if he couldn't hear the click that day, we were to infer that my heart was getting better. We didn't know if the murmur had anything to do with regurgitation. The chest pain also took on new significance though Austin had dismissed it as "de rigeur" for MVP. An enlarged spleen could be a sign of BE indicated by pain in the left upper quadrant of the body with radiation to the left shoulder. My chest pain resembled this description, but we could not know if it was from the heart or the spleen. We didn't even know if Dr. Austin had ever checked my spleen.

Although MVP was not listed in this huge book, there was a disease called Barlow's Syndrome about which several pages had been written.[6] When speaking of this syndrome, the author used the word, "prolapse". Was MVP the same thing as Barlow's syndrome we asked ourselves? Though we raised a lot of questions, we had no answers. Nor were we convinced that anything of such a seemingly serious nature as BE was going on. I had told Dr. Austin all about my tooth problem in November. He had shown no reaction whatsoever: ergo, the tooth was not the cause of the cardiac enlargement. Also his and Rhodes' insistance on the insignificance of MVP precluded any important illness.

The more information I gathered, the more I wanted, in order to solve the puzzle. On several occasions I had tried to call Dr. Austin but was never able to reach him, and he never returned my calls. One of these calls resulted in the news that my appointment had been postponed for a month to February 26, 1980 because Dr. Austin would be away on holiday. This disappointed and frustrated us very much.

The day of my periodontal surgery arrived. Apart from my exhaustion and unwell feeling, I was particularly tense, having driven for two hours through a heavy snow storm. This plus my anxiety over the cardiac enlargement and the unsettled questions did not add up to good self-control. Dr. Mentlik repeated the alternatives for me and the necessity of surgical exploration before a negative or positive prognosis regarding retention of the tooth could be made.

I did not want to have this surgery if the infection in my mouth could thereby spread to my heart, but I only vaguely understood how this might happen and didn't even know if this applied in my case. My tension was considerable, and, when I told him of my enlarged heart and my confusion over the need for antibiotics, tears began trickling unconsciously down my face. I was in no position to make a rational decision. However, Mentlik had his knife poised above my mouth. There were other patients waiting, and I must decide, he said, whether I wanted him to proceed. All I could think of just then was to ask that he contact Dr. Austin to see what he had to say. Mentlik agreed and went off to telephone. I felt somewhat relieved.

When he returned, I expected to hear that Dr. Austin had asked to see me before any surgery, having finally connected my tooth problems with my new heart findings. However, this was not the case. Mentlik was still prepared to go ahead with the surgery. I was extremely disappointed. It could only follow that I had misread the literature with respect to MVP and how cutting into an infected site could spread the infection. Mentlik's answer to my question, "What did Dr. Austin say?" was met with, not "He said that . . ." but "I'm going to give you a prescription for ampicillin which you will purchase after the surgery and take immediately at the pharmacy counter."

Even in my highly anxious state, the "I" seemed strange. Was Dr. Austin already on vacation? I would never know. Despite my doubts, I ultimately trusted that Dr. Mentlik had spoken with Dr. Austin. When I asked whether it was all right to take the penicillin after the surgery, Mentlik replied that it made no difference, an answer which I would have to learn on my own was an error. I was consumed with anxiety and confusion and, during most of the surgery, uncontrollable tears streamed down my face. Mentlik had to stop his work while his nurse dabbed at my cheeks. My discomfort even at my own behaviour was acute. I wanted to be in control of my own feelings, but the lack of information and straight answers made the whole fabric of my life appear to be coming apart at the seams.

After the surgery, Mentlik said he still could not tell whether the root of the tooth was cracked. I was simply crushed since he had insisted the surgery would reveal the problem and hence the means of correction. He then applied a bulky, uncomfortable dressing. I went to the nearest pharmacy where I gulped down the penicillin and tucked the prescription invoice into my handbag.

Several more visits to Dr. Mentlik followed during the months of January and February for changing and finally removing dressings. Afterwards, Dr. Mentlik announced that I'd have to wait a while to see the results. He said I could chew on that side again but there would be some soreness at first. Attempts to do so proved the tooth responded exactly as it had for eight months. For each of these visits, Mentlik prescribed a week of antibiotics following his inspection and probing of the tissue site. The most remarkable change in my condition was the cessation of the night time tachycardia. I no longer had to sit up to sleep.

By the time I saw Dr. Austin on February 26, the tooth was again showing visible signs of the hidden infection. A red bubble had appeared in the tissue at the base of the tooth. Dr. Austin conducted the fluoroscopy himself. Barium was not used though he had said, in his letter to Dr. Cory, that it would be. I stood with my back to a large tilting x-ray machine which Dr. Austin moved.

He pointed to a beating heart on the video screen and exclaimed confidently, "Well, well, your heart has returned to its normal size. But we'll get another echo just to see if everything is okay."

His conclusions made any questions irrelevant. I could not understand how he could make this decision from watching a moving picture. It seemed to me that an x-ray should be taken and compared for size with the previous one. But, when I asked him that, he only replied that x-rays meant more radiation. The fluoroscopy, he said, was sufficient for what he wanted to know. Dr. Austin then proceeded with his routine check of my heart. There seemed to be no reason to mistrust his judgement since, as far as I knew, he was now fully informed by a specialist in periodontics of my ongoing tooth problem. Surely, if he thought there was any connection with my cardiac symptoms, he would have ordered some tests before now! And, so, I neglected to ask if he had checked my spleen. But then this was hardly my responsibility.

However, I was to learn that I was way ahead of him. My husband asked to be present for our brief discussion after the examination, but Dr. Austin refused, as Rhodes had done. However, my husband would not accept this, and Dr. Austin had to give in. When we asked the cause of the cardiac enlargement, no matter how temporary, Dr. Austin's reply was that he didn't know. That shook us up a little. However, he added voluntarily, "When you were here in November, I did note a change in your murmur but I didn't think it was important at the time. Despite the enlargement, your heart remained within the normal limits." He paused and asked, "Did you have a fever at any time?"

"Yes, I did and still do. When I last saw you," I reminded him, "I told you that I was having ongoing dental work involving this tooth. All during it, I felt unwell with fever and sweating. I could never chew on that side because of a stinging pain and I'm still not able to do so. The problems began in April of 1979 when I had the endodontal infection and a fever of 105°F. I still don't feel well." This all tumbled out rather quickly because I was eager to impress upon him that I was not feeling well in the hope that he would, at last, give me some explanation and some method of improvement of my health.

At my request, he looked at the periodontal abscess, agreed it looked bad and advised I have the tooth "stabilized". When I asked what this meant, he said that was a matter for the periodontist or the endodontist. Once again he said nothing about antibiotics. But, this time, we had enough knowledge to raise the issue. His answer was, "Some MVP patients need them. Some don't. I don't believe there's much risk at all."

However, when another young, female doctor entered the room, he asked her opinion which was positive, and he agreed with her. When she left, we raised the issue of Dr. Mentlik's periodontal surgery and the use of ampicillin after the procedure rather than during. We also pointed out that this drug did not appear to be the drug of choice of the American Heart Association for dental prophylaxis. This much we had learned. Dr. Austin's response astonished us. He said he had no knowledge of the periodontal surgery, had never had any contact with Dr. Mentlik and had never prescribed ampicillin by telephone. He hunted through my file and verified that he had no note on this. We watched unthinkingly as he scribbled something in the margin of the page he had before him. Obviously, Dr. Austin was in total ignorance about my tooth problem and had never associated it with the cardiac symptoms I had conveyed to him.

"Did I have bacterial endocarditis?" I asked timidly, not at all certain I was asking something ridiculous and afraid of arousing his anger that I was even familiar with this technical term. It was a question we had both wanted very much to ask, but it seemed superfluous now in the light of his opinion that my heart had returned to normal.

Dr. Austin's response was startling. They say much can be read from a person's face. He blushed like a teenager and seemed startled as though this complication had never occurred to him or, if it had, he had rejected it in a MVP patient. He quickly regained his composure and, in the same jubilant, humorous tone he had used to announce the earlier fluoroscope results, he said, "Well, you don't have it now! Your heart size is back to normal." He looked just then like the cat that has swallowed the pigeon. "Bacterial endocarditis is extremely rare. I really don't think there's any risk for MVP patients."

"Well, what was the cause then of the cardiac enlargement?" I persisted.

"I guess it was the fever," he answered.

As usual, the interview terminated when he wished. His astounding opinions and his apparent unconcern clanged in our heads. A sudden inexplicable increase in cardiac size caused by fever from a root abscess that was still there while the heart had returned to normal! This seemed a bit incredible. Our confidence in the miracle workers was slipping slowly but surely.

5

The Patient as Teacher

The undesirable side-effects of approved, mistaken, callous, or contra-indicated technical contacts with the medical system represent just the first level of pathogenic medicine. Such clinical iatrogenesis includes not only the damage that doctors inflict with the intent of curing or of exploiting the patient, but also those other torts that result from the doctor's attempt to protect himself against the possibility of a suit for malpractice. Such attempts to avoid litigation and prosecution may now do more damage than any other iatrogenic stimulus.

Ivan Illich: *Limits to Medicine — Medical Nemesis: The Expropriation of Health*. (London: Marion Boyars, 1977), p. 41.

My situation steadily deteriorated. I was tossed back and forth between doctors and dentists over the next two months. No one seemed to know how to treat a patient with an abscessed tooth, murmur, chest pain, fever, tachycardia and unusual fatigue, all signs, I would learn later, of bacterial endocarditis (BE). At no time did any doctor or dentist suggest a blood test to see if there was bacteria in my bloodstream. To them, BE was a rare disease wiped out long ago by modern medicine. Instead, they treated the abscess with oral antibiotics, changing them when results were not apparent.

The periodontal abscess erupted, exuding blood and pus. My temperature remained low grade, ranging from 38.5°C to 38.9°C. I felt generally exhausted, and physical exertion produced drenching sweats and shortness of breath especially when I climbed stairs or hills or performed physically demanding household activities. The fluttering heart beat was frequent and the chest pain intermittent. And, yet, I never felt so unwell that I could not continue to function. The feeling I had was similar to that I experienced with a heavy cold, a general aching all over but without the sneezing and runny nose.

Extraction of the tooth now seemed urgent. This was not easily accomplished. The date of my final check-up with Dr. Mentlik was March 18, 1980. An attempt to get an earlier appointment was unsuccessful. I, therefore, went to see my husband's dentist, Dr. Blair, and outlined briefly what had happened to me. He was completely unfamiliar with MVP and refused to extract the tooth until I had seen Dr. Mentlik three weeks later. I feared that my heart, which had supposedly returned to its normal size, a fact my husband and I doubted, would enlarge again or my murmur deteriorate if the poisonous tooth remained in my mouth. I told Dr. Blair this and asked if I should take antibiotics until I saw Dr. Mentlik. He agreed and took an x-ray. To my astonishment, his x-ray clearly revealed a longitudinal root fracture which he pointed out to me. There was also considerable inflammation around the apex of the root and in the jaw bone. He gave me a prescription for oral antibiotics and I left.

When I telephoned Dr. Mentlik again to press for an earlier appointment, I told him about the longitudinal root fracture on Dr. Blair's x-ray. Dr. Mentlik denied that he had said the crack would not show up on x-ray. "But you did!" I protested vigorously. "Both you and Cohen said a fractured root would not show up on x-ray. You said you could only know this with surgical exploration and, then, even after the surgery, you claimed you did not see a fracture."

His denial angered me. I asked him to recheck his x-rays, but he only argued that what he and Dr. Blair saw were simply two different things. Then he refused to extract the tooth. That was not his job. The tooth looked stable as far as he was concerned, and he had many patients with chronically infected teeth with murmurs worse than mine. When I said Dr. Austin believed the tooth should be stabilized, Mentlik agreed but insisted Dr. Blair could do the extracting.

But Dr. Blair refused until Mentlik saw me. I waited, confused and anxious, and, when March 18 arrived, I brought Dr. Blair's x-ray for comparison. I insisted on seeing my x-rays. Two of Mentlik's four x-rays showed the same evidence of a vertical crack beginning in the dentine and veering off diagonally. With Dr. Blair's evidence before him, Mentlik was obliged to agree that his x-rays revealed a vertical fracture line. Mentlik then revised his earlier opinion at the time of surgery about the dire consequences of extraction and now emphasized strongly that I would not notice the loss of the tooth. Nor would anything disastrous happen to the other teeth. My sense of impotence and even betrayal were so great that I lacked the spirit to protest. Somehow, I knew deep in my heart, it would not accomplish anything.

I returned to Dr. Blair who once again refused to extract the tooth. This time he wanted a written order from Dr. Austin that the tooth must be extracted. On March 31, 1980, I wrote asking Dr. Austin for this decision. Our suspicions that I had been incompetently treated were multiplying. Mentlik's prevarications, the inconsistencies in his and Austin's stories troubled us greatly. We began to question the entire dental treatment. When I last saw Dr. Cohen, he had voluntarily offered to return part of my money for an unsuccessful root canal treatment. In the light of everything, this now struck us as unorthodox, a self-serving tactic to suppress my complaints. Likewise, Dr. Mentlik's refusal of payment for the last two visits now suggested a guilty conscience. Our most burning question was why a cardiologist would consent to periodontal surgery on an infected tooth without antibiotic protection in a patient with an inexplicable cardiac enlargement. Our reading had thoroughly convinced us that, according to the American Heart Association's recommendations of 1977 [1], the latest at that time, Mentlik's and Austin's antibiotic was not the drug of choice. The dosage was inadequate and the instructions to take it after the surgery incorrect since, to assure optimum blood levels during the procedure, antibiotics should be taken before not after surgery. Mentlik's instructions could only apply to a patient with a normal heart who was taking the antibiotic, not to prevent a systemic bacterial endocarditis, but a local infection in the oral cavity.

On April 1, 1980, I wrote to the Royal College of Dental Surgeons (RCDS) outlining my entire treatment. Like my letter to Dr. Rhodes, this letter was not accusatory. It raised my questions and asked for their evaluation of the work of the three dental practitioners involved, Slapek, Cohen and Mentlik. Their letter of April 8, 1980 indicated they were investigating the matter and requested that I let them know if I had lodged the complaint with anyone else. My husband and I did not know what that meant. The irony is that they were already thinking a legal suit might be launched against the dentists, a move that we had not even imagined.

In my letter to the College, I described Dr. Blair's findings and said that he would not remove the tooth until he had received written permission from Dr. Austin. That permission did not arrive until the third week of April and, even then, Dr. Blair once again refused. It was now the College which must give him permission and it had asked him to wait until the investigation was completed. This caused me enormous anxiety. I imagined an extremely long wait. As it turned out, it was many months but I did not wait for that. Even though I had made no complaint about Dr. Blair, he was furious that I had mentioned his name to the College. When I stressed the necessity for immediate extraction, he refused even to look at the tooth. He must await his orders. In his efforts to justify his refusal, he denied that 38.5°C was a fever. This was the normal temperature of babies he said. From this, I was to infer that I was behaving in a childishly emotional way over a minor problem. But I feared further complications because I had stopped the antibiotics since March 18. However, Dr. Blair wouldn't prescribe any drug without the College's permission.

I contemplated finding another dentist, but the effort of explaining everything seemed overwhelming, and the College, of course, would not approve. There was another reason for my hesitation in going to another general dentist. From my reading of the medical literature, the only safe way to extract the tooth was in hospital with intravenous antibiotic coverage which would be far more powerful against bacteria than oral antibiotics. Extraction of an infected tooth seemed extremely dangerous in an individual who felt as unwell as I did and who was experiencing symptoms that could be indicative of BE. A chronic infection could thus become acute.

My husband discussed my situation with Dr. Cory who felt that I had some low grade systemic infection, though he made no attempt to find out what it was and said I should be taking antibiotics. Dr. Cory prescribed 300 mgm. of penicillin V four times a day until the tooth was removed. The periodontal abscess which continued to ooze blood and pus was really an opening or fistula through which the purulent matter from the root infection could escape. I had several episodes of severe tachycardia which drove me to the hospital for an electrocardiogram, but, the attack was over once I arrived. A doctor in emergency looked at my tooth. I told him of my murmur and previous cardiac enlargement. He said that I was developing immunity to the penicillin and replaced it with cloxacillin. None of these doctors appeared to understand the purpose of oral antibiotics, that they cannot penetrate abscesses in the roots or sockets of teeth or heal infection in bone.[2] This was something I would learn later. At that time, I did not even know how antibiotics worked.

The situation had so deteriorated that I pulled the panic button. I talked with Dr. Austin's secretary to explain why Dr. Blair would not extract the tooth and insist on an appointment within the next few days. Dr. Cory advised me to put everything into the hands of Dr. Austin. In the event that he refused to admit me for the extraction, I called Dr. Blair. Curiously he asked to see me immediately. As soon as I was seated in his chair, he announced, "I'm taking that tooth out right now! The College said if you kept complaining, I was to extract it." The rough, angry manner in which he said this did not, of course, inspire confidence, and extraction without intravenous antibiotic coverage was beginning to appear unthinkable since oral antibiotics had not made me feel well. I did not even know if such treatment was available in a dental office. Dr. Blair simply scoffed at my suggestion of such a precaution and launched into an angry monologue. Cases like mine, he said, would cause him to lose business and he feared he would have to return money in the event of an unsuccessful root canal treatment. I wondered if the College had informed him that Dr. Cohen had offered a reimbursement and that this was to become the rule in cases of endodontal failure. Dr. Blair staunchly defended Dr. Cohen's work. What complicated problems would he encounter in patients with murmurs like mine he asked? I began to wonder how many patients Dr. Blair had with murmurs, either unidentified or of MVP, which he had been ignoring. To contact the cardiologist in these cases wasted his time he complained. The number of patients he could see would be reduced. And would he have to give all these MVP patients prescriptions for antibiotics? And if he didn't, would he be sued in the event of infection? A simple root canal procedure, he exaggerated, would now become highly complicated and risky and he would soon lose the greater part of his business to the specialists. After his tirade, he ordered me to go, saying he was washing his hands of the entire mess and Dr. Austin could look after me from now on. I was stunned, overwhelmed by the whole situation, and stumbled weakly out of his office.

I was given an appointment at TMSC for April 29th at 1:30 p.m. After talking with Dr. Blair, the College had contacted Dr. Austin. What followed next was more of what Dr. Blair had dumped on me, only more threatening and shocking. Austin was extremely annoyed that I had written to the RCDS about my tooth problem. Austin was one of the professors at the College who taught the dentists about the relationship between the teeth and the heart. Everything the dentists had done, he insisted, was correct. An angry discussion followed concerning the events of 1979 and 1980. I complained that he had ignored my account of symptoms of fever, sweating, exhaustion, SOB, tachycardia and chest pain and that he had not related these symptoms, or the cardiac enlargement and change in murmur to the prolonged root abscess. To prove he had, Dr. Austin began reading out loud to me his November 27th letter to Dr. Cory, a copy of which he had given me. Of course, there was no mention whatsoever of dental work, antibiotics or the suspicion of BE. When Austin realized this, his response was to tell me that our patient relationship was no longer "satisfactory" and I could look for another doctor.

A feeling of impotence washed over me and, with it, fear but, somehow, I vaguely understood that he bore some responsibility for my illness and then rejected his obligation to correct it. "I have a right to health care, to the treatment facilities at this hospital," I replied trembling. "I have a fever, a severe dental abscess and possibly further enlargement of my heart. You have no right to drop me! I want you to do something about my problem now!"

"Oh, you want me to play daddy," he answered somewhat more jovially. He assured me then that he had never yet dropped a patient. This response angered me. It was consistent with his attitude on my first visit when he had prescribed propranolol, not for my rapid heart beat, but for my anxiety. Now, he once again appeared to be adopting the role of psychiatrist rather than cardiologist and was treating me as an hysterical, neurotic female who must relate to her doctor as daddy.

This outburst was followed by an attack on our healthcare system. "I wouldn't have these problems," he said angrily, "if I went to the United States. I'd be free of control. A lot of doctors are leaving Canada. I don't get paid for teaching at the dental college. I'd make a lot more money south of the border and what thanks do I get for the care I give here?"

I had the distinct feeling, which I had had many times since the beginning of my illness, that I was, somehow, to blame for the calamities that had befallen me. But was Austin afraid that my contact with the dental college would, somehow, implicate him? Did he suddenly feel he had taught the dentists incorrectly with regard to antibiotics and MVP? Did his fear, in fact, begin earlier when I had raised the issue of BE?

His next comment seemed to imply that my situation had caused a change in his views about the risks to MVP patients. "I'll remind the dental students about the need for antibiotics with dental work for MVP patients," he said and then examined me. I had the feeling that his thoroughness was compromised by his anger since he checked my spleen only after I asked him to do so, at which point he showed me how this organ should be palpated and pronounced that it was not enlarged. "Well, I don't see any signs of BE," he concluded.

It was evident then that he was not going to admit me to hospital to extract the tooth and I, therefore, pressed. "Is it true that a chronic subacute endocarditis can linger for months unsuspected and even recur after a seeming cure?" He agreed, and, when I asked him to check my temperature, this seemed to be the factor which tilted the scales because he admitted me immediately to rule out BE and to extract the tooth with intravenous coverage.

The treatment I received in hospital and the investigation of the IE were suspect, but I had no way of evaluating my care at that time. As of my 1:30 p.m. appointment, I ceased taking the oral antibiotic. But Pen V has a 24 hour half life and would still be in my bloodstream until some time on Wednesday and could render the samples negative. The blood sample collected immediately after my visit with Dr. Austin and the two on the second day of hospitalization, May 1, 1980, were said to be negative. An intern, who collected one of these last two samples, dropped much of it on the bedclothes. The sample of blood taken immediately after the extraction grew alpha hemolytic streptococcus viridans, a common microorganism that resides in the mouth at all times, is a frequent cause of tonsillitis and is implicated in many cases of BE. The argument that this blood sample was positive only because it was taken after the extraction when bacteria would shower the bloodstream is not acceptable because there was no way of knowing whether the strep. viridans that was grown from my blood was not already in my blood stream and had been there for many months. Taking a blood sample immediately after extraction will always produce a positive culture. Later, I would ask if Dr. Austin, in fact, took this blood sample at that particular time simply to confuse matters? He could not be faulted for saying that a positive sample taken immediately after extraction does not mean IE. But the argument crumbles when we consider that the first two blood samples were, in all likelihood, negative because of the penicillin I had taken for a week prior to my hospitalization.

Dr. Austin told me that two doctors would be in charge of my care. I never saw these two until they came to see me on the morning of my discharge to announce I could go home at 1:00 p.m. The only doctors I saw were the intern in charge of my care and the intern who took the third sample of blood when he listened to my heart and a resident in internal medicine when complications from the IV vancomycin developed. It was as though I was there merely to serve as a dummy to assist the medical students.

Dr. Austin had ordered the vancomycin, 1 gm. IV every 6 hours, to start after the extraction on the Friday, May 2. This, I would learn much later, was questionable; my coverage should have begun prior to the procedure. The vancomycin was to continue until 12 p.m. on Sunday just before discharge. This drug caused extreme pain in my wrist which swelled up to twice its size. But, as far as I knew, that was what one suffered with intravenous antibiotics. Though I complained to the nurse when she was taking my pulse, she only dropped my left wrist and took my pulse in the right. She said that the pain was because the antibiotic was not going into the vein at that moment, but, when the next dose was administered, I would not feel this pain. I looked up to see that the plastic antibiotic bag was, indeed, empty. Long afterwards when I had gained more information, I realized how ridiculously inaccurate, how professionally irresponsible and inhuman that reply was. I was recently hospitalized for an unaccountable fever. A very competent nurse explained to me that swelling of an IV site meant that the needle had punctured the vein and the antibiotic was entering the interstitial tissues, thus causing swelling and pain and would, in fact, retard the circulation of the medication.

I endured the excruciating pain in my arm as long as I could, but, by late Saturday night, my wrist and forearm had grotesquely swollen. My heavy, fat limb lay paralyzed on the bedclothes as if in punishment for demanding special, preventative medicine for a condition so unimportant as MVP, while tears began rolling helplessly down my face. The nurses would do nothing without a doctor's orders. I asked to see a doctor, a very difficult request in a hospital if you are a MVP patient. When the resident finally came, he refused to take out the intravenous line and, only much later, after many complaints, did he transfer it to the other arm. It, too, began to pain and swell several hours afterwards though not as badly as the left arm since the antibiotic treatment ended at noon the next day.

Immediately after my discharge, I saw Dr. Cory who explained that the vancomycin had caused phlebitis, an inflammation of the vein wall. He gave me phenylbutazone for several weeks, but, long after this drug was discontinued, there was a sharp, prickly pain and the veins remained rigid and distended, especially in the left arm. Nevertheless, I responded to my hospitalization with naive emotionalism, thanking Dr. Austin for his care which had amounted to about fifteen minutes in all, ten when he appeared at the extraction of the tooth and about five when he came into my room to check the effects of the vancomycin on me. I imagined Dr. Austin had done everything possible to rule out subacute bacterial endocarditis.

At my follow-up visit two weeks after my discharge, he strove to convince me once again that the change in my murmur was unimportant. His attempt to allay my fears succeeded; I was temporarily blinded to his mistakes. But I had known years of childhood poverty and the deprivation of medical care. When I finally got this care, my instinct was to feel guilty and grateful simultaneously as if health care were a privilege I hadn't deserved instead of the undeniable right that I and many others, in my position, were entitled to.

6

Judge and Jury

It is a matter of common knowledge that members of any county medical society are extremely loath to testify against each other in a malpractice case . . . Anyone familiar with cases of this character knows that the so-called ethical practitioner will not testify on behalf of a plaintiff regardless of the merits of his case. This is largely due to the pressure exerted by medical societies and public liability insurance companies which issue policies of liability insurance to physicians covering malpractice claims . . . Regardless of the merits of the plaintiff's case, physicians who are members of medical societies flock to the defense of the fellow member charged with malpractice and the plaintiff is relegated, for his expert testimony, to the occasional lone wolf or heroic soul who for the sake of truth and justice has the courage to run the risk of ostracism by his fellow practitioners and the cancellation of his public liability insurance policy.

> The Honorable Jesse Carter of the Supreme Court Bench of California in David E. Seidelson. "Medical Malpractice Cases and the Reluctant Expert." (Nov. 16, 1966) *Catholic University Law Review* 16: 158-186.

After my discharge from TMSC on May 4, 1980, I felt gratitude for finally securing some help. However, I did have serious doubts that IE had been thoroughly investigated. These doubts would be shown to be sound when, six years later, I would at last have a look at my hospital records. In a letter I asked Dr. Austin if the enzyme, penicillinase, had been added to my blood cultures to destroy the oral penicillin which would have made my blood negative for bacteria. This is usually done in cases when oral antibiotics have been administered prior to culturing the blood. Austin never provided me with this information, and I did not see him again. It appeared that my blood cultures were kept only for the few days I was in hospital because I was released on the basis that there was no IE since my blood was, at that time, believed to be negative for bacteria. However, I knew from my reading that cultures should be kept at least three weeks to allow for slow-growing organisms.[1] As well, to assure optimum blood levels of the drug, prophylactic treatment should be started prior to, not after, the extraction.

The use of the drug, vancomycin, raised several questions. It was known to cause phlebitis and was ordinarily reserved for curing life-threatening staphylococcal infections and only when nothing else worked. It was not normally used in a prophylactic capacity. At the time of my hospitalization, Goodman and Gilman, summing up the current attitude to vancomycin, said, "There is presently very little indication for the use of vancomycin because of the availability of other effective and less toxic agents, such as the penicillins" and "therapy with vancomycin should be reserved for the management of disease produced by staphylococcus aureus."[2] My bacteria was said to be strep. viridans. At the present time, vancomycin is still used mainly for staph. aureus and in cases of penicillin sensitivity. During my hospitalization, my husband asked Dr. Austin why he used vancomycin and he replied that he thought I had penicillin sensitivity because my temperature remained elevated while I was on oral antibiotics. Later I would learn that, in all likelihood, my temperature did not decrease because the oral penicillin was inadequate to eradicate the bacteria from the valve. I have taken penicillin many times since for dental prophylaxis, and, on no occasion, has my temperature risen. This indicates that the penicillin I had been taking was ineffective against the microorganisms on my valve. Nor have I ever had an allergic reaction to this drug.

Dr. Austin had assured me that my change in murmur, during my cardiac enlargement, was insignificant and that "my prolapse would now settle down" without any residual valvular effects. I doubted this miraculous cure because I continued to suffer from fatigue, weakness in my leg muscles and SOB with vigorous activities I had carried on easily before. In the past I had been an avid sportswoman, skiing, cycling, playing tennis and performing daily yoga. I had even walked two and three miles a day when I worked on my house. I could not accept the exercise intolerance as normal.

I discussed my health situation with Dr. Cory. As in the matter of the cardiac enlargement, he read me relevant portions from Dr. Austin's letters. Dr. Cory always prefaced this act with "I should not be doing this. These letters are not meant for you." However, eventually he would hand over the entire file to me, telling me to photocopy whatever I wanted. It must be stressed here that, if I had not asked for this "additional" information, Dr. Cory would not have given it to me. And, that I asked presupposed that I had enough knowledge to form the suspicion that past events were responsible for my present health. Patients, in general, assume, out of great respect and trust, that the doctor will convey everything there is to know, not "everything" the physician determines is in the patient's best interests to know or is in the doctor's best interests to divulge. Dr. Cory may also have readily given me this information because he felt genuinely bad that I had suffered such complications or because he had begun to recognize his own responsibility. In the province of Ontario, patients do not have legal access to their medical records, and, in most cases the physician, if asked, will refuse access. Other doctors have not allowed me to see the personal information they have accumulated on my body. Access is entirely subject to the whim of the doctor involved.

Any doubt that something significant had happened to me and any guilt for having made a mountain out of a molehill completely dissipated the moment I laid eyes on Dr. Austin's letters. The dramatic change in his opinion was enough in itself to convince me something serious had happened of which only he had knowledge. Prior to my illness, in March of 1976 and December of 1978, Austin consistently described my murmur, in his letters to my GP, as "intermittent late systolic", "a rather innocent sounding mid-precordial systolic murmur" or a "mid-systolic sound". The murmur was confined to a specific area over the heart and did not radiate to other areas of the body, such as the back or neck, as a more prominent murmur would do. Likewise, Dr. Rhodes had referred to my murmur as "mid-systolic . . . at the apex" with "a late systolic click". As well, Dr. Austin's echocardiogram showed "mild mitral prolapse" while Dr. Rhodes had not confirmed the presence of prolapse, not because the machine was old as he said, but because my prolapse was so minimal.

The typical late systolic murmur of MVP begins in mid to late systole and can be introduced by a mid to late systolic click according to the *Merck Manual of Diagnosis and Therapy* written by doctors for doctors.[3] In Dr. Austin's opinion, this mid-late systolic murmur was "innocent", that is, posed no risks of IE and, thus, I did not require antibiotic protection during dental procedures. "I don't believe they (MVP patients) need prophylaxis against infective endocarditis", he stated in 1976 and, again in 1978, "I do not believe that the risks of infective endocarditis in these mild mitral prolapsers . . . is really significant." His was an opinion, I learned later, that was not shared by the medical profession at that time, even in his own locale, as common heart textbooks such as Hurst's confirm as early as 1974: "It is an error not to provide appropriate prophylactic antibiotic therapy for dental work or surgery in patients with valvular or congenital heart disease and those with mitral regurgitation due to prolapse of the posterior mitral leaflet."[4] For an opinion to be enshrined in a textbook of the status of Willus Hurst's, it must be the result of years of research and discussion and have been universally accepted by the medical profession.

Dr. Austin seemed to believe that the only symptom in MVP that required attention was anxiety neurosis. The treatment was reassurance, in his view, and he said I could have an annual assessment "if it made me feel better". In his letter of December 12, 1978 to Dr. Cory, Dr. Austin made it clear that he really needed to see me only if "significant cardiovascular problems" developed. However, when such complications did develop, he rejected them as insignificant because of his fundamental philosophy that MVP was a harmless condition. Though he informed Dr. Cory in a letter of November 27, 1979, that the cardiac enlargement might be caused by "increasing mitral regurgitation at the mitral valve site", Austin failed to relate his suspicion to the oral infection, the symptoms I had described or the change in the murmur that he had heard. Ultimately, he stuck to his old view that there were no risks in the MVP syndrome.

The most important of Dr. Austin's letters was that of April 9, 1980 which contained a markedly different opinion. In the space of four months he had changed his mind sharply. He no longer described the murmur as "innocent" or "benign", and my mitral regurgitation was now "important" enough and "the duration of my mitral murmur" long enough that antibiotic protection during dental procedures was imperative. Clearly, Austin was backtracking. "Most individuals," he declared, "with the benign form of mitral prolapse and with only a click and no evidence for *important* regurgitation may not require antibiotic prophylaxis (ABP) during dental surgery or any dental treatment that might create a bacteremia." But, in speaking of myself, he said that "such treatments do require antibiotic prophylaxis because of the duration of her mitral murmur." What Dr. Austin meant was that I did not need the antibiotic protection when I had only a late systolic murmur but now that I had a longer murmur with "important" regurgitation I required such protection. Now there is a risk where once there was none. It is an admission that the cardiac enlargement, brought on by some infective process, had increased the regurgitation and transformed an "innocent" murmur into a significant one. To say the LSM did not require ABP was a very serious error according to the medical literature at the time.

This April 9, 1980 letter, which was also Dr. Austin's order to Dr. Blair to extract my tooth, was, in essence, a complete reversal of his former opinion. In the past he had not viewed my dental problems as in any way related to my heart, but, now, four months later, rather than make use of completely reliable, preventative antibiotics during dental interventions in MVP patients, he took the extreme stand that no preservation attempts should be made in any case. "From the medical point of view it is not appropriate to try and maintain or preserve teeth and risk the potential problems of a bacteremic situation," he said. Not only is this an unnecessary stand in most cases but it is also clearly an example of closing the barn door after the horse has fled.

Dr. Austin's letter offered even further evidence that he now believed that I had suffered a damaging infective process. He informed Dr. Cory that he wished to see me at "six monthly intervals with clinical exam, x-ray and echocardiogram studies for a year or two" until, as he put it, my mitral prolapse would stabilize itself, presumably return to what it was. This meant he believed that "significant cardiovascular problems" had developed. Seeing me was thus no longer a matter merely of reassurance to lessen an anxiety neurosis; my health situation now demanded it.

Dr. Austin's April letter also represented his report to Dr. Cory of my follow-up visit on February 26, 1980. It was strange that he took over a month to reply when he had replied immediately at the time of the cardiac enlargement. But what was most astonishing about his letter was that he made no reference to the fluoroscopy examination he had personally done on February 26, 1980 but spoke of a heart x-ray that he said indicated my cardiac size had returned to normal. My husband and I knew I had not had a chest x-ray that day, only a fluoroscopy and echocardiogram. In fact, when I asked Dr. Austin if a heart x-ray would not be more valuable for comparison purposes, he replied that he did not want to expose me to further radiation after the fluoroscopy. His answer was the same at the time of my hospitalization on April 30, 1980. Thus, a follow-up x-ray was never taken for comparison of my heart size before and after the febrile illness. And, yet, he was now demanding x-rays every six months!

Ironically, Austin was correct about the radiation exposure, and we could never understand why he chose fluoroscopy. In Hurst's heart textbook, Weens and Gay state that "roentgenograms appear entirely satisfactory for the evaluation of cardiac size and configuration."[5] According to the Merck Manual for physicians, "Cardiac fluoroscopy has limited diagnostic value and gives the patient a relatively large dose of radiation," much more, in fact, than a normal x-ray. Fluoroscopy is normally used to detect cardiac problems other than size, for instance calcification of either valves, pericardium or myocardium or pericardial effusion, that is the accumulation of excess fluid around the heart.[6]

Why did Austin use the fluoroscopy instead of the x-ray? Using a fluoroscope is like taking a movie, the x-ray being seen immediately on a video screen, at least that was the way mine worked. Since he conducted the test himself, Austin did not need to consult a radiologist and, in fact, the hospital would later inform me that Dr. Austin had not provided a written report. In other words, there was no proof that I had actually had this test. What was Dr. Austin trying to verify by fluoroscopy? Was he, in fact, not looking for cardiac size at all and, instead, was looking for pericarditis or a pericardial effusion or even valvular calcification from an episode of rheumatic fever? Curiously, there was no barium swallow for the test as he had indicated there would be in his letter to Dr. Cory. The barium swallow highlights the esophagus, stomach and gastrointestinal tract and may be used for fluoroscopic study of the heart, though it is considered inferior to the chest x-ray for assessment of cardiac size and configuration according to cardiology textbooks and the Merck Manual of Diagnosis and Therapy. What did the moving picture of a beating heart tell Dr. Austin? What was he looking for? Chest pain of an esophageal origin? The supposed globus hystericus, or lump in the throat, of neurotic patients with MVP? That day, February 26, 1980, two things were clear to us for certain: I did not swallow barium and I did not have a chest x-ray. Therefore, from whence came the x-ray, that later vanished, which showed the return of my heart to its normal size?

Austin forwarded a copy of this April, 1980 letter, containing his reference to this February 6, 1980 chest x-ray and his statement that I had had no IE to Dr. Blair with the general recommendation that teeth should not be preserved in such cases as mine. This constituted the written permission Dr. Blair had asked for to extract my tooth. Dr. Austin had also forwarded a copy of his letter to Dr. Mentlik. It was this letter, provided either by Dr. Austin or Dr.

Blair, which the Complaints Committee of the Royal College of Dental Surgeons would ultimately use to arrive at their decision of whether or not the dentists had acted negligently in my case.

After my discharge from TMSC, I waited for the meeting with the Complaints Committee. Right from the beginning, I had been unhappy with the work of the dentists. This was the reason I had written to the College on April 1, 1980, eight days before Dr. Austin's letter to Dr. Cory containing his final opinion on what had happened to me. When I learned I was to have a meeting with this Complaints Committee, about which I knew absolutely nothing, I asked a casual acquaintance of mine, who was a lawyer, just what all this meant. My informal discussion led to an official meeting in his office and, eventually, to this lawyer's offer to act on my behalf to speed up the results of my meeting with the Complaints Committee. My earlier desire was to retrieve the money I had spent on not only unsuccessful dental manipulations but also on interventions that I suspected had caused a febrile illness that I could not, as yet, identify with certitude but that was clearly related to a change in my murmur and a deterioration in my health. These initial questions I asked of my lawyer eventually resulted in his making additional demands for damages, though small, $2500, from the dentists' insurers. My purpose became, however, to obtain what was most important to me: my medical records that would eventually vanish.

However, to the members of the medical and dental professions even such a harmless exercise as my initial query letter about my treatment was automatically interpreted as the first step toward full-blown malpractice litigation against my dentists. This was the reason the Complaints Committee asked, "If you have lodged this complaint with any other organization, we would appreciate being informed." At that time, the truth of the matter was that malpractice litigation was the furthest thing from our minds. In fact, neither my husband nor I realized that the word, "organization", used by this official body, could only refer to a legal firm. And, even though my so-called case would drag on for years, no official step would ever be taken against my dentists. And though Dr. Austin's name had never even been mentioned in my letter to the dental college, on the day of my hospitalization, he had expressed anger that I had written, not to his college but to that of the dentists.

However, my lawyer was unable to tell me anything about such a meeting with the Complaints Committee of the RCDS. He was unable to answer any of my fundamental questions such as whether or not the three dentists would be present, what kind of questions the Committee would ask me and whether or not the dentists would deny the evidence on x-ray of a cracked root, as Mentlik had done in my personal communication with him. I wanted to know if the Committee would be examining the x-rays and how would I prove that Slapek had put that awful "tin can" on my tooth. Would I be charged with "libel" because of my letter? This last pitiful question only testified to my profound ignorance in such matters.

We knew no more about the law than we had known about medicine.

We did not know that this lawyer had no experience in medical matters of this nature. We never asked. We were "babes in the woods" when it came to legal and medical matters. In fact, we didn't even know there were lawyers with expertise in medical malpractice or that there were very few in Toronto. This lawyer's advice was not to have legal representation at this meeting because the Complaints Committee would regard this as antagonistic. Thus, on my arrival, I would find Slapek, Cohen and Mentlik with their lawyers in tow to ensure that they didn't say anything that would make them appear negligent. They were armed, so to speak, to the teeth, with legal assistance, with knowledge, with my entire files which I had never been allowed to look at, all the evidence of how treatment should be conducted and what went wrong with mine, all the x-rays, notes, dates and their interpretation of purposes of appointments. I was alone with little or no knowledge of what had happened to me, nothing more, in short, than memories of a painful illness and a few receipts for antibiotics and for visits! But even then this little evidence I had would conflict with statements made by the dentists as to the dates and purposes of appointments.

We had never imagined suing a dentist or a doctor; they could do no harm. No paranoia propelled me to gather any evidence to substantiate my claims of their negligence prior to this meeting. I would realize later that my lawyer should have obtained my dental records prior to my meeting with the Complaints Committee. Without this proof, my complaints would be regarded as unsubstantiated, particularly in the matter of the cracked root.

In the fight to legalize abortion, the pro-choice argument has been that women should have control over their own bodies. This should be the cry of everyone who makes use of the services of doctors and dentists. Patients, without personal health information, without evidence of what was done to them, without knowledge, are totally out of control. And all personal health information must be obtained at the time that this information is being collected from the patient. That patients do not have a legal right to this information makes it impossible to have a truly fair investigation of what went wrong. Many members of the legal profession have complete faith in the integrity of doctors and dentists and, so, they do not bother to obtain this material and, once any action is commenced, there is little or no likelihood that doctors or dentists will release any of this personal health information to a lawyer. My lawyer, tragically, would never succeed in obtaining dental records from any of my dentists after my meeting with the Complaints Committee.

The medical and dental professions police themselves; they are free of criticism by the lay public. Their Colleges are invested with the responsibility of governing their graduates in their respective professions. These institutions have the right within law to grant and revoke licenses. They investigate the negligence of their members and decide upon whether their responsibilities were carried out appropriately. In effect, the Colleges have the power of judge and jury. As set out in an official Act, the Colleges have sole responsibility for establishing, maintaining and improving or updating the standards of

knowledge and skill in their respective professions, the standards of quali-
fication and practice and the professional ethics of their members.[7] But local
standards are not world standards and, if the Colleges do nothing to raise the
standards of the profession to that of the rest of the world or, if they set standards
which they do not enforce, then treament will be inferior and will vary from
doctor to doctor or from dentist to dentist.

At my meeting with the Complaints Committee, I told my story, and the
panel of three judges, all dentists, asked me questions. If I had little knowledge
of the nature of my injuries, I had even less of what constituted good dental
work or how important that was to the MVP patient. When Cohen stated
he had done his work well and had not cracked the root, I could not contradict.
When Slapek said she had made the crown properly and that she had warned
me that certain people could not tolerate crowns, I could not contradict by
stating what a proper crown should have looked or felt like. When Mentlik
claimed that he had correctly dealt with the abscessed root and claimed that
there were people with murmurs and teeth more badly infected than mine
who suffered no ill results, I could offer no proof to the contrary. It was my
"bad luck" he said. What the patient does not know, the dentists on the
Complaints Committee will not provide. An issue not raised by a patient is
an issue avoided.

The Report of the Complaints Committee, dated September 12, 1980,
contained the verdict of the three judges. My testimony, in most respects, was
superfluous. In fact, I need not have been present at this meeting. The
Committee ordered Dr. Slapek to return the $300 for the crown. Did this mean
it considered Slapek's ill-fitting crown to be improperly prepared? Or did it
mean that I no longer had the crown, not to mention the tooth, and so, why
should I pay for it? At the time of my periodontal surgery, Dr. Cohen offered
to return my money for the endodontal work. I did not accept it at the time
because I wanted to ask further questions about this treatment. Dr. Mentlik,
without any prompting from me, did not charge me for the last two visits
with him. Such behaviour on the part of these two dental practitioners only
made me more suspicious that something was amiss. However, the College
interpreted Mentlik's offer to return some of the money as a "gesture of
goodwill" and Cohen's as "a matter of policy". No suggestion of error or
negligence was attached to such offers. I did not agree with this assessment
but was unable, of course, deprived as I was of any dental information
whatsoever, to bring forward any argument to substantiate my allegation that
either of these dentists were responsible for the cracked root, the aveolar abscess
and the prolongation of an oral sepsis that, as I will show in this book, resulted
in the enlargement of my heart, the deterioration of a mild MVP murmur
and, ultimately, all the signs of heart failure.

In the matter of the cracked root, the Complaints Committee declared
that none of the practitioners was responsible. "The fracture of a devitalized
tooth," they said, "can occur without negligence on the part of the treating
dentist." Dr. Lowry was excused because, the Committee stated, he was obliged

to use excessive force to achieve retention of the crown. It must be remembered that the adhesive compounds at the hospital were out of date and he had difficulty making the crown stick. Though my feeling was that adhesive, not force, glues the crown to the remaining natural tooth structure, I agreed with the Committee since my stinging pain dated from the time of the endodontal work.

However, after this meeting, I would learn that much evidence existed in the dental literature that "devitalized teeth", teeth deprived of their nerves and thus blood supply, if prepared properly, are not as vulnerable as the Complaints Committee tried to convince me. This is understandable when we realize that vital or living molars, the "crushers" and "grinders", withstand enormous pressures over a lifetime of mastication. Proof that they can submit to extraordinary pressures without cracking is suggested by anthropology studies. Researchers, for instance, have examined lead balls which prisoners at Fort Ticonderoga in New York had bitten out of shape at the time they were being severely tortured. 1600 pounds of pressure were required to distort these same lead balls in the way human teeth had done.[8] This goes a long way toward proving that enormous pressure is necessary to crack the materials in a human tooth, be it crown or root.

Though teeth, deprived of their nerves and blood supply through the endodontal process, may not be as strong as healthy, living teeth, such as those described in the Ticonderoga study, the Committee's argument was a weak one which most dental researchers reject. Dr. Harold Gerstein, author of an endodontics text book, says, when speaking of devitalized teeth, that "fractures are often excused based on purported brittleness of enormous magnitude although the true cause of failure was inadequate restoration."[9] Gerstein confirms that "the correctly reconstructed pulpless tooth should be no more susceptible to masticatory failure", one of the chief causes of cracks, "than its vital counterpart."[10] As well, hard foods, such as nuts or apples, are not lead balls. Leading endodontists have proven that treatment is successful in 90-95 percent of cases.[11] It is, therefore, difficult to accept the Committee's opinion that such a rare event as the root cracking would be caused by the brittleness of the tooth or that this could happen immediately to an endodontally treated tooth. And, it was, of course, the "illusive" crack that was at the basis of all my trouble and lead to the prolongation of an extremely septic situation which is hazardous for a MVP patient.

A few years after this meeting, I had endodontal treatment on an identical lower, second molar on the right side. In the light of this, the question of trauma, not caused by iatrogenic error, becomes even more difficult to accept. The treatment of this tooth included extensive amalgam restoration, insertion of pins to hold the filling in place, application of a porcelain crown and subsequent endodontal work which necessitated drilling through this porcelain crown and refilling the tooth, later removal of the crown, further reshaping of the tooth structure, insertion of a stainless steel post and, finally, replacement of a second porcelain crown. Despite all these traumatic interventions, the root did not crack and there was no alveolar abscess! At no time did the endodontist ever declare, as Cohen had, that lower second molars were extremely difficult, almost impossible to treat.

There is another valid argument against cracking happening from masticatory failure. Teeth, like bones, become more brittle naturally with the aging process through loss of calcium, whether these teeth have been endodontally treated or not. For instance, in one extensive study of 256 fractured teeth, the mean age was fifty.[12] In another prominent study, cracks occurred in 30 percent of patients who were sixty and over, 28 percent aged between fifty and sixty and 22 percent between forty and fifty while only 20 percent were, like myself, under forty.[13]

The Committee accepted Dr. Cohen's statement as truth that "on a recall appointment, October 9, 1979, the tooth was comfortable." This statement had the effect of disassociating the cracking of the root from the endodontal treatment. However, I never once reported a "symptomless tooth". What I reported on that occasion was a mild stinging pain when I chewed, an ache in my jaw and a feverish feeling that increased with mastication. Cohen explained that there was extensive inflammation from the original pulp infection which would take up to a year to heal with signs of the inflammation remaining on x-ray for as long. In other words, this inflammation in my jawbone, if it proceeded from the original pulp infection, was self-limiting. The crown, he vowed, would improve the situation. But it did not. The same symptoms existed right up to the time of the extraction.

If, in fact, the crack occurred as a result of mastication, this could not have happened at any time prior to the fixation of the permanent crown because I did not chew on that side of my mouth. A masticatory accident could only have happened after the fixation of the permanent crown when I attempted, according to the advice of both Slapek and Cohen, to eat all manner of foods, but found that the extreme malocclusion caused sharp pain and very soon I abandoned all effort to chew on that side. The stinging discomfort and aching jaw, however, existed after the fixation of the crown as before.

Much proof exists that vertical root fractures are caused by the dentist. My x-ray showed that my fracture was vertical rather than horizontal and did not extend into the crown. This fact, in itself, is extremely significant since vertical fractures of teeth, involving only the root, not the crown, are virtually non-existent, unless iatrogenic in origin. Cracks, most dental experts agree, usually occur through the crown.[14] Dr. Wechsler, an endodontist, says, "it is generally agreed that injury usually results in horizontal fractures, whereas treatment-induced fractures are of the vertical type."[15] Negligence can arise from a lack of skill in filling a root canal with gutta percha after debriding or cleansing it of necrotic debris. This filling material, long, thin rods of a pinkish-gray colour, is made from the purified juice of latex of various trees of the family sapotaceae. Specialists in endodontics emphasize that it is the "excessive force used in the lateral condensation of gutta percha" that constitutes the negligence[16] and that "these internal forces begin at the apex and travel along one wall of the root canal."[17] Vertical, not horizontal fractures, can result if the endodontist uses too much force when inserting an instrument called a finger spreader into the canal in order to laterally condense the gutta percha and seal the canal tightly. The line that appeared on my x-ray was clearly vertical and did not extend into the crown.

After the debridement and filling of the canal with gutta percha and prior to the fixation of the crown, a permanent filling of stainless steel or some other appropriate substance, which acts as a post, should be inserted into the root canal to assure the tooth will be more resistant to fractures during mastication. Slapek omitted this step. One of the reasons for her omission was the fact that I had, contrary to Cohen's protestations, reported such discomfort to her after the root canal treatment, that she did not want to further irritate the area. The omission of this post could have contributed to a masticatory failure if, in fact, the crack was related to that.

However, the most important fact to underline is that all these dentists were dealing with a MVP patient who was at great risk of IE. Vertical root fractures, according to all textbooks and articles I read on the subject, have a hopeless prognosis and extraction is imperative if a systemic bacteremia is to be avoided. The majority of endodontics specialists such as those I have referred to, Meister, 1976, Weine, 1976, Wechsler, 1978, Grossman, 1981 and Gerstein in 1983, all agree the prognosis for vertical root fractures is very poor.

The x-rays of Mentlik and Cohen clearly showed a cracked root, but both dentists denied this until I laid eyes on the x-rays. Mentlik advised periodontal surgery was necessary, not as a direct means of saving the tooth, as he reported to the Committee, but as an investigative procedure to confirm the existence of the "suspected" root fracture because he could not see it on x-ray. At no time ever did Mentlik or Cohen inform me that vertical root fractures were hopeless and that the tooth must be extracted, and, at no time, did Mentlik ever give me a choice between extraction and periodontal surgery as an "effort to retain the tooth", regardless of the opinion he expressed before the Committee.

Mentlik's x-rays clearly showed the crack, as did Blair's, and yet Mentlik advised this unnecessary and dangerous surgery in a patient with MVP, fever, change in murmur and enlarged heart. But were these x-rays submitted to the Committee for examination? It was hard to believe they were. If the Committee had looked at all the x-rays of all the dentists, how could it approve of periodontal surgery on a tooth with a hopeless prognosis since the periodontal surgery would not have saved the tooth? Why did it not criticize the dentists for attempting to preserve the tooth once this was known, especially in a MVP patient who had cardiac complications? For what purpose did the Committee conceive the surgery was done? To please the deluded patient? Either the members of the Committee did not have adequate knowledge about the dangers of such interventions in a MVP patient or they simply accepted as truth Cohen's and Mentlik's representation of the situation as without danger.

The warning that vertical root fractures occur most frequently during the lateral condensation of the gutta percha was also contained in the manual used at the University of Toronto where Cohen taught at that time.[18] In fact, throughout his career, Cohen demonstrated considerable interest in vertical root fractures and had even written a paper on the nature of the problem. By his own admission, he was an expert at identifying vertical root fractures and clearly advocated extraction as the only method of treatment for a vertical root fracture. Cohen said that, when a root is fractured during endodontal debridement (cleansing) and obturation (filling) of the root with gutta percha, the tooth is immediately uncomfortable. Mine was even though he claimed I reported the tooth symptomless. It is logical too that such a fracture superimposed on a pre-existing abscess would cause even greater discomfort.

With all his knowledge and experience, why would Cohen advise me to go ahead with the crowning and then the periodontal surgery? This is a mystery to me. Was it self-protection? If the discovery of the cracked root were to be made much later after the endodontal treatment, six months or so, then it would be very difficult to pinpoint the cause of the crack since "brittleness" or masticatory failure could then be blamed. The effect would be of sufficient distance from the cause as to obscure or throw that cause into doubt. Was this the reason, therefore, why Cohen, like Mentlik, said that he could not definitely see the crack on x-ray which he took a few days before the periodontal surgery? The crack had shown up clearly on Blair's x-ray, but Cohen said he only "suspected" a crack and sent me on to Mentlik who would tell me the crack could only be verified by periodontal surgery. Even if his x-ray had not shown the crack, Cohen should have, according to his own research, realized that my symptoms, stinging pain on chewing, were identical to those of his patients he had written about. In fact, he, himself, said in his paper on vertical root fractures that he often performed periodontal surgery when he suspected a cracked root for, as he put it, no other reason than that he had nothing better to do. It appeared that, when his business improved, as surely it had when I arrived at his office years later and he was operating four chairs at once, he no longer had time to perform periodontal surgery and thus made me wait while he rushed to ask Mentlik, on the next floor up, if he could do it. Sending me on to Mentlik could only have meant another delay, like the crowning, a postponement of the inevitable discovery of the cracked root. If Mentlik made the tooth a little more comfortable by scraping away the inflamation and sterilizing the area, as he described in a letter to Slapek, then the tooth could, as he claimed, "remain in place" at least long enough to divert attention away from the cause. Meanwhile, my heart and spleen enlarged. I had fever, tachycardia and chest pain and my valves were undergoing further insidious changes.

What is also so curious is that Cohen said in his paper that periodontal surgery was infallible in exposing root fractures, yet, Mentlik claimed, even after the surgery, that the crack was undetectable. In fact, he claimed the tooth was loose and that this was the source of all my trouble. It is not surprising, therefore, that Mentlik was extremely upset when I confronted him with the evidence of the crack on another dentist's x-ray and forced him to re-examine his x-rays in my presence. His only avenue of escape then was to attempt to make me doubt my own senses by protesting that what Blair and I were seeing on x-ray was not a crack. When he could not convince me of this, he resorted to bribery, refusing to accept payment for his surgery and his last appointment.

One of the questions I had asked both in my letter and of the Committee was why either Slapek or Cohen had counselled retention of the tooth in light of the severe pulp infection with which the whole problem began. This was a question the Committee answered by saying the patient demanded that the tooth be saved. There was no demand; there was only the presentation of a choice. No choice, however, should have been given to a patient with MVP which was known both to Slapek and Cohen, especially when ABP was not used. According to endodontic research, chronic partial pulpitis, an inflammation in the root canal, with accompanying necrosis or decay of nerve tissues in the canal, chronic total pulpitis or total pulp necrosis, as in my case, are definitely untreatable. No work should ever have been commenced on my tooth. According to Dr. Grossman, in the majority of these cases, "the microorganisms survive and, if virulent", the author says, "multiply rapidly and reach the periapical tissue where they continue their destruction to produce an acute alveolar abscess" or less virulent microorganisms may remain in the root canal and, gradually, leak out toxic products of metabolism and decomposition into the surrounding periapical tissues to produce a chronic abscess that manifests with milder symptoms and eventually a visible fistula or opening in the periodontal tissues through which the purulent matter from the canal is forced out.[19] This explains why I eventually developed a periodontal abscess which exuded blood and pus months before extraction of my tooth. An acute infection became chronic and a local infection became systemic with resultant damage to my mitral valve.

For a MVP patient there was grave danger, unbeknownst to any of the dentists involved, in this ongoing septic situation. Since bacteria from dead tissue could leak out of the root canal into the surrounding periapical tissues, a systemic bacteremia could develop. It is also highly possible that the endodontal work, itself, could have forced bacterial products out of the canal into the tissues, further exacerbating the pre-existing alveolar abscess. The University of Toronto Handbook on Pre-Clinical Endodontics states the objects of root canal procedure as "the total removal (debridement) of organic debris (necrotic pulp tissue, food, inflammatory exudate, bacteria and bacterial products) from the root canal system" and warns that "seepage of tissue breakdown products and bacterial toxin into the periapical tissue is the source of periapical inflammation."[20] If the endodontist is careless or lacks skill, he or she may err by pushing instruments beyond the "apical foramen", the narrow anatomical constriction at the apex of the canal root through which the nerves and blood vessels of the healthy pulp connect systemically with the blood circulation and are nourished, and, thus, these tissue breakdown products are forced out of the canal root to contaminate the surrounding tissues and bone.

Endodontal textbooks warn that, in susceptible patients, this can lead to the systemic infection of bacterial endocarditis. In animal research, it has been dramatically illustrated that such infection can be initiated by first introducing hemolytic streptococci into the root canals of monkeys that have had endodontal treatment, forcing the instruments beyond the apical foramen of the teeth and sealing known microorganisms into the canals.[21] Bender et al have shown that no blood stream bacteremia exists when instrumentation is confined to the root canal.[22] To avoid this error in instrumentation the endodontist must constantly verify the length of the root canal throughout treatment because, during the process of debriding and shaping the canal, tooth structure is removed, changing the length of the tooth canal. If the file is too long, it will pierce the apical foramen, and, if too short, the endodontist may leave necrotic pulpal remnants inside the root canal, thus initiating chronic inflammation, leakage of bacterial toxins and an eventual aveolar abscess.[23] Since, in between appointments, my tooth had to be opened and drained because of a sensation of pressure and aching, it would appear that the infection was beyond the endodontist's power to eradicate, and the pulp remnants not completely cleared from the canal or forced out into the tissues and bone were creating further contamination.

It was thus negligent on Slapek's part to have sent me on to Cohen for further work on this tooth especially in the light of my murmur which she completely disregarded. The next person with the opportunity to bring this unnecessary, dangerous process to a stop was Cohen who ought to have exercised a judgement superior to that of a general practitioner. Rather than tell me the truth, that such teeth should never be endodontally treated because the prognosis was hopeless, according to the dental literature, he led me to believe that lower, second molars were difficult to treat but that he, alone, was especially good at working on them. If the procedure were unsuccessful, it would not be his fault, either in skill or in judgement, but only a failure related to the "nature of the beast" as doctors are fond of saying. He implied that his "special" skill could work miracles whereas the truth was that no amount of skill could repair such a risky situation. Neither of the three practitioners possessed more knowledge than the lay person about how the teeth could affect the heart in a MVP patient. It is very easy for professionals to shift responsibility to the patient, claiming that she wanted the work done even though no patient could possibly, given the little information I had, make an informed and, therefore, correct decision.

IE could have been caused at any stage then of the entire treatment or with the initial acute pulpitis. All dentists involved should have been alert to this possibility. Slapek, who examined my teeth regularly, should have been particularly careful, since she was dealing with a MVP patient, to spot any sign of a root canal problem or a possible pulpitis and prevent it with early endodontal treatment.

In the Committee's view, nothing had happened to me. The whole issue of oral sepsis related to IE was dismissed. The Committee's attitude towards the use of ABP with MVP patients was equivocal when, in fact, it should have been absolutely clear. This Committee represented the Royal College of Dental Surgeons and, therefore, the standards of the dental profession. In August of 1979, the RCDS issued a Dispatch[24] to its dentists reminding them to conform to the recommendations of the American Heart Association (AHA) then in effect and adopted around the world, for the use of antibiotics with MVP and mitral insufficiency. Though my endodontal work took place slightly earlier than August 1979, this Dispatch was a "reminder" prompted by the death of a patient from subacute bacterial endocarditis (SBE) related to dental surgery. It follows that there must have been a previous identical warning prior to this release. As well, the remaining treatments, endodontal check-up, crowning and periodontal surgery all took place after this directive went out from the RCDS to its members.

The instructions for the administration of ABP and the drug of choice are set out in these AHA recommendations, a copy of which was included in the RCDS Dispatch. In fact, the standard in this regard was certainly well established by the governing body of the dental profession in the city of Toronto. The University of Toronto Dentistry College, where Mentlik and Cohen taught, was using a textbook for first year students, *Clinical Pharmacology in Dental Practice*, printed in 1978 which, like the RCDS Dispatch contained in its appendix the AHA's recommendations for antibiotic prophylaxis for MVP patients on pages 471-475.[25]

Further proof that my Toronto dentists should have been aware of their College's and Faculty's standards and of the common association between IE and dental procedures and the necessity for protection exists in the fact that Dr. A. Brown[26] and Dr. Richard Ellen,[27] who taught in the University of Toronto Dentistry Faculty at that time, had published articles, prior to my treatment, in *Ontario Dentistry* in 1977 and in *The International Dental Journal* in 1978 on the subject of the prevention of bacterial endocarditis. Brown reminds dentists in Ontario, and presumably the rest of Canada, about the usage of antibiotics in susceptible patients and warns that there is great confusion among practicing dentists despite these clear cut recommendations. Indeed, there was confusion regarding ABP and MVP. Neither Brown nor Ellen, abiding by the AHA recommendations, advocates the use of Ampicillin, as Mentlik used. Nor did they, in keeping with the AHA recommendations, advise that this protection can be commenced after the dental manipulation. And both Brown and Ellen referred directly to the AHA Recommendations that clearly showed MVP patients with mitral insufficiency were known to require such protection.

Brown also cautions dentists of the ineffectiveness of bacteriostatic, as opposed to bactericidal, drugs such as tetracycline. As I described earlier, on a recall between visits, because of stinging pain and aching in my jaw, Dr. Cohen did further work and gave me one tetracycline. He was totally unaware of the inadequacy of this treatment. Bacteriostatic drugs, as Brown says, control infection, though one tetracycline would be totally ineffective, but do not kill it and would "do more harm than good". Cohen had obviously not even updated himself on what drugs were available for use with dental manipulations or how to use them to prevent IE.

The Committee criticized Drs. Cohen and Slapek for not having consulted their records regarding my murmur nor having contacted my cardiologist to find out whether my murmur required antibiotic protection. Austin would have, of course, according to his records, said MVP didn't require protection. However the dentist has an independent obligation in the light of the RCDS Dispatch, the teachings at the Dental Faculty and the information currently in his dental journals. To conclude, as the Committee did, a statement to the effect that all heart murmurs do not require antibiotic coverage and that the dentist should consult the patient's physician to see if the murmur should be covered is to suggest that the dentist, in full knowledge of the kind of murmur being dealt with, could disregard the standards of his governing College and follow those of a single doctor. In effect, such directives as the Dispatch are nullified. Furthermore, all members of the Committee, as well as the dentists, knew what kind of murmur they were dealing with. Rather than unequivocally state the standard of the profession with regard to MVP and ABP, the Committee appeared thus to contradict it.

In fact, one of the dentists on the panel had specifically said to me that all murmurs did not require antibiotic prophylaxis with dental manipulations. When I had asked if he were referring to MVP murmurs, he answered yes. Such a statement created doubt in my mind about what I knew from the medical literature on this subject and led me to believe that there must be a kind of MVP murmur that didn't require antibiotics or that some other pronouncement had come out which had nullified the recommendations of the AHA with respect to MVP and mitral insufficiency. This dentist also suggested that I wear some type of bracelet or tag indicating I required antibiotic prophylaxis with certain dental procedures so that I could be differentiated easily from other MVP patients who did not. This suggestion was clearly intended to lay blame on the patient rather than the dentists who had not consulted their records about my murmur and were unaware of the standards of the governing body of their College and the rest of the world. This member of the College's Complaints Committee was contradicting his own College's standards.

What was most disturbing was the Committee's acceptance of Mentlik's testimony about antibiotic coverage for his MVP patient. He was exonerated on the grounds that he had contacted my cardiologist, a highly questionable aspect, as I have shown, and on the grounds that he had provided antibiotic coverage as recommended by my cardiologist **prior** to the periodontal surgery. At that meeting, I challenged Mentlik's testimony by saying that he had given me a prescription for antibiotics to be taken after the surgery, specifically at the counter of the nearest pharmacy, and that I could prove this by the prescription receipt which is numbered and can thus give a fairly close estimation of the time of the day when the prescription was filled. Why would

I have asked Mentlik to call Austin at the commencement of the surgery if I had already taken the appropriate preventative dosage and why would I wait until I was sitting in the chair to do this? Why would I wait to fill the prescription at a pharmacy in Toronto on the same day as the surgery when my husband was a pharmacist, if Mentlik had given me instructions to take this medication prior to the surgery? If Mentlik had called Austin as he had purported to do, why would Austin have given an inadequate dosage of a drug clearly not considered the most effective by the AHA standards which medical doctors also follow? And why would either doctor or dentists not know the proper regimen and instructions for taking this drug and the proper amount of the drug which was inadequate? Obviously my version of the events was not believed.

Neither Mentlik nor Austin knew that to be most effective the antibiotic must be taken not less than 30 minutes nor more than one hour prior to the procedure to assure optimum blood levels at the time of the surgery when bacteria will enter the bloodstream. To provide antibiotics after the procedure defeats the whole purpose for which this protection was intended. Dentistry textbooks refer to these AHA recommendations and stress the necessity of providing the protection just prior to the procedure. They also stress that it is the absolute responsibility of the dental practitioner to be thoroughly familiar with these guidelines for the administration of antibiotics and to be aware of any revisions that are made at a later date. The opinion of Dr. Richard Ellen emphatically underlines the necessity of giving the antibiotic before the procedure. He pointed out that animal studies show "streptococci to colonize damaged heart valves faster than antibiotics can eliminate them from the blood" and that "colonization of vegetations on heart valves occurs within minutes."[28] It is obvious that performing the surgery when the patient is not covered would be extremely dangerous since the microorganisms would have had an excellent head start. Why would both specialists, cardiologist and periodontist, not know the recommended regimen when it is the same for patients with rheumatic heart disease, the most commonly known indication for such protection? Surely both Austin and Mentlik had patients with rheumatic heart disease and would have to be thoroughly familiar with the guidelines regarding the use of antibiotics! The only answer is that my dentists, not to speak of Austin, were totally unfamiliar with not just the procedures regarding MVP patients but obviously with the use of preventative prophylaxis even with rheumatic heart disease patients. This could mean that there are a lot of unprotected patients.

If the Committee had reviewed my x-rays and had taken note of the acute pulpitis, how could it approve the commencement of any treatment whatsoever or the continuation of that treatment in a patient with a sudden cardiac enlargement? How could it believe that the endodontal work had failed because of the brittleness of the tooth when prominent researchers unanimously agree that, in the case of endodontics, "the degree of success enjoyed is probably the best found in any phase of dentistry, much higher than that in periodontics and other phases of reconstructive dentistry" and "this degree of predictability has been the factor most responsible for the acceptance of endodontics by the general practitioner, who is acutely aware of the fact that treated teeth may be counted on to perform any function in the oral cavity that an untreated tooth performs in a tremendous preponderance of cases".[29] How could a regulatory body invested with the power of licensing and maintaining the standards of the profession believe the statements of these dental practitioners or agree with an absolutely unjustifiable sequence of events?

There were a number of other discrepancies in the testimonies of the dentists which were taken as truth while my evidence was not. For instance, these dentists gave incorrect dates of certain visits and omitted others. The periodontal surgery of January 7, 1980 was not referred to anywhere in the report. "Some restorative work", which was not defined, was given as having been done on January 30, 1980 and that I first reported problems to Cohen on that date and was then recommended to Mentlik for this "restorative work". I saw Cohen a few days prior to the periodontal surgery, which he rushed out to arrange; I did not see Cohen after the surgery on January 7, 1980. I saw only Mentlik. This is an example of the inadequacy of this investigation. It seemed that the only answer to any of my objections lay in the fact that the personal testimonies of the practitioners involved were accepted as truth and anything the patient had to say was not.

The Committee pronounced that, despite all my symptoms and changes in my murmur and cardiac enlargement, that I had never had IE. This final opinion was based solely on the opinion provided by Dr. Austin in his letter of April 9, 1980. That letter was the linchpin upon which everything else turned since that was my most pressing question, whether or not I had had IE as a result of dental interventions without antibiotic coverage. Austin had written this letter one month prior to my hospitalization at TMSC. Apart from the fluoroscopy and the echocardiogram, the print-outs of which would vanish mysteriously, Austin had done no tests for IE. In particular, he did no blood tests at the time of my report of symptoms. In fact, until my meeting with him on February 26, 1980, he had not even suspected IE, and, yet, he stated unequivocally, with virtually no proof whatsoever except that of the echocardiogram, and even when he did not know the cause of the change in my murmur and my cardiac enlargement, that I had never suffered from IE. This was pure opinion without proof. The Committee used Austin's statement to conclude that the dentists' manipulations without antibiotics had, in no way, caused an IE. There was no onus upon this institution to provide reasons for its judgement. The medical and dental professions, because they are regarded as unquestionable authorities, do not have to provide reasons to corroborate their opinions.

7

Conspiracy of Silence

Personalities enter in, friendships, bias, previous favours modify, intimate contacts persuade, and an unwillingness to cast the first stone asserts a strong effect. Thus it is that although members are usually the first to be aware of a fellow member's dishonesty and unfairness, they are often the least likely to accuse or indict.

Dr. John Birkhardt at a National Congress on Medical Ethics in Knoxville, Tennessee in Howard and Martha Lewis. *The Medical Offenders* (New York: Simon and Schuster, 1970), p. 65.

The meeting with the Complaints Committee only served to convince my husband and me that we wanted an evaluation of Dr. Austin's care. In particular, we wanted to know if what I had experienced added up to IE and what exactly was the nature of the damage done to my heart and its valves as a result of the cardiac enlargement, fever, tachycardia and alveolar abscess that had been present for over a year.

Dr. Cory would not discuss Austin's treatment except to say that I was entitled to a "better" explanation of the mechanisms of infection and fever in relation to the cardiac enlargement, something he, himself, was unable to offer. An appointment was arranged with a Dr. Warren of The Metropolitan Hospital (TMH). However, during my visit with this cardiologist, I realized quickly enough that this doctor also had an inappropriately biased attitude toward MVP. In his view, MVP was a distinctly female disorder and its symptoms as imaginary as premenstrual cramps. He declared with hearty chuckling that doctors called MVP "the slick-chick syndrome" because the "gals" were tall and slender. With all that had transpired, his smart-alecky attempts to deflate the importance of MVP hardly impressed me. I freely discussed my complaints about Dr. Austin's treatment and asked Dr. Warren if he would examine my medical records in an attempt to give me an answer as to what kind of illness I had suffered, whether or not it was IE, why my murmur had changed to one of important regurgitation, why I was breathless when I climbed stairs or hills and why I had SOB with sports I could carry on before with ease. Tennis left me red faced and panting after about ten minutes and, now, when cycling I had to walk my bicycle up hills. Dr. Warren was very good-humoured but refused outright to do this, saying it was totally unnecessary to examine Dr. Austin's records. He knew this "venerable" colleague very well and assured me that he would have spotted any problem. After a quick clinical examination, Warren took an x-ray, told me he saw no sign of cardiac enlargement and only a typical murmur of MVP. At this point in time, I believed naively that doctors, if they found fault, would openly criticize their colleagues' treatment. It would take some time to shatter this delusion.

Dr. Warren's report of September 24, 1980 to Dr. Cory could not possibly represent an objective, second opinion. There was some subtle evidence that he was protecting himself against an accusation of bias or what is termed in medico-legal cases a "conspiracy of silence". Though I had clearly discussed Dr Austin's treatment, Dr. Warren claimed he did not know which doctor and hospital had investigated the IE. The only logical explanation for his denial of these facts had to be his desire to establish in writing that he had given me an unguarded, unprejudiced opinion, uninfluenced by any personal relationship with the colleague who had treated me.

Dr. Warren went even further than Dr. Austin's statement that there was no IE. My "splendid recovery", Warren reported to Dr. Cory, "would be almost impossible if she had genuinely had endocarditis." In other words, I did not die; nor was I in acute cardiac failure, neither of which need happen immediately, as Emanuel Libman, whose work I will discuss later, demonstrated so convincingly in the past, and, oral antibiotics may have controlled the bacteria enough that some spontaneous healing, leaving damage to the valve, took place. Dr. Warren also doubted that there had ever been any cardiac enlargement and was not convinced that I had tachycardia, either in the past or during my illness. My description, he said, was "not the typical subjective description of paroxysmal atrial tachycardia" (PAT) of which MVP patients complain. What did he mean by this comment? That my account was untrustworthy because I had used the word tachycardia and had not described my rapid heart beat in quaint, metaphorical terms, like "the flapping of a bird's wings" or the "flopping of a fish in water" but instead had usurped the private language of the medical profession? Dr. Rhodes, however, had said in a letter to Dr. Cory, prior to any of these events, that he was convinced my past episodes were "true bill P.A.T." and, long ago, my GP had called these episodes atrial fibrillation according to his medical records. Warren's final comment that I was an "unusual lady" appeared to mean that I was a "neurotic" lady.

Dr. Warren gave Dr. Cory the promised thyroid test results, which were negative, but never submitted the results of the blood sample he had taken for the viral antibody test to determine if there had been any "intercurrent infection", as he put it, which might be related to my heart. His conclusion was that my MVP required no follow-up since this condition was totally benign. In fact, he reported that my murmur was the same, late systolic, as before the infection, thus contradicting even Dr. Austin's view that my murmur had changed significantly in becoming longer. It was not surprising, therefore, that Dr. Warren said nothing about the use of prophylactic antibiotics.

It was beginning to look as if oral infection had meant nothing whatsoever and was entirely unrelated to my cardiac manifestations, in short that the Complaints Committee had been right in exonerating the dentists of any blame in regard to the precipitation of a bacterial infection. After this visit, nothing about my illness or my condition, it seemed, would ever be explained. In rapid succession, palpitations, chest pain and, now, SOB with activities I had engaged in with ease in the past became mere "nuisances". Symptoms, which I had not experienced before, were suddenly classified as common features of MVP that still did not, in the view of the doctors, affect the prognosis. I might be limited in what I could do but not in how long I would live or how healthy I would be.

Such a contradiction, of course, rekindled the earlier desire to have a child. Subconsciously, I wanted to believe the opinions of Drs. Warren and Austin, that there was no permanent cardiac damage, were accurate. But, somehow, my doubts could not be suppressed. The realization that I was a victim of medical incompetence was gaining strength and, with it, my determination to get some answers that I believed I was entitled to. I decided to try for a third opinion.

Through a family member, we were given the name of a Dr. Sam Cofman at Richview General Hospital. My visit with him took place six days after that with Dr. Warren, on September 29, 1980. Dr. Cofman was younger than either Austin, Rhodes or Warren, and, therefore, I hoped he would be more up-to-date, co-operative and informative. This first visit consisted of clinical examination, electrocardiogram and history taking. I felt that criticizing Dr. Austin personally to Dr. Warren had not earned me an objective opinion and I, thus, decided to withhold the names of the doctors and hospital involved unless Dr. Cofman specifically indicated he could not give me an opinion without this information and my TMSC records. However, early in the discussion, it became evident that withholding these names only antagonized Dr. Cofman and I felt compelled to give them.

The long questionnaire which I filled out for Dr. Cofman did not deal with the unusual such as I had experienced, that is fever, dental problems, SOB, PAT, and, in our discussion, he repeatedly endeavored to make me stick to answering a long list of general questions that he presumably gave every MVP patient. Everything I said he attempted to relate to his fixed opinion of MVP. For instance, when I mentioned that my SOB first began during the fever and dental work, he said that this connection could not be established with any validity. In other words, my account, in fact my own senses, were being interpreted as false. He insisted that the chest pain I experienced was caused by nothing more than the emotional stress that resulted from all the dental problems and my general lack of wellbeing at the time. Of course, I couldn't deny that I had been stressed by my illness. Every symptom he held to be longstanding rather than of recent origin. My symptoms had nothing to do with my dental problem and were merely typical of MVP. This was exactly what Warren and Austin had said. The cumulative effect was equivalent to a denial that I had ever been ill.

After the question period, Cofman examined my heart and gave me the five line, well-worn textbook description of MVP that Rhodes, Austin and Warren had given me, its benignity, its predilection for females, its excellent prognosis and its lack of complications. We discussed the matter of pregnancy, and he assured me that MVP posed no problem and that there was no sign of cardiac enlargement or of any lasting effects upon my valve of the illness I described. Like Dr. Rhodes, he cautioned that propranolol must be discontinued during pregnancy.

And, on the subject of the antibiotics with dental work, he said that doctors were still undecided but added that I could use them for dental procedures that drew blood. Our interview came to a close with his final reassurances of the complete benignity of MVP and his suggestion that I return for an echo at some time in the future to confirm that I even had MVP.

"Benign" was the word used right from the beginning when I was first told I had MVP. Because Dr. Cofman had so emphasized that every symptom was typical of prolapse, it seemed fruitless to ask him to review Dr. Austin's x-rays and echocardiogram print-outs. Nevertheless, in spite of Cofman's reinforcement that changes in the MVP syndrome were either insignificant or non-existent, I was not relieved because I knew I had not felt this way before my illness. Furthermore, I knew what I had read in Dr. Austin's letters. These denials of my experience were so distressful that I was tempted to return to Dr. Austin. He, at least, was now alerted to complications in the MVP patient, had now stressed the use of antibiotics and had indicated that my situation needed close watching. While others had said nothing had gone wrong, Austin's reversal of his former attitude constituted an admission that something had. His knowledge was, of course, at my expense, but some health care was better than none.

However, when I saw Dr. Cory several months later to discuss my visit with Dr. Cofman and look at his report, I was just as shocked as I had been when I had first laid eyes on Dr. Austin's letters. In his letter to Dr. Cory, Dr. Cofman stated unequivocally that he could not possibly be certain of what was going on in the past without examining my films and echoes from TMSC. "I don't yet have her permission to review the records from TMSC and obviously to gain a clear insight into just what might have been going on as far as the change in heart size, etc., at that time, one would want to see the chest x-rays and also at least review the summaries . . . I would not have thought that she has cardiomegaly and would suspect that the prolapse does not produce a hemodynamically significant degree of mitral regurgitation. This will be supported or rebutted by assessment of chest x-ray and echocardiogram, of course." And, again, at the close of his letter, he repeats, "Finally, should it be your wish and hers that I undertake her cardiologic follow-up in light of the circumstances . . . I would agree to do this but I would have to review the previous records. The outstanding questions relate to the significance of the "cardiomegaly" which was a transient finding apparently unassociated with symptomatology."

It was clear from this report that Dr. Cofman regarded the past "circumstances" of my case as unorthodox enough to require cardiologic follow-up, despite what he had said to me. It was also clear that, without my x-rays and other test results, done when I was ill, he believed he could give neither a complete nor accurate explanation for the cardiac enlargement. Nor could he, without this important evidence, give an opinion of just what had happened, whether my cardiac enlargement was associated with my symptoms, then and now, an association he seems to be acknowledging Austin did not make. In other words, he was not at all certain that I did not have IE. Furthermore, his closing remarks that his acceptance of me as a patient was contingent upon reviewing those specific documents dramatically underlined their importance in resolving my medical dilemma and in assuring me the best in future care. However, on the basis of the opinion he had given me verbally, I had not asked if he would like to review them. However, the impression is created in his letter that he had asked but I had not yet given permission. It had become increasingly apparent that there was a significant discrepancy between the written medical record, which the patient was never allowed to see, and the verbal explanation which the doctor gives the patient.

After our first meeting, in his letter to Dr. Cory, Cofman stated that I had a "typical" murmur of MVP, one which he described as "late systolic in the squatting position and is almost holosystolic with no audible click in the standing position." Of great importance here is the nature of the "typical" MVP murmur which I have already described. The prefixes "pan" and "holo" are synonymous and come from the Greek word for "all". Thus a pansystolic or holosystolic murmur (PSM or HSM) is one that can be heard throughout all of systole. According to Robert Jeresaty, the PSM in the MVP syndrome is associated with severe prolapse which causes the mitral valve leaflets to separate early in systole.[1] Most of the studies I had read indicate that a PSM is not typical but is found in only ten percent of the MVP population, increasing to as much as 25 percent in older patients, and appears to be a factor of the aging process.[2] Did I now have this PSM on standing as a result of previous events? Was this the change that Dr. Austin had heard during the infection? He had said that he could not hear the click, "the noise", at the time of my cardiac enlargement when there was an increase in regurgitation, that it was being covered by the murmur.

I suspected that there must be specific auscultatory signs that would pinpoint the onset of sudden, significant regurgitation. One of these was the splitting of the second heart sound. The normal second heart sound has two components, A_2 and P_2, associated with but not necessarily representing aortic and pulmonic valve closure. Whether disease is present or not can be determined by the time interval that separates these two sounds into distinct audible components. According to what I had read, splitting that is audible during expiration is the result of patho-physiologic mechanisms. Dr. Cofman had said my second heart sound was split but he had not said whether this was during expiration or inspiration though Dr. Rhodes was later to say it was during respiration which I can only understand to mean both expiration and inspiration. I wanted to know the significance of this finding because I had read that "Persistent and audible expiratory splitting of S_2 is an uncommon finding in mitral regurgitation in the adult. When it occurs it is almost always associated with acute mitral regurgitation . . . audible expiratory splitting of S_2 is occasionally associated with the late systolic murmur syndrome (i.e.MVP) when the mitral regurgitation is significant."[3] This auditory phenomenon, not heard in my heart before, might therefore explain my exercise intolerance and, because it was a sign of sudden acute regurgitation, it could also be proof that the onset of more severe regurgitation began, in fact, during my illness, not before, and was likely the cause of the excessively rapid heart beat at the time.

I decided to return to Dr. Cofman and, approximately one month before my visit, on or about February 17, 1981, a Tuesday, a day my husband and I always spent together in Toronto, I went to Richview Hospital and asked Dr. Cofman's secretary for the proper requisition for release of my past records. This form specifically requested the name of the treating physician, and I duly entered Dr. Austin's name in the space provided, as well as the hospital's name, TMSC. This was to emerge as a detail of considerable importance.

On the 16th of March, I had the chest x-ray and echocardiogram which Dr. Cofman had said would "support or rebut" the hemodynamic significance of my regurgitation and a second examination with Dr. Cofman. When he entered the room, he did not greet me cordially with "Hello and how are you today?" He was frigidly silent and immediately began the electrocardiogram. It is said that silence often speaks volumes. When people are angry, they drop their masks. He began his clinical examination, still not having said a word, and, when he was finished, he asked coldly, "What I want to know is why you came back to me?"

The suddenness of this brittle and curious question startled me. He did not give me a chance to answer. "What happened in the meantime?" he asked with obvious irritation. This comment, like the first, was not made out of natural bewilderment or concern at my delay in consulting him further or coming back sooner for the echo.

I told him the truth. "You gave me the impression that you did not believe I had suffered any significant illness that affected my heart. There appeared to be no point in returning to you. I then talked with Dr. Cory and learned that you were not at all certain and did, in fact, believe an assessment of my past records was essential to determine just what had happened to me in order to answer some of the questions I had asked."

He didn't comment, and his next admission angrily confirmed the complexity of the issue now facing me. "I just had a long talk with Dr. Austin."

I was astounded. My heart sunk. Obviously, from Dr. Cofman's emotional state, I could kiss the second opinion good-bye. I simply replied "oh" in a flat voice and, then, the instinctive response surged up. "What did he say?" I sensed, as I asked this, that Dr. Cofman would not tell me and, if he did, it would not be the whole truth. The substance of that discussion, so crucial to my wellbeing and rights, would remain a mystery forever, something that I could later, when everything was taken into consideration, only guess at. But I did wonder if it had anything to do with my complaints and my investigation of the dentists' work.

"We had a long talk about you," Dr. Cofman said. Then he was silent. I was bewildered and feared the worse. Why had he chosen to tell me this? Was he subtly trying to make me talk? From his unpleasant attitude, it was obvious that Austin had likely informed him of the "mischief" I was up to regarding the dentists. Again, I felt like a subordinate who had done something immoral or a disobedient child. I then told Dr. Cofman that I had returned because I wanted him to examine Dr. Austin's films and echoes. I reported what I had learned about the importance of these documents to his proper evaluation as he had indicated in his letter to Dr. Cory. Dr. Cofman's answer was shocking. "I don't have them. They only sent me the radiologist's summaries."

I was suddenly filled with despair at the prospect of never getting any answers. Still imprisoned in the delusion that the medical profession functioned solely for the benefit of the patient, I found it inconceivable that TMSC had not promptly fulfilled my request for the films. Cofman quickly added that he didn't need them anyway, and I, not realizing the full significance of this turn of events, reasoned that the summaries must be just as good as the actual films. After all, I was getting further than I had with Dr. Warren. Hope surged up; certainly these radiologists' reports would explain what had happened to my heart and why I now had these symptoms. And they would be proof for Dr. Cofman that my cardiac enlargement was genuine.

When I followed Dr. Cofman into his office, I made the grave mistake of not asking my husband to join us. But, then, if he had, the ensuing drama would not have taken place. No doctor would ever act like Cofman did in front of a man. There might have been a few insulting snipes of the Rhodes variety but certainly not the profoundly frightening, unprofessional behaviour I witnessed. Whether Dr. Cofman had my medical records or not, I was determined to ask my questions. When I expressed doubt that he would be able to give explanations without Dr. Austin's films and echo print-outs, Cofman stressed that he would, contrary to the opinion he had expressed in his letter to Dr. Cory. He folded his hands and waited silently for me to talk. By now, I had been reading the medical literature and knew the difference between a late systolic murmur (LSM) and a pansystolic murmur (PSM) and I understood things like tachycardia and infective endocarditis (IE). Familiarity with these medical concepts made it easier to discuss my health situation clearly. However, hearing a patient use medical terminology was the first unpleasant shock for Dr. Cofman. Like Rhodes, Cofman's face registered the same surprise and angry indignation rather than acceptance. And, like all doctors, especially when the patient is being critical, he would have felt more comfortable hearing me use words like "noise" in my heart, "swollen heart" and "infection", the shapeless scraps of language the medical profession forces upon the patient for use in talking about illness. I had learned the danger of this "talking down" from Dr. Rhodes who had never used the word, "infective endocarditis". If he had used this correct term, instead of the vague word, infection, and given us a brief explanation, we would have known the connection between the teeth and the heart.

I launched into my questions that centred on the deterioration in my health and its possible causes. The rapid changes in Dr. Cofman's physiognomy were startling. He was, to put it mildly, thunderstruck. A variety of emotions swept over his face, first shock, then outrage and profound incredulity that I dared to use his private language to question my treatment. I was the proverbial thief flaunting the stolen goods. Anger, that I could only guess had accumulated since his talk with Austin, flushed his face. He spread his big hands on top of his desk and pushed hard as though mentally forcing me out of the room. "I don't have to put up with this!" he growled, almost choking with the effort to swallow his rage. "You're just trying to trip me up. You know more about mitral valve prolapse than I do. I've changed my mind," he cried emphatically. I watched astounded as he clutched his chest dramatically and said, "You're making my heart beat fast. I don't want to listen to this. I don't want you as a patient."

Later in a letter to Dr. Cory, Cofman would, in fact, explain that he had changed his mind about accepting me as a patient specifically because my questions had greatly angered him. Dr. Cofman's behaviour was so shocking that I, somehow, became very calm and deliberate, intent on laying out all my concerns that had accumulated since the beginning with the initial endodontal infection and stressing my right to get at the truth about my illness once and for all. My timidity and fear at criticizing an authority figure vanished miraculously. The strength of being right surged up in their place. In a sense, Cofman represented for me an impregnable bastion of secrecy and, in fact, it was all the secrecy and misrepresentation that I had constantly encountered that drove me on to find the truth. Also urging me on was that bitterness I felt from having been so impotent before the dentists at the Complaints Committee meeting. I referred to my medical records and the literature I had read, plus Cofman's own letter, to substantiate my belief that my murmur had seriously deteriorated as a result of my illness, leaving me with a disability that could only increase faster than if I had never had an illness related to my tooth. What was this infection I asked? Was there a pericardial effusion, pericarditis, rheumatic fever or infective endocarditis? Why was I not given antibiotic prophylaxis as soon as my MVP murmur was identified? What caused my heart to enlarge? "I want to know," I insisted. Why was he, like Dr. Austin, telling me that changes in the MVP syndrome were insignificant? Had the valves escaped the vegetations and only the heart been affected? Did I have a myocarditis or a mural endocarditis then? Why would my heart enlarge and supposedly go down miraculously even before the tooth was extracted? Did my heart valves have changes that would not appear on echocardiogram?

Those medical words spewing out of the mouth of a patient struck him like bullets from a hidden enemy. And the fact that I dared to question, to criticize the treatment I had received, horrified him. "I don't have time to waste on you!" he shouted vehemently. "You have an entirely benign condition. I'm not interested in discussing it with you."

But I could not leave; I remained stubbornly rooted in my chair. I wanted answers. Why did I have such excessive tachycardia during the dental infection and the cardiac enlargement? Why couldn't I lie flat on my back at night? Why did I have to sit up to breathe, to stop the rapid heart beat? Was the chest pain from the spleen or the heart? My questions poured out. "Have you read Robert Jeresaty's book on MVP?" I asked. Dr. Cofman had not heard of this book and was unable to comment. "Jeresaty says that if the LSM of MVP deteriorates in a short space of time into a PSM, the likely cause is infective endocarditis. You said I have a PSM. I had an aveolar abscess for a year with fever, chest pain, cardiac enlargement, rapid heart beat, and change in murmur and, in hospital, strep. viridans was grown from my blood. What is the connection between this and my present symptoms?"

Cofman pushed back his rollered chair violently and sprung to his feet. He towered over me, a massive, immovable, white giant. "I'm not going to engage in an intellectual discussion with you. You have nothing the matter with you. Your prolapse is completely benign. You're making the whole thing your life's obsession."

In his eyes, I, not he, was the hysteric. "Oh, so you think I'm a case of cardiac neurosis in spite of everything that has happened!"

He didn't answer and moved swiftly to his door. I was obliged to follow. Short of physically manhandling me, he was throwing me out. Although his fists were clenched at his sides, he made a supreme effort to gather up his cool, professional demeanor that clung now in shreds, like clothing after a rape. I had attacked the unquestionable authority of the medical profession. My questions were subversive, dangerous to himself, to his colleagues.

It would take me a long time to get used to the idea that medical information about my own body could not be had for the asking no more than truth in our society, that I had no right to this information in the eyes of doctors and that the medical profession was not sworn to helping people but to protecting its members. Doctors are constantly coached by their professional organizations never to criticize their colleagues, never to make statements, as Canadian doctor-writer, Empson says, such as "My God who did that?"[4]

Just how strong is that protective instinct among doctors? I audited a Medical Jurisprudence course at the University of Toronto law school and was able to obtain from the Professor the Annual Reports, not available to the public, of the *Canadian Medical Protective Association* (CMPA) which insures the majority of doctors in Canada against malpractice litigation. Founded by the doctors themselves at the turn of the century, it is a "powerful and well managed protective organization"[5] that exists solely to defend the doctor against the patient. This organization encourages the conspiracy of silence by psychologically compelling its members to assist their "brothers" with testimony at trial.

On the 80th anniversary of this organization, the 1981 CMPA Annual Report reprinted the 1902 inaugural address published in the *Canadian Lancet.* It was to serve as a reminder of the purpose of this brotherhood. At its foundation in 1902, the indissoluable bond that unites doctors as "brothers" in a vow of mutual protection was idealistically defined in a quote from the Latin poet Horace: "Thrice happy those whose hearts are tied in love's mysterious knot so close, no strife, no quarrels, can divide and only death, fell death can loose."[6] These words of Horace are the sublime rhetoric of lovers, the mysticism and reverence of the sacrament of Holy Matrimony.

But in cold, hard language, the purpose of this organization uniting the doctors against the patient was clearly spelled out.

> In the first place, if an action for damages is brought against a member, he receives financial assistance. This makes him bold in resisting an unjust attempt to extort money from him. Another advantage is to be found in the fact that such an organization would go a long way towards preventing malpractice suits. Most suits of this kind are unjust and known to be so to the plaintiffs. If it was known that they would have the entire profession to fight instead of a single member thereof, they would count the costs with much more care before they embarked on their suits.[7]

That the Christ-like ideal, that no greater love hath any man than to lay down his life for a friend, should be distorted for the purpose of the conspiracy of silence is somewhat terrifying. "By assisting your fellow practitioners in the hour of their trouble," the foundation address advised, "you secure their sympathy and assistance in the hour of your own trial and anxiety."[8] The CMPA legal counsel frequently reminds its members at meetings, as it did in 1981, that the purpose of their organization has not changed since 1902: "the basic nature of the Association as a non-profit mutual help organization has remained unchanged."[9] And, in fact, a doctor's service to that organization is measured in terms of his faithfulness to that bond. An eulogy, marking the death of a Dr. Hooper in the 1971 Annual Report, provides a perfect example: "Never did he interfere with the work of other men and never did he withhold help which so frequently was sought of him".[10] This statement echoes Dr. Empson's remarks that a doctor should withhold criticism of his colleague's treatment of a patient. Knowing the purpose of this organization, and the fact that the substance of their meetings is the discussion of malpractice cases, the "help" extended can only be understood as the refusal to criticize and the willingness to give testimony in defense of a colleague who has a charge of malpractice laid against him.

Dr. Cofman's power to silence me had been as effective as if I had been thrown into some dark prison in some far off militaristic regime. It was the pattern for all future consultations with doctors. None would comment upon my past events and none would look kindly on my seeking information from the medical literature. This is their terrain and the patient who wanders into it is automatically an enemy.

As soon as my husband and I were alone after this meeting with Cofman, I broke down. Tremendous shock had prevented me from crying weakly in Dr. Cofman's office, but, at least, I was grateful for that. I had been able to ask my questions though I had not got any answers. But, now, everything gushed out, tears, criticism, outrage and fear. My husband was deeply distressed. I had believed innocently that I could ask any question I wanted of a doctor about my health, and, if he had an answer, he would tell me. I did not believe that my questions would cause a doctor to resort to such a violent display of anger. For many days afterwards, I was paralyzed with exhaustion. It was as though I had imbibed some poisonous chemical, some toxic pollutant in our atmosphere, that left me psychologically and physically lethargic. My faith in the socratic principles of our society had been profoundly and irrevocably shaken.

8

Vanishing Records

It's not exaggeration to report that there's more actual alteration of records, more "lost" reports, more "phony findings", more downright perjury in the medical malpractice case on defendant's side than in any other kind of law suit including the criminal case! What's more, otherwise respectable doctors countenance it . . .

Melvin Belli: *"An Ancient Therapy Still Applied; The Silent Medical Treatment"*. (1956) Villanova Law Review Vol 1: 250-289.

My depression did not last long. I was not the hypochondriac obsessed with her health that Cofman elected to see or the neurotic for whom Austin had provided the "anxiolytic" drug, propranolol. Neurotics shun action and change. They subconsciously want conflicts to remain unresolved so that they can continue on the familiar path of suffering and endurance. I wanted to solve the mystery of what had happened to me. In particular, I was beginning to realize that my experience with the medical profession went beyond the fact of a physical illness to encompass a kind of social sickness. Powerful people were standing in the way of certain basic rights, the right to personal health information which was important to me in the planning of my life. Neurosis, hypochondriasis have nothing to do with this matter. I was entitled to know what information had accumulated on my body, in the form of tests such as x-rays, echocardiograms, laboratory results and other documents of medical history and to submit this information to someone else's judgement.

After this interview with Cofman, we continued to take positive steps. In spite of everything, my husband and I still wanted to have a child. We continued with our investigation of the infertility question, even though two female physicians, completely familiar with my past events, now advised me against this. In that regard, it would have been of great peace of mind to us to know the nature of my illness. One of the reasons I had returned to Cofman was my desire to have co-ordinated heart and maternity care. However, it was obvious now that Dr. Cofman did not want to resume my care simply because I had asked questions and, in a letter to Dr. Cory, he confirmed this, giving as his reason that my questioning had made him "angrier and angrier". In view of my past events, the co-ordinated maternity and cardiac care seemed now even more important.

Dr. Cory didn't know of any other specialists to recommend to me. The problem, which we didn't realize at the time, concerned the whole question of MVP itself. Certain groups of doctors either did not regard this condition as a serious disorder complicated by certain risks and chose to tell their patients that it was innocent, and, therefore, that I did not need ongoing care or they realized, as Blair had, that, if I continued my investigations into a syndrome doctors were telling the public was benign but, in fact, was not, a whole Pandora's box would be opened. My case showed there were perhaps unexpected problems in this condition, and there was thus also the possibility of medical negligence. Knowledge of MVP was not something these doctors wished to share with the public, but I was bent on knowing just what MVP was all about.

I dealt with my situation by writing two letters, one to the Ontario Medical Association (OMA) to ask for the name of a cardiologist and the other to an American cardiologist whose name Austin had, ironically, mentioned to me. Though I felt it was necessary to explain my situation to the OMA I did not wish to reveal the names of the doctors I had seen. However, this was naive. The OMA would not co-operate unless I provided them with names. That I complied meant I totally misunderstood the nature of this organization, that it is the doctors' union and is supportive not critical. The association made no comment upon my situation and gave me, curiously, the name of a Dr. Peter Austin who was at the same hospital as Dr. Rhodes. To simplify matters, I will refer to my first and most important cardiologist as Dr. Austin, as I have already done, and to this second doctor as Dr. Peter Austin. Thinking that the obvious is often a decoy, I called the association to verify that there was no connection between the two Austins. How it could know there wasn't, unless they spoke with these doctors, was somewhat of a mystery to me.

My second letter to the American specialist, who had written extensively about MVP, secured me an appointment in August, 1981. It was at the time of my follow-up visit after my hospitalization that Austin first casually referred to this specialist. What troubled me so much later, when I had put all things together, was that Dr. Austin must have known but had not shared the opinion of this expert on MVP who advocated the use of antibiotics with dental procedures in a patient with MVP and a murmur. For the appointment with him, my previous test results were naturally requested. We were very eager to, at last, have an unbiased doctor outside of the country evaluate my past events and explain to me why I did not feel as I used to, why I now had ankle swelling at the end of the day and SOB with most activities that I accomplished with ease prior to my fever and endodontal infection. The change in my physical response convinced me I was not the same person.

Dr. Cory arranged for me to pick up my x-rays, echocardiogram print-outs and other hospital records at TMSC since they had not gone to Dr. Cofman in February of 1981 as they were supposed to have. My husband and I arrived at the Medical Records Department on July 14, 1981. The bureaucratic routine of dredging up my records would take approximately a half hour we were told, but we were very patient because we believed the gold was at the end of the rainbow. To our astonishment, the clerk returned immediately and said that there were no records for me.

"But Dr. Cory arranged for me to pick them up," I said in disbelief. "He sent a letter and telephoned." There had been a mail strike, and Dr. Cory assured me he would call. "There must be a mix-up," I lamented. We were utterly bewildered. The indifferent clerk went away, promising to dig further. As we blindly watched other clerks call on the intercom, metal cylinders containing documents tumble down a chute and other people come and pick up x-rays, we became more despairing and anxious. Where were our documents? A feeling of impotence that had been growing all along rose now to overwhelm us with frustration. When our clerk returned she had the manager of Medical Records with her. He apologized liberally but repeated the same story. To convince me, he showed me a file card. There were five entries with the kinds and dates of tests, three chest x-rays and two echocardiograms. The sixth entry was handwritten in black felt pen and indicated that these films had been sent on February 20, 1981 to a Dr. Korman at the Toronto Cardiology Institute (TCI).

We were shocked because we had never requested that my films be sent to this hospital where, curiously, Dr. Peter Austin was. Austin knew I had once been to that hospital because I had told him and again in a letter I repeated the fact that I had decided to come to him instead of Dr. Rhodes. I asked the manager to speak with Dr. Austin to ask him if he had my records or knew of their whereabouts. It just seemed natural to ask him since he had been involved in my care. That anyone else had them simply didn't occur to me. "Did Dr. Austin make this last entry in black felt pen?" I asked unthinkingly as I stared at the incomprehensible entry. "Why would my records be sent to the TCI?" I asked rhetorically. I calmed down and explained about the requisition I had signed requesting that my documents be sent to Dr. Cofman at Richview back in February of 1981.

Of course, the manager did not know the answers to my questions. He went away to call Dr. Austin who insisted that I had specifically requested that my x-rays and echoes be forwarded to Dr. Korman at the TCI and that he wanted nothing more to do with them. Requested of whom we asked ourselves? This bald-faced lie left me white and shaken. The manager assured me that he would do everything to locate these missing documents.

At this time I was staying at a girlfriend's place in Toronto. For the next few days, I tried to track down my records. I called the TCI. Korman had been mistaken for Cofman I reassured myself. A simple clerical error. Korman would gladly return the records. However, it seemed extremely improbable that the records had been sent to a different hospital. Korman at Richview was logical but not Korman at the TCI. My hopes sank when I thought of the conversation Dr. Cofman told me he had with Dr. Austin and the wretched events that had followed. My call revealed there was no "Korman" at the TCI and, furthermore, there never had been. I was stunned and frightened. What was I up against? It seemed that powerful forces were trying to prevent me from getting any information about my health because I had dared to question my treatment. It was this continuous mystery, this secrecy, that urged me to press on. When one feels impotent, out of control, one feels overwhelming panic, and, as I explained my mission to the manager of the film library, I had to fight this feeling of being engulfed by something totally unmanageable. What would happen, I asked, to records addressed to a doctor who was not on staff at that hospital? The clerk replied promptly that a notation would be made and the records would be returned immediately to the sender. The TCI had no record of ever having received my documents from TMSC.

The manager of Medical Records at TMSC had insisted that they did not keep a written record of the transfer of a patients' records because they couldn't record 400 calls a day. There was only the handwritten notation on the file card containing my list of tests to indicate the transfer of my documents. When I told the TCI Medical Records manager this, she said this story was "pure nonsense" and would represent "extreme irresponsibility". All records were very important in the event of a medical crisis. The TCI, she declared, received more than 400 calls a day and kept a written record of every transaction.

I called Richview and found a Korman on staff, but my hopes plunged when I learned he was not a cardiologist. His secretary told me Dr. Korman had never received my documents and, if he had by mistake, they would have been promptly returned to the sender. Again this Medical Records Library kept a written record, and the clerk verified that there had never been any exchange of films in my case.

I telephoned several other Toronto hospitals to ask about their procedure with regard to transfer of medical records. All swore that such test results could not get lost in the manner I described because, if they were not requested by a physician, they were immediately returned unopened to the sending hospital. Three facts emerged from my efforts. Hospitals always kept a permanent, official record of these transactions, not hand-written notes seemingly dashed off. There was no possibility of loss during transit by special delivery courier service and the requisition always went through the treating physician.

I made several other fruitless attempts to get help, even calling the OMA from which I had begged the recommendation of a cardiologist. The secretary of that organization told me there was nothing that it could do. I called the College of Physicians and Surgeons. The ordinary channels were open to me, a formal written complaint, a wait of several months and an assessment of my complaint by the Complaints Committee of the College, exactly as had been done in my case with the dentists. There was no time for taking such a formal route. My appointment with the American doctor was fifteen days away. A call to the Ontario Hospital Association confirmed that I should forward a written complaint to The College of Physicians and Surgeons and, if this was of no help, I could then appeal to The Health Disciplines Review Board (HDRB). I was given the name of the person to contact at the HDRB as well as the name of the Director of Patients' Complaints at TMSC.

In desperation I called Dr. Austin. I wanted to ask him why he had said that I had asked to have my films forwarded to a non-existent Dr. Korman. He was, of course, unavailable. His secretary reported that he had received no request from Dr. Cory, either by telephone or letter, to have my documents ready for me. But, curiously, a telephone call to Dr. Warren, whom I had seen on September 24, 1980 shortly after my release from hospital, revealed that he had received both the telephone call and the letter dated June 24, 1981, requesting that my records be available for pick up. His one x-ray was waiting for me at his office.

When I returned to the Medical Records Department at TMSC, the clerk showed us a black binder containing the radiologists' summaries of my x-rays and echocardiograms, what, in fact, Cofman had received. What we found in that binder astonished us. There was a buff coloured page with a warning scrawled in big letters that no further information was to be released without subpoena. This was meant for me. If I wanted anything I would have to hire a lawyer to act on my behalf. This handwritten note was in black felt pen and was signed by Dr. Austin and dated February 20, 1981, the date my records were supposedly sent to the fictitious Dr. Korman at the TCI. Of course, it was never intended that I actually lay eyes on this page. The clerk would have been given instructions to report to me that I was not permitted to have my records, and, not having any legal access, it was expected that I would simply walk away in anger. It struck me as significant that both the note on the records card and this note were in the same black felt pen.

Back in November of 1980, after my meeting with the Complaints Committee of the RCDS and in between my two appointments with Cofman, my lawyer had written Dr. Austin to ask him for a clarification of the mysterious telephone call from Mentlik regarding the prescription for antibiotics after my periodontal surgery. My lawyer was convinced I was entitled to a small amount in damages, and, evidently, the lawyer for the dentists had agreed to talk about an amount in the range of $2500. However, my interest in investigating had never been motivated by the desire for any money beyond the return of what I had spent. However, I had now come to the realization that, if my dentists were in error in not giving me ABP during all their dental manipulations, so, too, was Dr. Austin. And with continued opposition, my quest became one of using the legal system if I could, to tear down those unjust barriers that had prevented me from obtaining personal health information.

My lawyer's letter, of course, informed Dr. Austin that I was now engaged in some kind of legal action against my dentists, though it was in no way malpractice litigation since no writs had been issued. Curiously, Austin did not reply to my lawyer's November letter until almost four months later, towards the end of February, 1981. This was about the time when Austin would have received my requisition asking that my records be forwarded to Dr. Cofman.

When my lawyer finally received a letter from Dr. Austin, it was to advise that he had now found a note in his file to the effect that he had conversed with Dr. Mentlik and had prescribed ampicillin over the telephone for my periodontal surgery on January 7th of 1980. This was directly contrary to what he had told us on February 26, 1980 when he said he had no knowledge of the periodontal surgery nor of having prescribed ampicillin over the telephone. We would always remember seeing Austin scribbling something on a piece of paper as I asked about this telephone call. This letter of Austin's also came after Mentlik had lied at the Complaints Committee meeting in June of 1980 about giving me the antibiotics before the surgery.

The clerk did not understand Dr. Austin's order to have a subpoena and inadvertently allowed me to photocopy the five radiologist reports, but the empirical evidence, the x-rays and echoes, more valuable than these interpretations, was gone forever. In these reports, there was a very startling piece of information. The December 12, 1978 echocardiogram, prior to my fever and endodontal and other interventions, had shown "a trivial end-systolic mitral valve prolapse" while that of February 26, 1980, during my illness, when my heart, according to Dr. Austin, had supposedly gone down in size, read "excellent visualization of the cardiac valves and chambers reveals a holosystolic mitral valve prolapse". Dr. Austin had told us that my murmur had changed but that the change was unimportant. Did the first 1978 report correlate with the late systolic murmur I had prior to my febrile illness? And did the second in 1980 correlate with the change in murmur Austin heard in November of 1979 during my cardiac enlargement and the holosystolic murmur subsequently heard on auscultation by Dr. Cofman? It seemed logical that the greater the prolapse, the greater the regurgitation. But it would take me a long time to hunt down the answer to that question. Was this proof that my heart had not returned to its normal size at that time? Again, we would have to wait for that answer.

The Executive Director of Patient and Community Relations confirmed that, after Dr. Austin had personally done the fluoroscopy on February 26, 1980, he had the option of asking the radiologist to prepare a permanent x-ray film for the hospital and a report from the fluoroscopic test but had chosen not to do this. My earlier suspicions that he had chosen fluoroscopy so that he could preview my situation prior to having a permanent x-ray done seemed correct. Either he was able to tell from the movements of my heart with the fluoroscope test that it had not returned to its normal size or he knew, right from the beginning, that the cardiac enlargement would not reverse itself because of the sudden increase in regurgitation. Was the fluoroscope, therefore, just a ploy to give me the impression that there was proof my situation had corrected itself? We still had no explanation for the x-ray of February 26, 1980, supposedly showing that my heart had returned to its normal size, which my husband and I knew I had not had.

The Director of Patients Complaints provided us with another bizarre clue to the puzzle. She promised she would do her best to recover my test results though she insisted that x-rays had not disappeared from their hospital in fifty years. She pointed out that all test results and radiologists' comments were stored in the same large envelope called a "master bag". This whole package was forwarded to the new doctor when the medical records were requisitioned. "How then," we asked in bewilderment, "could Dr. Cofman have received the radiologists' summaries without the actual films?" She merely agreed this was a perplexing problem. Hospital officials, I was rapidly learning, did not have answers. Explanations were replaced with apologies. But, it was obvious, I'm sure, to her as it was to us, that someone had removed the x-rays and other documents before the master bag was sent to Cofman at Richview. Upon questioning, the Director said that the treating physicians were always consulted first before the patient's file was sent to another doctor. She also admitted that doctors at TMSC had uninterrupted access to patients' files. This meant they were not required to sign in or out for any document, and no record was kept of anything a doctor took out of a file.

On the matter of whether or not Medical Records kept a permanent record of documents that were transferred to other facilities, she attempted to convince me that they did, in direct opposition to the information given us by the manager of Medical Records. She then showed us a file card identical to the one the manager had shown us with one exception that astonished us. This was a new card, and the last entry, dated February 20, 1981, that had been written in black felt pen, showing that everything had been forwarded to Dr. Korman at the TCI, was now typed.

The Director then showed us another handwritten message dated February 20, 1981, on which the name of Dr. Korman was scratched out and Cofman written underneath. It said one bag, five films, 1:30 p.m. February 20, 1981, Richview, giving the incorrect impression that everything had been forwarded to Dr. Cofman.

Hopeful that Austin would have a change of heart and call me to tell me he had found my medical records in his office, I left instructions with his secretary for him to call me at my girlfriend's place, where I was staying, before 3:30 p.m. on Friday when I would leave for my last appointment with the Director of Patients' Complaints. Dr. Austin called at 6:30 p.m. Friday. His conversation with my friend, which she recorded, was very disturbing. The normal procedure, on finding an individual unavailable, is to leave a message or ask where the person can be reached, say thank you and hang up. Dr. Austin, however, questioned my friend extensively about my plans. The following conversation was constructed from notes I took when my friend called me at home in the evening to report on Dr. Austin's conversation and to apologize for her blunders in giving information.

Dr. Austin first asked what I wanted of him. My friend, of course, replied that I wanted my x-rays and echocardiogram print-outs. His response was to repeat that I had requested that these records be sent to Dr. Korman at the TCI. He then asked where I was. My friend replied that I had left and reminded him that he was supposed to have called before 3:30 p.m.

He ignored this and asked ,"Where did she go?"

"She had an appointment at the hospital."

"Which hospital?"

"TMSC."

"Oh, I guess she went to the Dentistry Department," he said.

This seemingly casual but incorrect supposition that I had gone to the Dentistry Department might be considered baffling. However, it could only reveal what was on Dr. Austin's mind. Four months had passed since I had seen Dr. Cofman. It had been in November of 1980 that my lawyer had first written to Dr. Austin to ask about the ampicillin prescription. And it was over a year since Dr. Austin had seen me. During that time, Austin had seen many patients. How could he remember me unless he had reason to do so? If he were innocent, had not intervened in my case and was not responsible for the disappearance of my records, he would never have asked these questions of my friend, much less assumed I was on my way to the Dentistry Department where he supposed I would be asking for my dental records for my legal undertaking. My legal action against the dentists and his own possible implication was obviously uppermost in his mind.

To my friend's response that I was meeting with the Director of Patient Complaints, Austin naturally wanted to know why.

"She wants her missing x-rays," my friend replied.

"Why does she want them?"

"She has an appointment with another cardiologist."

"Oh, that's right. Her appointment with Dr. Cofman did not work out."

This was shocking: Dr. Austin could only have known this fact if he and Cofman had conversed after our disastrous meeting. Austin's first call was the one that had made Cofman so angry. Yet, Cofman, like Warren, claimed, in his letter to Cory, that he knew nothing about Dr. Austin's treatment. Cofman stated only that I had had some cardiologic investigations in the past and that the nature of my questions had angered him. His anger arose because he perceived that he was being asked to evaluate a colleague's care, and he would not do that. The mysterious telephone conversation between Cofman and Austin suddenly became clearer. Knowing from my original requisition, filled out and signed at Richview Hospital, that I would be consulting Cofman, Austin had telephoned to find out why and to assure that Cofman understood I was a troublemaker.

"Who is she going to see?" Dr. Austin asked my friend who responded that I was seeing an American doctor on the east coast. She told me afterwards that she had mispronounced the name though her version very closely resembled the original. Dr. Austin terminated this conversation with another contradiction. He had, he said, received Cory's telephone call and letter, but the x-rays had already been sent out to Dr. Korman at the TCI. This was the information my friend conveyed to me the evening after the telephone call. Dr. Austin was frequently changing his story. Previously he had denied that he had received any such instructions from Dr. Cory and he had denied that he had received a telephone call from Mentlik but later said that he had.

Six long years afterwards when I had in fact undertaken litigation primarily to obtain my medical records, my Toronto lawyer would give me a copy of the TMSC hospital records. Among these papers would be a copy of Dr. Cory's letter, dated June 24, 1981, to Dr. Austin, asking for my medical records in time to go to the States. The existence of this letter verified that Dr. Austin had, indeed, lied in this matter as he had likely done in others. Dr. Cory's letter stated that I would be visiting another cardiologist, whose name was not specified according to my request, and would like to pick up my x-rays on July 14, 1981. At the bottom of this letter was the most valuable piece of information: a note in a handwriting very similar to that on the buff coloured page that demanded a subpoena before release of any records and similar to the handwriting that appeared on all other copies of letters from Dr. Austin to Dr. Cory which I had in my possession. The statement said, "Dr. Austin to see x-ray file ?, make copies." This note could only confirm Dr. Austin's ongoing intervention to prevent me from discovering the truth about my past illness and present health situation. The question mark is inexplicable unless it was simply a ruse to convey that Dr. Austin was not sure whether my documents had gone to another doctor at another hospital. The letter suggests that Dr. Austin had access to my medical records prior to my coming to the hospital to ask for them, that he arranged in some way for their removal to his safekeeping in response to Dr. Cory's letter and then fabricated the evidence that they had gone, by mistake to the fictitious Dr. Korman, at the time I had previously requisitioned them to be forwarded to Dr. Cofman. And this, without doubt, would make any normal person suspicious that something of major importance, some evidence, most likely of valvular vegetations, existed on those missing print-outs of the echocardiograms in addition to the evidence of the enlargement in my heart.

In looking back on the events, I could only ask had Dr. Austin contacted Mentlik, after our February discussion, about the ampicillin and then contacted my lawyer to provide the story that he had prescribed this drug over the telephone. To give some protection even after surgery was better than to give none at all. And this agreement enabled Mentlik to state that he had given me ampicillin prior to my surgery at the Complaints Committee meeting since he knew that Dr. Austin would back him up. It was certainly not unreasonable to suspect that there had been contact between these two parties, just as there appeared to be contact between Austin and Cofman for the purpose of stifling my investigation. The only unknown is the exact time when Austin actually removed my films etc. from the Master Bag. It would seem likely that he extracted them from the bag on receipt of the original requisition to forward them to Richview because he anticipated a malpractice suit against himself. Since I had already complained to the dental college, what was there to stop me from complaining to the medical college as well? Since Austin had unobstructed access to patients' files, it would not be difficult to remove the documents from the Master Bag before they were sent to Cofman. However, it is unlikely that Austin would have gone to this trouble just to hinder my legal action against the dentists. It had to be to protect himself, unless he saw his own fate inextricably tied up with that of the dentists. Only Dr. Austin, it seems, could have made the handwritten Dr. Korman entry since it was done on the same day, and with apparently the same black felt pen that was used for the subpoena note appended to my radiologists' reports. When he returned the master bag to Medical Records for delivery to Dr. Cofman, Austin could have given the clerk the name Korman, then changed it to Cofman to create confusion and make it appear to future observers that my records had got lost through a completely natural error in name. This handwritten note with the name scratched out, representing the transference of the original order from my requisition, was kept on file and suggests that the clerk never saw my requisition which clearly gave Cofman and Richview as the destination for my medical records. Clerical errors occur frequently, and no one would question them. A clerk would not contravene the orders of a doctor and look in the bag to see what was in there. And the hospital's practice was to destroy the original requisition.

The loss of these records prevented us from carrying on our legal investigation. All lawyers said it would be impossible to obtain the records after the apparent loss. We had never had any intention of proceeding beyond the process of discovery when I would have my lawyer ask Dr. Austin the questions I always wanted to ask him. Nor did we have a spare hundred thousand dollars to continue on to court. And, of course, we were unable to find anyone in the city of Toronto to contradict Dr. Austin's judgement that I had never had IE. The female doctor to whom my lawyer would pay a thousand dollars of my money to engage as Expert Witness would demonstrate not only unfathomable ignorance of the condition of MVP but of what was in my file. She would write that Dr. Rhodes had discussed "infective endocarditis" in great detail with me. How else could the "dumb" patient have possibly acquired such an understanding of this disease! She ignored all the copies of articles from the medical journals and my own article that I had my lawyer forward to her. Dr. Expert Witness would also state that I had "been warned many times by many people that antibiotic prophylaxis is necessary." She ignored the dates of these discussions, not warnings, which took place long after my dental work and that none of the doctors I talked with unequivocally committed himself to ABP with dental work, that, in fact, it was my insistence that made them capitulate, an insistence which they interpreted as evidence of a cardiac neurosis. This Expert Witness had neither my TMSC hospital records nor the most important documents that had vanished. Nor had she examined me herself. She regarded my cardiac enlargement as premenstrual fluid retention, my MVP as a completely harmless, innocent "anatomic entity" and my positive blood culture in hospital as "academic". My lawyer said it was impossible to find any other Expert Witness in the city of Toronto. The powerful doctors and the lawyers, "the hired guns of the rich",[1] of the same social and economic class, who, in the words of one American Law Professor, are "men of mystery and magic, members of a sacerdotal class in close communion with God",[2] looking down on us from their carved rosewood and leather thrones, crushed our lowly case as if one fragile piece of flesh, a heart valve, was as insubstantial as the petal of flower.

The loss of our records meant our visit to the U.S. doctor would be unsuccessful. Without the films and echoes showing the changes in my cardiac status, we did not believe we could obtain an "objective" opinion. The disappearance of my records appeared to us as a full blown act of aggression, our first real taste of how a powerful, protected group can eradicate opposition. I had been needlessly exposed to radiation and would be exposed to more as doctors insisted on further x-rays to prove that my heart was not enlarged. It would be impossible to prove, without sequential x-rays on the same machine, that my heart had actually returned to its normal, smaller than average size.

To be stripped of any means of righting a wrong is to be overwhelmingly stressed, an undesirable situation for any cardiac patient. In her book, *Stress and The Art of Bio-Feedback*, Barbara Brown says, "When changes in the social environment and social dynamics become stressful, it is largely because the information needed to adjust or resolve problems is incomplete, and thus mental projections about the social future continue to be uncertain. It is the uncertainty that keeps both the mind and body altered and prepared to take action against seemingly impending threats to wellbeing and security and survival."[3] Not knowing what kind of illness had affected my heart filled us with anxiety about my present and future health. The response of Warren, Cofman and Austin proved that access to future health care was threatened. Only if I remained quiet would I get care. All these doctors then had made me a prisoner of my own helplessness. We had simply asked questions we were entitled to ask. Now it was our turn to be angry.

An interesting study done in the United States at the University of Colorado[4] illustrates the dangerous effects on the body of total impotence. Two groups of caged rats were given mild electric shocks. Group I had a lever to stop the administration of electric shocks. Group II had no levers, but their electric shocks were stopped and started at the same time as those of Group I. The first group were unaffected by the repeated shocks, but the second group sickened and became severely weakened. The stress, not of the shocks, but of not being able to control them, caused a breakdown in the immune system of the rats thus leading to illness. The conclusion for human beings is that having control over one's life leads to wellness and the aim, therefore, of psychotherapy is to create in the patient "the feeling that he has control over things."

Norman Cousin's experience with illness in his book, *Anatomy of an Illness*, is essentially the human parallel of this animal experiment. In the introduction, René Dubos says that "The basic theme of this book is that every person must accept a certain measure of responsibility for his or her own recovery from disease or disability."[5] The book's popularity depends on people believing, like the rats, that they can control their wellbeing. People thus choose "treatment methods" over which they can have full responsibility, diet, exercise, jogging, vitamin supplements or laughter to create the feeling that they are in control of the means of producing or perpetuating healthiness. My lack of control began when I first asked questions of Dr. Rhodes about MVP and was refused answers. My impotency reached its climax with the destruction of my records which abolished all hope of any control. I could thus no longer "activate the levers" to stop the shock of uncertainty and anxiety.

Because Norman Cousins is a published author and lecturer, people listen to him. His personal beliefs thus gain credibility which is a kind of therapy in itself. He says his doctor encouraged him "to believe I was a respected partner with him in the total undertaking,"[6] including "sharing with the physician the responsibility for the choice of therapy."[7] But is it really possible for a patient less prominent than Norman Cousins to have a say in therapy, to be a "respected partner"? Being a woman meant that I received no respect whatsoever from the moment I stepped inside a doctor's office. Rather than assist, doctors actively prevented me from participating in my therapy. I first had to struggle to find out the dangers that awaited a MVP patient. No one identified them for me nor gave me the option to prevent them. My experience demonstrates that as long as the authorities continue to control the "means" to health, the knowledge, I would remain powerless, my voice solitary, muffled, a desperate cry in the wilderness.

9

MVP — Alias Cardiac Neurosis

Medicine has the authority to label one man's complaint a legitimate illness, to declare a second man sick though he himself does not complain, and to refuse a third social recognition of his pain, his disability, and even his death. It is medicine which stamps some pain as "merely subjective", some impairment as malingering, and some deaths — though not others — as suicide. The judge determines what is legal and who is guilty. The priest declares what is holy and who has broken a taboo. The physician decides what is a symptom and who is sick. He is a moral entrepreneur, charged with inquisitorial powers to discover certain wrongs to be righted.

Ivan Illich: *Limits to Medicine, Medical Nemesis: The Expropriation of Health*. (London: Marian Boyars, 1976), p. 53-54.

The disappearance of my documents verifying my illness marked the beginning of the discrediting of my medical history and therefore an attack on my credibility. Doctors now had a loophole that relieved them of the untenable obligation of criticizing a colleague, an act uniformly condemned by the profession itself. They could deny the cardiac enlargement ever existed or dismiss it as an x-ray technician's error. They could deny that I had ever had an illness, in particular IE, and insist that the pansystolic murmur (PSM) existed prior to my illness. The more evidence of a previous infective endocarditis (IE) would accumulate over the years, the more doctors looked for other improbable causes or diseases and the louder they cried that MVP was a benign syndrome without any risks.

In countries ruled by powerful, dictatorial groups, one of the most effective methods of suppressing dissidents is to accuse them of psychosis and incarcerate them in prisons that are quasi psychiatric restraining facilities. The medical profession imprisoned me in silence, bound and gagged me with the lesser but equally fraudulent charge of neurosis. All I had wanted right from the beginning was to have a few pertinent questions regarding my MVP answered. But, when I had quietly put these questions to Dr. Rhodes, he had become very angry, refused to answer them and even terminated our discussion.

My situation could be compared to that of patients in psychiatric facilities.

In an interview in *The Toronto Globe and Mail*,[1] ex-psychiatric patients referred to their treatment as an effort to "psychiatrize" and "tranquilize" them. Their chief complaint was that they were "victimized by a system that humiliates, degrades, invalidates and infantilizes." The reaction of doctors to questions about my past care stripped me of any power, rendered me as helpless and inarticulate as a child, and, in this powerless state, I was forced to accept whatever information I was given. The disappearance of my records invalidated my claims of inappropriate treatment and prevented me from ever knowing what evidence had existed on those x-rays and echocardiograms. To be deprived of my right to information was a true humiliation. My history then became suspect and I was further degraded by being accused of concocting stories. The more I searched for truth, so necessary to my physical and psychological wellbeing, the more doctors, like Cofman, branded me as neurotically obsessed with my health. The tactic to silence me was identical to that used with the psychiatric patients interviewed. When they sought information about their medical condition or took notes during consultations with their psychiatrists, their efforts were classified as "symptoms of mental illness."

It was Dr. Austin who first laid the charge of neurosis. In his letters to Dr. Cory, he attributed my symptoms to an obsessive, highly emotional and exaggerated fear for my heart. On my first visit, in response to his questions on my career orientation, I told him I was a French and English secondary school teacher, currently unemployed, and that I was working on a degree in music and giving piano instruction in my home as well as teaching a creative writing course two hours a week to senior citizens. Dr. Austin ignored everything I did and referred to me in his records as "this creative writing teacher". Why did he do this? I can only conclude that it was because he held the belief that creative writing teachers possess elaborate imaginations and could easily become tense or "anxious" about their hearts. My first report of chest pain at the time of my dental problems thus became evidence to him, not of infection, but of cardiac neurosis: "She is obviously in an anxiety state once again complaining of chest pain." The cause of my anxiety, he assumed, without any proof whatsoever, was the "continued worry" over "the family history of sudden cardiac death" which I had related to him only once in four years in response to his routine questions for his medical record.

In line with his view that my two previous episodes of rapid heart beat were nothing more than a few "harmless palpitations", my complaints of an increase in nighttime tachycardia with SOB that was only controlled in the upright position, led him to emphasize the benefits of keeping on with my "anxiolytic medication" of propranolol. Austin was assuming the role of psychiatrist rather than cardiologist. Thus, when I saw him for only the third time in four years, hardly the behaviour of a neurotic, on November 29, 1979, IE was the furthest thing from his mind, and all my symptoms, fever, chills, sweats, chest pain, cardiac enlargement, change in murmur, tachycardia, unusual fatigue and SOB in association with an abcessed tooth and numerous dental interventions without antibiotics signified nothing at all to him. His comment in his letters was "Her labile mental state suggested a pathological degree of anxiety on this visit beyond what we had noted in the past." Unconsciously applying the royal "we", his majesty all but declared that I required institutionalizing for psychological instability of a pathological degree.

The mind, "diseased" or not, is incapable of causing the heart to enlarge. Therefore, to what did Dr. Austin attribute the cardiac enlargement? He had suggested that an increase in mitral regurgitation could be causing the increase in cardiac size. But what was causing the increased mitral regurgitation? Austin was not concerned with this. In his view, the drug, propranolol, was "allowing a little cardiac enlargement" and, therefore, the regurgitation was secondary to the cardiac enlargement rather than the reverse. Cardiac enlargement must, therefore, be a side effect of propranolol. Mine was a mini-dose, only 60 mg. a day, and, according to Goodman and Gilman's *The Pharmacological Basis of Therapeutics*[2] or the CPS [3], which discuss the side effects of all drugs, there is no evidence that propranolol causes cardiac enlargement. Furthermore, the fact that my heart increased and decreased miraculously, while I was still taking propranolol, renders this argument totally absurd.

Dr. Austin's second explanation was equally improbable and completely lacking in proof. Because of the increased regurgitation, reflected in the change in my murmur, he jumped to the conclusion that I must have severe "myxomatous degeneration of the mitral valve". In order to appreciate this pathology and how it causes the valve to leak, it is first necessary to understand how the normal mitral valve functions. A correctly functioning mitral valve is one through which blood *does not* leak backward from the left ventricle into the left atrium during systole. For its smooth operation, the mitral valve depends upon the delicate co-ordination of six anatomic parts: chordae tendineae, annulus or ring that anchors the valve, posterior left atrial wall, papillary muscles, leaflets and left ventricular wall. Two scalloped leaflets, anterior and posterior, close and hermetically seal the mitral valve preventing the reverse flow of blood into the atrium. Thin, strong, fibrous cords or tendons, called chordae tendineae (from the Latin) hold the valve leaflet in place. The majority of these chordae tendineae arise from the tips of the heads of the finger-like papillary muscles which are embedded in the walls of the ventricles. The papillary muscles of course are involved in the pumping function of the ventricles. The thin chordae form a network of dividing, subdividing and interconnecting threads which attach to the fibrous bands of the free edges of the valve leaflets and to the ventricular surfaces of the leaflets. Other chordae arise directly from the left ventricular wall and attach to the posterior atrial scallop of the mitral leaflets. In photographs of the excised valve, the whole mechanism resembles an inflated parachute.[4]

Dr. Joseph K. Perloff describes how these parts of the normal mitral valve function during systole.

Left ventricular systole begins with contraction of the papillary muscles. The vertical forces exerted by the contracting papillary muscles move the leaflets into apposition. As the intraventricular pressure rises, the free edges of the cusps firmly coapt, mutually supporting each other along a comfortable margin of their atrial surfaces, and firmly sealing the orifice. The remainder of each leaflet bulges like a parachute toward the left atrium. The annulus not only serves as a fulcrum for the leaflets, but during ventricular systole decreases its circumferential size, thus reducing the area that the leaflets are required to bridge. Even so the surface area of the leaflets is about two and one half times the area of the orifice, thus providing a comfortable reserve. As the left ventricle ejects, its apex and the mitral orifice approach each other. Shortening the vertical axis of the left ventricle is accompanied by synergistic contraction of the papillary muscles so that an appropriate vertical anchoring force is applied to the chordae tendineae, that prevents eversion of the leaflets.[5]

This description explains why some doctors claim that everyone has mitral valve prolapse, in that the normal mitral leaflets bulge during systole towards the left atrium. The difference is that normal leaflets remain in firm apposition so that there is no reverse flow of blood into the atrium. If the tissues of any of these parts are diseased, this delicate, precise mechanism is disturbed. Mucoid or myxomatous degeneration is a progressive disease that affects the connective tissue that is part of the valve's composition. This disorder is believed to be the cause of the prolapsing valves. Researchers have studied the cellular components of prolapsed valves and have found that the sturdier, more fibrous connective tissue of prolapsed valves is replaced in varying degrees by spongiosa or myxomatous tissue. As the word suggests, spongiosa tissue is stretchable because it contains excess mucopolysaccharides. "Loss of this normally dense, collagenous supporting structure (fibrosa)," according to Ariela Pomerance, a British histopathologist, "would clearly allow stretching of the cusp (leaflet) by normal variations in intraventricular pressures and would result in the characteristic voluminous, ballooned leaflets."[6]

The existence and degree of this mucoid or myxomatous tissue can only be determined by direct observation at surgery or autopsy and, often, only with microscopic study of the valvular tissue. Hill and co-workers from the Department of Cardiovascular Surgery at St. Thomas' Hospital in London, England are among many of the researchers who have pointed out the chief pathological features found in prolapsed valves at autopsy. They describe leaflets that are expanded and thickened, ballooned, heavy and floppy and chordae tendineae that are "attenuated, weakened and prone to rupture."[7] But, other workers, Mills et al from the University of North Carolina School of Medicine in the United States, have observed chordae tendineae that are short and thickened.[8] Redundant, hooded, voluminous, furled, and pleated are some other adjectives commonly used by researchers to describe the abnormal appearance of prolapsed valves. When we know how the normal mitral valve functions, we are better able to visualize how such defects could interrupt the smooth performance of the mitral valve by a "valvulo-ventricular disproportion in which the mitral valve is 'too big' for the ventricle."[9]

Austin's conclusion that I had myxomatous tissue deterioration was, therefore, pure speculation on his part. According to the leading histological experts, this process is linked to aging. It is rarely found in young people, especially those who have minimal prolapse which would be manifested by a click and a LSM as I had prior to the infection. In fact, the condition, MVP, came to be regarded as "benign" because its deterioration is so slow. Significant deterioration does not take place in the space of a year or even three years. Ariela Pomerance, who has extensively studied and compared the histology of prolapsed valves in animals and man, emphasizes the striking relationship to age. "In man too it is seen most often in the elderly but this fact is more an expression of the long natural history than an indication that aging itself is the aetiological factor."[10] The average age of the patients in Pomerance's studies was 73.6 years and, at death, none were under fifty with the highest incidence being in the age group eighty to ninety years.

Other researchers have observed that this myxomatous tissue is not seen in patients under forty and that the degree of it increases linearly with age from the fifth through to the eighth decade [11] and that it affects about five percent of the population over age fifty.[12] The evidence that the myxomatous process is slow acting and correlates with age is logical if one realizes, as do Davies, Moore and Braimbridge of Britain, that the collagen content of the human valve declines with age in the same way that collagen in the outer skin of the body, the face in particular, loses its elasticity as one ages. "The clinical course suggests that this process may begin very early in life and progress extremely slowly if at all, or begin late in life with more rapid progression over a few years."[13]

There is yet another significant reason for rejecting Dr. Austin's conclusions. Though MVP is purported to occur in four times more women than men, some studies have shown that "severe and clinically significant myxoid changes occur more frequently in men than in women," according to some researchers, because the aortic valve, rather than the mitral, seems to be more affected by the myxomatous process though it is not concluded that men, therefore, suffer from aortic valve prolapse more than mitral.[14]

As well, the more progressive and severe form of myxomatous tissue deterioration, which is called Marfan's disease after the physician who studied it, is found in people with skeletal abnormalities.[15] Although MVP shares this same tissue abnormality, the valves in Marfan's disease deteriorate more rapidly. Patients with Marfan's disease have pronounced physical abnormalities, heads that are longer than broader, dislocated lens, an armspan greater than height and a high arched palate.[16] It would be obvious to even a lay person that I had none of these physical aberrations.

Without our records we did not believe we could get an unbiased opinion and, so, did not want to make a long journey to the United States, a journey that would take all of our holidays. Instead of peace and relaxation, our vacation would be spent in anxiety and effort. Now that the objective evidence had vanished, the only proof, apart from the radiologist's reports, of my cardiac enlargement and change in murmur was in Dr. Austin's psychologically damning letters with suggestions of psychosis in the words, "labile mentality" and "pathological anxiety". Doctors do not listen to patients; they listen to other physicians. And, if I did not bring these letters, there was no evidence that my present condition had not existed before my illness. Furthermore, in his letters, Dr. Austin does not describe my symptoms of fever, rapid heart beat etc., or make any reference to the fact that my murmur changed while my heart was enlarged at the time of my illness, despite the radiologist's comments on the echocardiographic picture, and declares, without any blood tests, that I did not have IE. A doctor reading these letters would assume that Dr. Austin had done blood tests and ruled out IE.

However, when I attempted to cancel the appointment by telephone, explaining why I did not have the past films and echoes, I was told I did not need them and should come anyway. Though I shuddered at the thought of showing Dr. Austin's letters with the humiliating comments on my mental state, a faint hope and the desire to trust in the good sense and humanitarian instincts of the American doctor made us consent to go. But, when we finally met with him, it was immediately apparent that "the tenor of my questioning", to use Dr. Cofman's phrase, was guaranteed to arouse this doctor's hostility as well. But why was this so? I asked my questions calmly and politely as I had of Dr. Cofman. Although I, myself, was unaware of the cumulative effect of my questions, it would be obvious to any doctor that these questions were of a medico-legal nature, what might be asked of an "an expert witness", that is a doctor who might be called upon to testify about another doctor's care. Compatible with my increase in knowledge was an inevitable increase in the directness of my questions relating to cause and effect.

"This is what happens when patients read the medical literature," the doctor remarked abruptly when I had finished reciting my medical history.

What was "this" that was happening? Patients making useless long journeys? Patients wasting important doctors' time? Patients criticizing their doctor's care? And, ultimately, patients attempting by devious means to get another doctor to testify against a colleague in a malpractice suit? I could not, of course, respond to this remark because I didn't know what it meant. All that I could gather from this seemingly unrelated comment was that my questions had, despite my coming all this way, angered this doctor just as they had every other doctor I had encountered.

However, we hadn't come all that way to be evasive or thwarted. I had, by now, laid Dr. Austin's poisonous letters on the desk, and he was thumbing through them. When he had finished, I said, "You have made the statement that a benign LSM can become a PSM. The causes, you say, in an article you wrote, are IE, slow deterioration, that is not rapid over the time period of a year and in the presence of ongoing dental manipulations as in my case or through chordal rupture which can happen spontaneously or as a result of IE but which is almost always verifiable by echo. I would like to know if the change in my murmur from a LSM to a PSM in the space of six months, given that I had an abscessed tooth, was caused by IE." I listed my symptoms at the time.

"You've read the article haven't you!" he said, not looking up. To me this could only mean that he was not, at the very outset, going to give me an answer. However, I persisted. "But, I want to know from a specialist if it applies to me," I said with a sinking feeling, "or if there is some other cause for my present symptoms of SOB with activities I used to perform easily, ankle swelling and increased muscle fatigue. None of these things were present prior to my dental infection.

"I can't comment," he said with finality, "on what happened to you in the past. I didn't examine you then."

So ended the conversation after travelling almost a thousand miles. In his examination, he listened to my murmur with the phonocardiogram. Phonocardiography, used simultaneously with electrocardiography, allows the cardiologist to hear the cardiac sounds at the same time as they are depicted graphically. In effect, the phonocardiogram can pick up vibrations a cardiologist might miss on auscultation. A non-invasive test, it can demonstrate the various features of the first and second heart sounds, S_1 and S_2. Phonocardiography is of particular importance in establishing the timing and shape of murmurs, specifically whether the murmur is late systolic or pansystolic and whether the sound is crescendo-decrescendo or plateau. From these and other graphic depictions, the phonocardiogram can give information about left ventricular function and mitral regurgitation.[17]

When he was listening to my murmur with the phonocardiogram, he commented that he was unable to hear the click and that it was likely buried in the murmur. In our conversation that followed, he said that I had "moderately severe regurgitation". He paused and then changed that to "minimally severe".

To us this was not encouraging since we assumed this expert on MVP knew a great deal about the disorder. To us, severe regurgitation, with whatever qualifying adjective, must eventually lead to cardiac enlargement as the mitral regurgitation increased and, ultimately, to heart failure. In the first monograph of MVP ever published, Dr. Robert Jeresaty outlined five stages in the progression of prolapse:
1) silent prolapse
2) MSC without a murmur
3) MSC and LSM (what I had before my infection)
4) PSM (the result of IE, gradual deterioration and chordal rupture)
5) severe regurgitation, floppy valve and heart failure.[18]

I appeared to be in the 4th of five stages, or one step away from heart failure albeit that might be a process of ten or more years. However, this American specialist's attitude discouraged questions and, so, we did not ask anything further. He then looked at the one x-ray I had brought, Dr. Warren's, which was taken one year after Dr. Austin's crucial x-ray, and said that he saw no evidence of an increase in heart size. Without Austin's sequential heart x-rays, it was, of course, impossible to see that my heart, which was initially described as undersized, or, in Austin's words, "tiny", could, when it enlarges, remain within the normal limits. Drs. Hurst and Span, in a chapter of *The*

Heart entitled, "The Etiology and Clinical Recognition of Heart Failure", point out that "the normal range of heart size is great. Accordingly, a heart, the size of which was previously near the lower limits of normal, may undergo enlargement and still seem to be within normal size limits."[19] It was once again emphasized for us that, without past x-rays for comparison, there was no way of knowing whether the increase in heart size in 1979 over 1978, recorded on the missing x-ray, had in reality been only temporary.

We returned to Canada with the knowledge that the regurgitation had increased significantly and was now "minimally or moderately severe". But we still did not know the cause of the deterioration. That information was not likely ever to be confirmed by any doctor because of the legal implications. I, of course, discussed all this with Dr. Cory. Previously, when I had told him that my records had vanished and that I had nothing to take to the States, he gave me my file, saying I could copy whatever I wanted for my visit. As usual, he allowed me to photocopy the American doctor's letter describing my visit.

Once again, the contrast in the doctor's personal communication and the written record was profoundly disturbing. "Moderately or minimally severe regurgitation" was recorded as "minimal mitral insufficiency". Minimal and severe are not synonymous. Nor is "minimal" equivalent to "minimally severe". My symptoms of shortness of breath, marked exercise intolerance and ankle swelling, he described as "Minimal non-disabling symptoms". "Non-disabling" to a doctor, I had to surmise, means a patient is not confined to bed or house. The fact that one can't climb hills or stairs, hike, swim, play tennis or cycle as one used to do without SOB or even take long walks or other milder forms of exercise without fatigue is insignificant.

This prominent specialist said he saw no sign of IE or deterioration of the mitral valve. But, logically, there are no signs of IE once that infection is under control. The increase in prolapse and regurgitation in a short space of time are, per se, the signs that an infection has taken place but this cannot be known without a continuous medical history which I no longer had. However, if doctors hold the view that any change in a prolapse murmur is completely harmless, then they will not find any evidence of IE. According to his letter, the echocardiogram showed "pansystolic sagging" which is synonymous with the "pansystolic prolapse" that was documented on February 26, 1980 on echocardiogram and which had contrasted sharply with the previous year's "trivial end-systolic prolapse" and LSM which were documented prior to the onset of illness.

In his letter, the American doctor questioned the accuracy of the echocardiogram in demonstrating regurgitation. But studies have shown that the degree of prolapse on echo correlates with the length of the murmur heard on auscultation. It is widely believed among doctors that a PSM heard on auscultation signifies severe regurgitation with only a few notable exceptions according to O'Rourke and Crawford in 1976[20] and repeated in 1984 by Cheitlin and Byrd.[21] Since a PSM correlates with PSP (pansystolic prolapse) on echo, it, therefore, follows that echo, by showing the degree of prolapse, can indirectly show the amount of regurgitation. It is now at the time of this writing, of course, fully accepted that the echocardiogram can measure the amount of regurgitation and with more advanced Doppler technology even show it in colour.

This correlation was proven in the studies done by Dillon and co-workers at The Indiana University School of Medicine as early as 1971.[22] It was observed that when prolapse of the mitral leaflets occurred at or near the beginning of systole, the murmur heard on the phonocardiogram was correspondingly longer. Regurgitation was simultaneously shown by cineangiography. When there was no prolapse on echo, there was no sound of a murmur either by auscultation or phonocardiography and no visual evidence of regurgitation by cineangiography.. These researchers used certain pharmacological tests as well. Their patients inhaled amyl nitrite, a substance that decreases the volume of blood in the left ventricle, increases its contractile force and moves the click and murmur earlier in systole. The anterior and posterior valve leaflets then separated earlier in systole and the separation lasted longer as did the murmur heard on phonocardiogram. Since the leaflets allow the reverse flow of blood earlier, it then seems logical that more blood is being shunted back into the atrium. Later studies prove that this is exactly what is happening.

Dr. Robert Jeresaty's paper published in 1971, "The Syndrome Associated with Mid-Systolic Click and/or Late Systolic Murmur", confirming the studies by Dillon et al, showed by angiocardiography that this longer, louder murmur, the pansystolic murmur, which begins earlier in systole and coincides with early separation of the mitral valve leaflets, indicates more severe mitral insufficiency. He said, "Of some interest were five patients with no click, but with a pansystolic murmur, louder in late systole and mitral regurgitation on cineangiography. The insufficiency through the ballooning mitral valve was more severe and the murmur was louder in these patients than in the others in this series. We postulate that, as the ballooning increases, mitral insufficiency occurs throughout systole and the click may become masked by the loud pansystolic murmur."[23]

In fact, this is exactly what was found in my case. In his letter, the American doctor said, "I heard a ? late systolic click which was not recorded by phonocardiography and may have been "buried" by the recorded murmur." As further proof that my mitral regurgitation had increased in severity, he heard a (PSM) in the reclining position when I lay on my left side, as well as in the upright position. Dr. Austin had heard, prior to my infection, an intermittent late systolic murmur. Only three months prior to seeing this American doctor, Dr. Cofman in his letter to Dr. Cory had said he had heard a PSM in only the upright position. It seems that his hearing was impaired by his anger. Otherwise, it could only be said that my murmur had further deteriorated in the three months to become a PSM in the resting position.

The import of this letter was that I had a common garden variety of heart disease, MVP, and that I was exaggerating my past illness and my present symptoms which were referred to as "non-disabling". It seemed, too, that doubt was cast upon my report of the cardiac enlargement because I did not have the x-rays. The doctor wrote, "Unfortunately, the films were not sent to me. They had been requested." I had carefully explained why I could not bring the films. It seemed that my testimony of their disappearance was inadequate, and the implication was that they existed and were simply not procured because they would disprove my story. And, without these documents, this specialist said he could not render an opinion as to the "validity" of the change in heart size just as Cofman had said. The missing films were thus crucial. Without them, doctors claimed that my past events, such as the cardiac enlargement, were possibly fictional and my entire illness in their opinion questionable. "I have no explanation for the transient increase in heart size that was reported two years ago," this American doctor said. "It is possible that this was a spurious finding." In other words, he is saying that possibly this aspect of the patient's history may be a technical error as in the angle of the x-ray or a radiologist's misinterpretation.

The final recommendation to Dr. Cory was that some kind of counselling might be necessary if I continued to be concerned, i.e. continued my investigation. "I have tried to reassure this patient as much as possible. If she persists in her unwarranted concern about her cardiac condition, it would be helpful to obtain some kind of counselling." I can only infer that this means psychiatric counselling. Such a statement echoes Dr. Austin's "labile mentality" and "pathological anxiety". And, of course, many times after this visit, we thought of Dr. Austin's conversation with my friend about my visit to the United States and just what the repercussions might have been. It seemed that the red herring of cardiac neurosis would divert the attention of the doctors I saw away from the real problems of MVP, or perhaps the workings of the conspiracy of silence, operative in both Canada and the U.S. and probably in every country where malpractice is deemed a threat, could even lead a doctor to deny the opinions he had expressed in his own published writings. Why else would this American doctor who had written that the pansystolic murmur meant moderate to severe mitral regurgitation write to my GP that it meant minimal mitral regurgitation in my case?

After this visit, we were back at square one with no hope of periodic follow-up of my heart. There was, still, however, Dr. P. Austin recommended by the local medical association. In view of the difficulties I had experienced in acquiring ongoing care, he represented literally a last resort. When I did see him in October of 1981, his diagnosis was so astonishing as to arouse our immediate suspicion of a "snow job". Contrary to the opinions of every doctor I had seen, Peter Austin claimed that I did not have MVP!

A cardiologist's job is to listen to heart sounds, all day long in fact. Very shortly in his career, he would have listened to thousands of hearts. How could this doctor have expressed such confusion over what he heard in my heart? The murmur he heard, he said, was a functional, systolic ejection flow murmur that was not due to mitral regurgitation. Presumably he meant by this the so-called "innocent" systolic ejection murmur associated with ejection of blood from the ventricles which has been attributed to turbulence at the aortic root or base of the aorta and aortic valve. The sounds of murmurs for the sake of identification are described in musical terms. The "innocent" systolic ejection murmur is said to be crescendo-decrescendo in shape, quite unlike either the LSM of MVP or the PSM of MVP, or other pathologies that cause this regurgitant murmur throughout systole. The LSM is crescendo in shape and the PSM is plateau in shape or uniform in pitch.[24] Back in 1972, the specialist I had seen had said my murmur was functional, not really even a murmur, but a sound of turbulence caused by dilatation of the aortic root, a fact that had never been supported by subsequent cardiac auscultatory examinations or by x-rays. What this opinion seems to suggest is that doctors, like Peter Austin, are still confusing the murmur of MVP, whether LS or PS, with this kind of ejection murmur. Here was a specialist in a big hospital in a sophisticated city like Toronto in the eighties making the same mistake as a doctor ten years ago!

But was this cardiologist even more confused? There are other kinds of ejection murmurs that are distinguished from the innocent kind described above. These are distinctly pathological. They begin in mid-systole, as the LSM of MVP does, and are related, not to the mitral valve, but to abnormalities in either the aortic or pulmonic valves, usually stenosis or narrowing of the valves, or again to a dilatation of part of the aortic or pulmonary artery.[25] These murmurs in sound are crescendo-decrescendo or diamond in shape. They are usually regurgitant murmurs, according to the Hurst heart textbook,[26] and are definitely not innocent ejection murmurs. It can only be presumed that Peter Austin did not know the distinction between these kinds of ejection murmurs or, if he did, chose to say mine was the innocent kind not caused by regurgitation.

Peter Austin unknowingly said something else in his letter to Dr. Cory which verifies my history. He said he could not hear a click and, apparently, this was the reason he rejected a diagnosis of MVP since the click is said to be a classic sign of prolapse. In its mild forms, when a late systolic murmur is present, the click does indeed identify the MVP. However, when the murmur has deteriorated, as mine had, a moderate to severe pansystolic murmur will bury the click, the identifying sign or hallmark of MVP. This was what Dr. Austin had said at the time of my illness. Subsequently Dr. Cofman and the American doctor also said the click was buried by the long, loud pansystolic murmur and it is what is said in numerous articles. However, if a doctor does not want to make the statement that a mild prolapse has deteriorated, that a mildly regurgitant LSM has become a severely regurgitant PSM, or if he is simply unskilled in the listening techniques of auscultation, he will have to find another explanation for the sound he hears. Or perhaps Dr. Peter Austin was confused because of my rapid heart beat, which averages 90 beats per minute in the resting position. A rapid heart beat is usually found in the presence of severe regurgitation and can make it difficult for a physician, especially an unskilled or careless one, to identify what he is hearing.

If I had read nothing about MVP and other murmurs, I would have been in a hopeless quandary after this diagnosis. First of all, it is baffling that a cardiologist would say that the murmur he heard was non-regurgitant. Such a conclusion clearly gave the impression, for the medical record, that my condition had either improved since the dental infection or that I never had, at any time, a murmur that predisposed me to the risk of IE and, therefore, my story of having had IE, cardiac enlargement and all the other signs, was fictional. Furthermore, once again, Peter Austin's conclusion smelled of the red herring of neurosis. He was ultimately saying that I had nothing the matter with me at that time, and, therefore, my continued questioning of my past events and my complaints of related symptoms were evidence of a cardiac neurosis.

Were these opinions of Peter Austin, therefore, error or a manifestation of the workings of the conspiracy of silence in order to suppress my investigations? There were other curious opinions expressed by him. Still uncertain about what he was hearing, he said that he would do tests to rule out IHSS (idiopathic hypertrophic subaortic stenosis), an altogether different heart disease. This was the differential diagnosis Dr. Austin had once made in his first letter to Dr. Cory. At that time, in 1976, Austin had also said my murmur was not regurgitant, likely because he simply did not know or believe that the LSM of MVP was a regurgitant murmur or he simply interpreted it as "innocent" as it had been erroneously regarded for over one hundred years. Furthermore, Austin, like Peter Austin, said he would do additional tests to rule out IHSS. Curiously, this heart disease is described as a cardiomyopathy or a disease of the myocardium or muscular wall of the heart, as opposed to a valvular disease. It can be identified by the patient's history, is characterized by marked hypertrophy or enlargement of the left ventricle and can be easily recognized by electrocardiogram which Dr. Peter Austin did. It is usually also accompanied by a moderately severe murmur of mitral regurgitation.[27] Such a diagnosis was entirely incompatible with my clinical findings and history. And, once again, why would Dr. Peter Austin say the murmur of IHSS was non-regurgitant in contradiction to the opinions expressed in well known textbooks such as Hurst's?

Dr. Peter Austin's whole assessment was highly questionable. Strangely, he wrote to Dr. Cory that he had me perform the valsalva maneuver. This is a maneuver defined as a "sustained, forced expiration against a closed glottis or some other suitable external obstruction to air flow."[28] I did not perform such a maneuver or any other routine maneuvers used to uncover MVP such as squatting or lying on my left side. Dr. Peter Austin listened to my heart while I was lying flat on my back. Furthermore, he said the valsalva maneuver decreased my murmur. But it is well known that the MVP murmur increases with the valsalva maneuver just as it does with the inhalation of amyl nitrite, inspiration or standing and is reduced with squatting and recumbency.[29]

In my opinion, to create the impression that a specialist would have confusion in distinguishing MVP from other entities is to excuse diagnostic errors as inevitable. Scientific accuracy cannot be achieved. Peter Austin's argument regarding the use of antibiotic prophylaxis for MVP brought this home even more forcefully. He said "I told her that in patients with definite prolapse and good mitral regurgitation I recommend prophylactic antibiotics" but, in my case, he said "I would conclude that it is a functional or ejection flow murmur and I would not conclude that it was due to mitral regurgitation." Therefore, he did not recommend antibiotic prophylaxis for any procedures in my case and pleaded that this was "a medical decision based on the state of the art rather than a scientific decision because we do not have enough data to make firm statements in this regard." According to him, not only was my condition confusing but the medical profession was confused about the use of antibiotic protection with MVP. He was saying that, at the time of my illness and his examination, there was no uniform opinion on the use of antibiotics with MVP. With this kind of letter in my medical record, there is a defense for Austin. Peter Austin's opinion demonstrates that there are colleagues of the same professional standing as Austin's in the same locale, Toronto, who still do not accept that MVP with a murmur requires antibiotic protection. Austin's error in this matter clearly becomes a difference of opinion which other colleagues share, and his standard of medical care is equivalent, from a legal point of view, to the standard of care of his locality, and, therefore, acceptable as good practice.

After much discussion with Peter Austin in which I attempted to persuade him of the importance of antibiotic prophylaxis, he finally agreed I could have this protection but stressed that, in his opinion and that of the entire medical profession, it was unnecessary. Eventually he capitulated and said, in his letter to Dr. Cory, "I told her that in her particular case, it probably would be reasonable to do so." "Reasonable" does not mean mandatory. This suggests he is endorsing the antibiotics, not to prevent the risk of damage to my valves or death, but just for me. As he put it, "I have always made the statement to patients with mitral prolapse that they should leave my office reassured . . . I am not sure this lady was reassured . . . I hope I have helped her deal with some of her problems constructively." Translated this means that he granted the antibiotics for the same reason Dr. Austin had given me propranolol, as an "anxiolytic" medication for a patient with a cardiac neurosis. All MVP patients require is "reassurance". If they do not accept such reassurance, they are not dealing "constructively" with their benign condition; they are behaving destructively or neurotically.

This opinion expressed in 1981 is the same that I have consistently received and that others have received even now, in 1989, at the time of this writing. It was becoming manifestly obvious that doctors considered MVP a neurotic condition suitable for the psychiatrist's couch and that antibiotic protection was dispensed at the whim of the examiner. If the patient needed reassurance, then ABP with dental work was provided as a reassuring medication to calm fears. Dr. Peter Austin's efforts were designed to make me doubt that such protection would have prevented the cardiac enlargement and whatever infection it characterized. My husband and I recognized a deliberate attempt to dissuade us from criticizing Dr. Austin for his errors in not providing antibiotic protection and in not testing my blood once there were clinical signs of an infective process.

My meeting with Dr. Peter Austin closed with the astounding revelation that he did not take patients on a regular basis and, so, was unwilling to give me follow-up care. This was very peculiar because my sole reason for writing to the OMA had been to secure the name of a specialist who would give me ongoing care. We came away from this visit feeling cheated out of the help we had requested and deserved.

10

Mounting Evidence

You couldn't be too outspoken during rounds either, you couldn't call a spade
a spade and come to an agreement with each other. You couldn't even say
a patient's condition had worsened . . . Everything was discussed in
euphemisms and half-allusions, sometimes even in substitutes, or else in
a way that was in direct antithesis to the truth . . . Then they all went into
a small room and sat down round a table. The names mentioned during
the rounds now came up for discussion once again, but the general impression
of improvement and recovery that an outside listener might have gathered
during the rounds was now completely exploded and disintegrated.

Alexander Solzhenitsyn: *Cancer Ward*. (New York: Farrar, Straus
& Giroux, Inc., 1969), pp. 357, 360.

One month had passed since this confusing visit with Dr. Peter Austin. We
had driven up against an unscalable wall. We now doubted whether medical
science had answers to anything. Why after two hundred or more years of
study of the human body and thousands of books and articles was there still
so much inexactness. We had to admit defeat and carried on with our family
life much as before. I taught music and began preparing in earnest for my
Associate Degree in Piano.

The season changed, and the leaves fell from our three black walnut trees,
leaving only the hard, green fruit hanging defiantly from the barren branches.
Our friends told us we should gather the delicious black walnuts to eat, but
all our attempts, even with a hammer, failed to crack these stubborn nuts.
We read somewhere that nothing short of driving over them in a car with
chained tires would crush their incorrigible shells. Like the black walnut,
exquisite delicacy defended in its ugly, dark shells from the attack of the culinary
artist, truth escaped us, imprisoned in the mighty fortress of the medical
profession.

However, I found I did not have the physical stamina I possessed prior
to my illness, and, when I played vigorous passages of music or demanding
technical exercises, my arms tired more easily. I was generally much more
tired than I used to be and had muscle fatigue and SOB when I climbed stairs

or hills. During a routine physical examination, I asked Dr. Cory to check my spleen because I continued to have annoying upper left chest pain. To my surprise, he said my spleen was enlarged. He agreed that this seemed to be additional evidence, like the PSM and the cardiac enlargement, that I had suffered from some serious illness or still had an underlying bacterial infection that should be investigated. Researchers point out that "accidental cures" of IE, as a result of the use of oral antibiotics, happen regularly because of "our present antibiotic ambience"[1], the tendency to dispense antibiotics for even minor infections without first assuring the presence of bacteria in the bloodstream. While I had been given two or three short courses of antibiotics intermittently after my periodontal surgery and when I had a visible abscess, I did not know if this were enough to eradicate an IE and I feared that my enlarged spleen might mean I still had a chronic SBE or a relapse of an old infection. It was disturbing that Dr. Peter Austin had recently checked my spleen and found no enlargement.

The spleen is the largest lymph organ in the body. Because it produces antibodies to assist in the fight against disease, it plays an important role in bacterial infection. Its chief function is the removal from the circulation of aged red blood cells, leukocytes and platelets at the end of their life span. The spleen literally ingests or eats cells and, by this process of phagocytosis, it gobbles up bacteria as well. In man, only a very small amount of blood, twenty ml. of red blood cells, is normally stored in the spleen. Thus, if the spleen enlarges or becomes congested with blood, the patient has some blood disorder or an infection.

"Few, if any abdominal organs can be palpated,"[2] according to the *Atlas of Medical Anatomy*. In particular, the spleen should not be palpable because it lies in a very protected position beneath the left dome of the diaphragm, the ninth and tenth as well as eleventh posterior ribs. With inspiration, the spleen descends but "should not be palpable, even with the most energetic maneuvers on the part of the doctor to lift it forward with the hand behind the ribs posteriorly, or with postural contortions on the part of the patient. If the spleen can be felt, it means either that it is three to four times larger than normal or that a normal spleen is being displaced anteriorly . . . by a retroperitoneal cyst or tumour."[3] Prior to the advent of technology and "the machine", palpation of the body had been the time-honoured diagnostic technique for identifying diseased organs by virtue of enlargement of that organ.

Splenomegaly has long been recognized as one of the major signs of IE especially in conjunction with fever, an organic heart murmur or a change in a previously existing murmur. It was strange that, since my discharge from hospital, my temperature had remained slightly elevated between 99° and 100° F. From my reading of the medical literature I knew that IE could exist up to a year and longer, and that splenomegaly, in the right context, was a sign of chronic low-grade or subacute infection.[4] Contrary to what doctors had led me to believe, patients did not necessarily die immediately as a result of inadequate treatment or no treatment at all. Prominent British researchers at St. Bartholomew's Hospital in London, England say that "Organisms of low virulence and identical in the laboratory may in one case cause valve rupture and heart failure within six to eight weeks from the onset of symptoms, whereas in another the disease is a true "endocarditis lenta" (slow) with febrile symptoms often for over a year, without embolism or progressive valve damage and with a good response to treatment."[5]

Dr. Cory and I discussed the possibility of IE. Although the one blood test he ordered was, as I suspected, negative, he believed that further investigation was required. But to whom did I turn? Both Rhodes and Warren considered Austin either a respected colleague or friend. Warren was aware of my complications but had scoffed at the idea of IE and had refused to look at Dr. Austin's records. As well, he doubted the past cardiac enlargement. Cofman had thrown me out because I dared to criticize my past treatment. And Peter Austin claimed I didn't have MVP and, only one month ago, had said my spleen was not enlarged. Furthermore, he did not take new patients. Rhodes, it would appear, was the only one who knew nothing of my complications and the possibility of IE since I had not seen him since 1978. I, therefore, chose to see him.

It was approximately three and a half years since my first visit. I told Rhodes only the bare essentials of the past complications and the appearance of new symptoms, swelling of my ankles and abdomen, shortness of breath and the enlarged spleen which Dr. Cory felt should be investigated. Dr. Rhodes showed no surprise, interest, nor annoyance. It was as if he had heard it all before. He listened to my heart and checked my spleen. He made no comment on the change in my murmur, and, to our astonishment, denied that the spleen was enlarged. He then dismissed me with the reassurance that my condition had not changed. In fact, he wrote Dr. Cory immmediately to say that I had a LSM, little mitral regurgitation and that I was no worse than in 1978, contrary to the opinions of Austin himself, Cofman, the American doctor and Dr. Cory who had once reluctantly agreed that he, too, heard a PSM and that this change, which he recorded in his records, meant my condition had deteriorated.

The question that disturbed us most was why a general physician could feel the spleen and a specialist could not? A cul de sac was opening up before me. A call to Warren revealed he was on holiday. His associate, Dr. Tatler, agreed to see me, and, without hesitation. I filled him in on my past complications and he agreed with Cory that my spleen was enlarged. He immediately hospitalized me in order to rule out IE. Both Tatler and Warren were at TMH. Both cardiologists were on staff with Dr. Austin at the same university. Dr. Mentlik, the periodontist whom I was suing, also taught at that institution and was on staff at TMH. It was not a situation made comfortable by anonymity.

While in hospital at TMH, at my initial bedside visit, four doctors — an internist, a resident in cardiology, an immunologist and Tatler — confirmed the splenomegaly by palpation. An intern disagreed. A liver-spleen scan was done. This scan involves the injection of a radioactive isotope which emits radiation, beta or gamma rays. The reticuloendothelial cells of the spleen trap this substance. Detectors scan that area of the body, picking up the number of gamma or beta particles and transforming them into a visual image, made up of spots or dots, on a video screen. A permanent photograph is made of these images. If there is a tumor or cyst in the organ, more or fewer particles of the radioactive tracer accumulate in that spot than in surrounding tissues and the resultant dot image is brighter or dimmer. Scans of this nature are primarily used to detect such growths or the amount of blood in the organ. Thus they can determine enlargement associated with vascular congestion, the rate that liquids pass through the organ and any changes over a period of time.[6]

However, there are dangers in nuclear scanning as in any test that involves radiation. The organ being investigated is particularly sensitive to absorption of this radiated substance. Though the long term effects of ultrasound are not known, it would seem safer because radiation is not involved and doctors, whom I later spoke to, prefer it for another important reason. The margin for error is less.

The machine, supposedly more sensitive than human touch, triumphed! The scan showed no enlargement and was negative in every other respect even though six doctors had unmistakably felt the spleen, one of the "most protected of the body organs".[7] How did these doctors explain this curious event? Because I was so thin, Tatler said, the doctors had actually been feeling my left kidney which was congenitally displaced lower than the right. I had too little knowledge to protest.

I raised some other issues. In the matter of the cardiomegaly I asked if Dr. Tatler had compared his x-ray of my heart with Dr. Warren's of September 1980. Tatler replied emphatically that this was not necessary because my heart was now a normal size. The argument of the "tiny, normal" heart of 1978 did not interest him. He was bent on convincing me, once and for all, that I had not suffered from IE in the past, that I had not suffered any illness that affected my heart. IE was extremely rare, he said, and MVP was "benign". Half the patients he saw, he declared, have MVP. I addressed the issue of the documented change in my murmur. His explanation only confused me. Prolapse was a "dynamic thing", he claimed, that was changing constantly. One minute or one day it might be late systolic, the next completely pansystolic. Though his echo showed pansystolic prolapse, Tatler said that had nothing to do with how much prolapse there actually was or the amount of regurgitation. He was invincible, and I had the impression I would never be able to find a doctor in the city of Toronto who would contradict him no matter how unsound his explanation.

The intern who had disagreed with the splenomegaly prepared my discharge summary from the other doctors' notes and his own. It was full of inaccuracies from beginning to end. Two isolated, impressive episodes of rapid heart beat in 1976 became four to five episodes of palpitations a month in that year. While I described the heavy labour I was engaged in, this fact was not mentioned. No description was given of the cardiac enlargement, the rapid heart beat associated with it, nor of any of the other symptoms I had during my illness. One click became "multiple clicks" which had never been recorded by anyone. This same intern had also noted "a soft, palpable thyroid", but there was no indication that there was any problem with my thyroid at that time nor subsequently after my discharge according to numerous tests. To top it all off, he reported that I had used antibiotics during the many dental manipulations, not after them.

However, certain laboratory results that could have pointed to a lingering, chronic IE or a past infection were totally overlooked. The internist had noted swollen cervical nodes. My haemoglobin was low normal; platelets were lowered; neutrophils were on the upper limits of normal and rheumatoid factor (RF), an auto-antibody that attacks one's own antibodies, was slightly elevated. Later, I would learn that infectious disease experts such as Brunson and Gall claim that "The factor (i.e. RF) is present in about seventy-five percent of patients with well-established disease."[8] An elevated RF, though found classically in rheumatoid arthritis, is also found in the so-called auto-immune diseases. In particular, it is "found in the serum of the majority of patients with SBE (subacute bacterial endocarditis) most of whom lack joint disease," that is rheumatoid arthritis, and it is evidence of "prolonged duration" of infective endocarditis.[9] I had no clinical evidence of rheumatoid arthritis at that time, nor later, according to subsequent tests. These modest abnormalities were, however, totally ignored by all the doctors at TMH. And, once again, there was the, by now very familiar, accusation of cardiac neurosis in the intern's repeated references to my "anxiousness". Like the psychiatric patients I described, to ask questions means one is anxious and obsessed with one's health and, therefore, psychologically unstable.

Because I preferred to forget everything after my discharge, I did not see Dr. Cory until about three months later, when, to my acute distress, he insisted my spleen was enlarged and that a kidney could not be mistaken for the spleen. In the *Atlas of Medical Anatomy*, the kidneys are described as "deeply placed against the posterior abdominal wall. The right kidney, situated somewhat lower than the left, can sometimes be palpated between two hands during deep inspiration."[10] But, even then, the authors say, there is a special technique for palpating the "right" kidney. One hand is placed on the back and must push a particular muscle, the quadratus lumborum, forward while the other hand is placed on the anterior abdominal wall below the tenth rib. The mass in question was felt on the left side of my body, and no such examination, as Langman and Woerderman describe, was ever attempted on me.

I became more convinced that the splenomegaly was the sign of a previous infection when I saw a letter from the internist, Dr. Hall, who had examined me at my bedside. The letter had been sent to Tatler with a copy to Dr. Cory. Dr. Hall favored the human diagnosis over the machine and stated that the splenomegaly could be a "hold over from a previous infection". However, Dr. Hall's notes were not meant for my eyes. He said he would follow this up if Dr. Tatler was in agreement. Obviously the cardiologist was not since no further investigation was done during my hospitalization.

According to writers who specialize in immunology, "slight splenomegaly persists for several years after a straightforward attack of glandular fever" and does not revert completely in cases of hemolytic anemia even after cure.[11] Why, then, could it not remain enlarged for some time after IE?

The big question now was what was Dr. Cory going to do? He was in a quandary because he did not know where to send me since he believed I required further investigation. My husband and I, of course, were very upset. The spectre of the self-interest and protectionism of many members of the medical profession troubled us. Patients, it seemed, could be pawns sacrificed in the closure of the powerful protective ring around a doctor who had erred. Dr. Cory, who knew about my attempted litigation against the dentists, agreed that my complaints were likely the reason why four Toronto hospitals had "ganged up on me" as he put it. But he did not want to get involved and steadfastly refused to criticize his colleagues.

There was only one doctor I could possibly turn to. After my discharge from TMH, my lawyer had given me the name of a Dr. Cabot, an internist, in another city because I had not been able to find medical care in Toronto. Also it had become evident to my lawyer that Dr. Austin was as responsible for the deterioration in my health as the dentists. Dr. Cabot was my lawyer's idea of an "expert medical witness" if I should decide on pursuing malpractice litigation against either Dr. Austin or the dentists.

On my first visit to Dr. Cabot, I had recounted my dental and medical history in the belief that he frequently "rented himself out" as an expert medical witness. I laid specific emphasis on the negligence of Dr. Austin and the dentists. But, gradually, during our conversation, it had become clear to us that my lawyer had never contacted Dr. Cabot and that he knew absolutely nothing about my case. Nor had he ever testified in a malpractice suit, and, in his subsequent letter to me, he indicated unequivocally his unwillingness to assist me in any way with a legal suit against his colleagues.

Because I had told Dr. Cabot everything and had criticized my past care, I felt uneasy about recontacting him. However, he found my spleen enlarged and immediately hospitalized me in April of 1982. This hospitalization caused me anxiety primarily because I believed the investigation would not bring me any further information and that no cause would be found, certainly not that of an active chronic infection, since I did not feel as unwell as I had during the dental manipulations. By now, I suspected, too, that no doctor would admit, in the event that there was no active infection, that the splenomegaly must then be evidence of a previous IE. Such an admission would be equivalent to accusing Dr. Austin of negligence in having missed such an infection in the first place.

Dr. Cabot felt that I had signs of chronic, active infection, in particular in the slight temperature elevation and the clubbing of my fingernails which is a classic sign of IE. Dr. Cabot explained that in "clubbing", the nails are rounded and bulging with loss of the normal nail angle and softness or sponginess, a sort of edema, around the nail bed. From his examination of me, he said, he would have to rule out causes other than IE for this clubbing. But what would come of his suspicion?

The highlight of my hospitalization was the quicky "courtesy call" from the cardiologist, Dr. Adami, who was in the midst of preparations for his holiday but would, I was told, generously squeeze me into his busy timetable. In keeping with current Canadian attitudes to MVP, I was never quite regarded as a cardiac patient. In fact, I had to ask to see the cardiologist. But, in reality, the visit turned out to be a psychiatric session, and the infectious disease investigation became nothing more than background music. His visit went a long way towards establishing that, in Canada, the heart of an MVP patient requires little or no attention.

Dr. Adami hurried into my room, telling me at the outset that he had little time since he was leaving the city soon. He began by examining my heart. It was noteworthy that he did not put me through the various postures associated with an MVP examination to uncover the click. Dr. Cabot had told me he heard a loud PSM in all the positions and that he could no longer hear the first heart sound. In the presence of a loud pansystolic murmur, the click is rarely heard. My husband and I viewed Cabot's findings as evidence that something had gone wrong.

Afterwards, Dr. Adami, who had seemed in such a hurry, sat in the chair by my bed, crossed his legs, pyramided his fingers and waited quietly for something. I was reminded faintly of other doctors I had seen, particularly Austin and Cofman. When I said nothing, he handed down the five line description of MVP which others had given, describing my MVP as I had heard it described on numerous other occasions before any complications. His voice was calm, measured and velvety, and I longed to feel as comfortable, as confident, that nothing had gone wrong.

Dr. Adami was familiar with my history, including Austin's absurd psychiatric evaluation in which the significant facts were embedded. What I didn't realize at first was that he was gearing up for a discussion not of my heart but of my head. When he was finished his description, I feared that any question I would have, in the face of such a positive diagnosis, could only be regarded as evidence of anxiety and would likely contribute to a diagnosis of neurotic behaviour. Neverthless, I felt compelled to ask.

"What about the loud pansystolic murmur which Dr. Cabot says he can hear when I lie flat on my back? He also said he can't hear the first heart sound."

"That's true. You have a long systolic murmur." He was silent, and it was obvious he would add nothing further.

"But," I protested, "I had a brief, intermittent late systolic murmur before the abscessed tooth."

Dr. Adami registered some surprise and discomfort at my familiarity with his private language. But, very soon, I was forced to make the same realization

I had made many times before. Dr. Adami was not going to comment on the past. A perfect analogy might be that of a woman who goes into hospital to have some varicose veins removed and wakes up from the anesthetic to find her leg is amputated. She goes to another doctor to find out what went wrong. Her records mysteriously disappear. She goes to another and another doctor, but the conspiracy of silence makes them all say they didn't examine her in the past. They don't know that she had varicose veins. She could have had cancer. They don't even know if she had two legs because they didn't see her before the operation. It does not matter that she shows them a picture of herself with two legs before the operation. Perhaps the angle of the camera was incorrect, and a double exposure resulted. Dr. Adami, using this unassailable defense, maintained he did not know whether or not I had a pansystolic murmur before my infection even though he had seen the letters in my file which clearly documented a LSM.

"It doesn't matter," he insisted in liquid tones, "you have a mitral valve prolapse murmur and it is a completely benign murmur." His voice became whispery, caressing, as though he were trying to subdue an hysterical patient while the orderlies attempt to put on the straightjacket. "There's really nothing wrong with a prolapsed valve."

"But all degrees of prolapse and of murmur are not the same," I protested, feeling overwhelmed by his inflexible attitude. "If the murmur changes from late systolic to pansystolic, something has happened to cause this deterioration."

"That is not deterioration," he said in hard tones as he flexed his pyramided fingers indifferently.

I was exasperated, and a sick feeling settled in the pit of my stomach. "Have you read Dr. Robert Jeresaty's book on MVP?" I asked, trying to remain calm.

"No," he replied flatly with no interest whatsoever.

"Dr. Jeresaty says unequivocally that a sudden change from a LSM to a PSM is caused by IE or spontaneous chordal rupture without IE. My echo didn't show chordal rupture." Dr. Adami said nothing. I went on. "Do you agree then that I had IE that could have healed spontaneously or with all the oral antibiotics that I was given after there were signs of an aveolar abscess and that, as a result, I now have a pansystolic murmur with more severe regurgitation, ankle edema, which Dr. Cabot has noted, shortness of breath with exercise as well as left-over signs of clubbing and splenomegaly?"

"My dear," he insisted firmly, "there is no such thing as spontaneously healed endocarditis and oral antibiotics are totally ineffective. You must have a long six week course of intravenous antibiotics."

"But that's not true!" I exclaimed beside myself. "What about all the references to spontaneously healed IE in the medical literature especially those of Emanuel Libman! Many patients have had an IE which their doctors overlooked. They went on to heart or renal failure and died anywhere up to ten or more years later."

I was angry at this denial of medical evidence, of all the work of past researchers, and, subconsciously, I resented the use of the belittling term, "my dear". If I had been a man, I would have escaped this patronizing form of address. "You would have been dead by now if you had had bacterial endocarditis," Dr. Adami uttered with enormous conviction. "Your chances of getting it are extremely slight. It is a very rare disease and the chances of an MVP patient contracting it are almost negligible." These last words he seemed to bite out with a machete-like chop.

The mistaken opinion of Dr. Adami and of other doctors I had seen was that IE is immediately and uniformly fatal unless intravenous antibiotics are promptly instituted. Or, they expect such a patient to be in acute congestive heart failure. Hence, doctors would say there was "no evidence of endocarditis" or that my "splendid recovery" showed it was unlikely I had ever had the disease. To express the opposite opinion would be tantamount to saying that Dr. Austin had been negligent.

Contrary to the opinion of these doctors, spontaneous cures of IE date back to the turn of the century, long before the introduction of antibiotics. Therefore, it should not be surprising that IE could be controlled or eradicated with oral antibiotics. In the first fifty years of the 20thC, Emanuel Libman published numerous articles which offered convincing evidence of spontaneous cures of IE. Libman manifested exceptional dedication, persistence and a remarkable facility for making penetrating, original observations overlooked by less astute colleagues. His contemporaries showed great respect for his judgement. Louis Hamman said of him, "first being especially interested and experienced in the diagnosis of bacterial endocarditis he recognizes many mild cases which would escape the notice of average observers. Second, he is more indefatigable in the search for bacteria in the blood stream. Third, his technical resources are superior to those of the average laboratory."[12]

Libman's investigations of IE are extremely valuable because they spanned both the pre and antibiotic eras. Contrary to the opinions of modern doctors, like Adami and Warren, on the rarity of the disease, Libman, who had observed hundreds of cases of the disease throughout his long career, said that physicians must discard the notion that IE is an unusual disease and that the prognosis is uniformly hopeless. "The cases became so numerous," he lamented, "that not all could be accurately followed up for a proper length of time."[13] Of most interest to me were the "mild cases" Libman described. Adami and other doctors had insisted that IE would be so violent an infection that a doctor could not overlook it. In describing these mild infections, Libman said,

> It is curious . . . there should exist so many cases which must have had a bacterial infection, have recovered from the infection and have certain clinical pictures from the changes brought about during the infective period. We must assume that in these cases the period of bacterial infection was very short as compared to the cases which we see with bacteria in the blood or very short and very mild. When one sees cases of the disease with bacteria demonstrable in the blood go about for weeks with hardly any symptoms, it is not difficult to believe that some patients with a mild or short infection

may not feel sick enough to ask for medical attention or present such mild clinical pictures that they are not put to bed.[14]

From these mild cases, Libman made some remarkable observations and conclusions. He estimated that, in about twenty to twenty-five percent of the cases in the pre-antibiotic era, the patient lost the infection spontaneously, but true recovery, without damage to heart or valves, he found to be rare. It occurred in only about three percent of cases.[15] Positive blood cultures confirmed the infection which often dragged on for as much as eighteen months. Of the rare cases of complete cure, Libman said, "It is of interest to note that these patients did not even show any myocardial insufficiency beyond that which had been present before the infection."[16] This means that the infection had not changed the murmur.

In the majority of these mild cases, the patients, whose initial, acute infection had spontaneously disappeared, passed into what Libman called the "bacteria free" (healing or healed) stage when blood cultures were negative and "residua or sequelae", that is damage, from the previous infection were "clinically manifest",[17] that is a deterioration in the patient's murmur. Almost all such patients eventually succumbed, sometimes even years later, to congestive heart failure (CHF) resulting from further damage to their heart and its valves and/or renal failure from the effects of lesions in the kidneys. Libman proved, at autopsy, that the hearts and valves in these cases showed characteristic signs of endocarditis lesions, the small lesions representing the milder infection. Mild attacks were often followed by one or more attacks with ultimate death from increasing valvular damage. Frequently, Libman stressed, recurrence might be mistaken for a first acute attack but, at autopsy, lesions in all stages of healing, some completely healed, were found alongside fresh vegetations from the current acute infection.[18] The longer the patient survived in this stage of negative blood cultures, the greater the healing and thus the fewer bacteria, found in the vegetations at death.

Of great interest to me was the fact that many of these patients retained clinical signs of their former infection for some time after. These signs were clubbing, splenomegaly, elevated temperatures, slight proteinuria, joint pains and sternal tenderness.[19] During my infection, I had many of these clinical signs, and my sternum or breast bone was tender to the touch. Libman described the case of a tailor who did not see a doctor during his acute infection. This man observed that his fingers became progressively clubbed over several months, but, as the infection receded, the clubbing began to regress. An autopsy proved the existence of his longstanding endocarditis in the lesions that still contained bacteria.[20] Libman, like modern researchers, observed that splenomegaly existed for several years after such an infection. In one case, the patient's spleen decreased in size over a period of three years to become, as in my case, "just palpable".[21]

Libman's contemporaries, Horder, Weiss, Hamman, Friedberg, who co-authored a book on IE with Libman in 1941, and the famous Canadian, Sir

William Osler, all made the same observations and came to the same conclusions. In 1885, on the occasion of his Galstonian lectures, Osler described chronic cases like those of Libman that were prolonged over periods of a year or more with intermittent low grade fever.[22] Horder remarked in 1909 on the duration of many of the subacute cases, six to eighteen months and even two to three years.[23] And Hamman, writing in 1937, confirmed the frequency of cases of the type Libman observed of patients dying in second and third attacks after having recovered from the first which had gone undetected by the physician.[24]

His contemporaries regarded Libman as a giant in IE research. Hamman writes, "I must admit that Libman's results are more in accord with evidence obtained post mortem than are the usual results of other physicians. This is strong corroboration of the truth of his observations if, indeed, any corroboration is needed for the observations of so distinguished a student in the field."[25] Hamman brought forward evidence of his own which, like Libman's, emphasized that many doctors fail to identify bacterial endocarditis in the clinic and that many of these patients recovered and lived on with the valvular defects brought about by the disease. From all the cases Hamman cites, a pattern of characteristics can be assembled, beginning with an infection related to teeth, followed by a short period of one to three years of relative stability and, then, return of symptoms with shortness of breath finally ending in overwhelming infection with cardiac and pulmonary failure.

The response of the doctors I encountered to Libman's idea that a mild IE could heal spontaneously was invariably the same: scorn or ridicule. The past had nothing to teach them. Libman diagnosed with his medical knowledge and skill; they diagnose with the aid of sophisticated, technological equipment. However, in 1952, forty years after Libman's startling observations on the healing of mild IE, *The American Journal of Medicine* chose to reprint his 1912 article. This was obvious proof of the relevancy of Libman's studies today. As well, the reprint was a warning to modern doctors that this disease can be overlooked. Very few modern papers on IE do not refer to Libman's work. Modern animal experimentation for the study of the healing process of IE, which I will refer to later, also relies on the studies of this famous researcher. For doctors truly interested in IE, Libman's studies are significant. In fact, the phenomenon of MVP has renewed interest in IE and possibly even alerted doctors to a disease that they might otherwise ignore because they believe it has been eradicated with antibiotics. No stronger proof could be had of such mild cases as Libman describes, where the patient makes no complaint of any symptoms and the doctor finds no clinical signs, than that of the tennis player whom I discussed in my introduction. Only at autopsy could this young woman's IE be proven.

From my reading of this older literature, I was convinced that I had suffered from an acute attack of IE of short duration at the time of the initial endodontal infection back in April of 1979 and that this was followed by one or more mild relapses during the prolonged dental manipulations without antibiotics or I had an ongoing subacute case. In Libman's day, I probably stood a better chance of my mild case of IE being diagnosed. However, in the eighties, even though I related my symptoms to my cardiologist and even though he found clinical signs on examination, he chose to ignore them. In essence, he refused to learn from the past. The result was that I did not benefit from years of study and the accumulation of knowledge about this disease.

I found it difficult to accept Adami's opinion or that of any other doctor that I had seen because I had read Libman's work. In it was an explanation for my present health situation. If IE could heal without treatment, then surely it could heal assisted by some oral antibiotics, though, in either case, there would be damage to the valve. His studies explained why I now had signs of what I would later discover was the beginning of heart failure just as in Libman's cases. Like his patients, I had evidence on clinical exam of a previous infection, clubbing, splenomegaly, an increase in the pre-existing valvular defect in the longer murmur and, possibly, kidney damage in the increasing urinary protein and nocturia that would take place over the next few years.

There was no assurance from this hospitalization that I was free of an underlying chronic infection, and I realized this as I attempted to discuss confusing aspects with Adami. When I introduced the issues raised by Libman's studies, Adami was scornful and outrightly rejected every suggestion I made. He would not agree that my present clinical findings were evidence of a previous infection or that they indicated a low grade, chronic active infection because my cultures were negative. But I knew that many of Libman's cases had negative blood cultures, and active IE was disclosed only at autopsy. In particular I wanted to ask him about the echocardiographic results that confirmed a change in the appearance of my mitral valve, thus pointing to healed or healing vegetations. Before my dental infection, the radiologist's report from the TCI showed no evidence of prolapse and TMSC's report showed "trivial end systolic prolapse". Such descriptions correlated logically with the minimal regurgitation of a late systolic murmur recorded by both Rhodes and Austin at that time.

After the infection, Warren had said my echo showed "thickening" of the mitral valve but he did not consider this as a sign of a previous IE. Five subsequent echocardiographic reports from RGH, TMH, the American hospital and this hospital where I now was, as well as TMSC, had shown pansystolic prolapse. This was a point of great significance to me. I knew that pansystolic prolapse (PSP), unlike late systolic prolapse (LSP), could not be considered typical of MVP because research showed it corresponded with pansystolic regurgitation, or regurgitation, usually obliterating the first sound as in my case, throughout the whole of systole, regardless of the underlying condition. In his book, Jeresaty explains that only the mid-systolic dipping or buckling seen on echo should be considered specific for LSP and, thus, MVP because "a pansystolic sagging can be encountered not only in idiopathic MVP but also in ruptured chordae tendinae resulting from endocarditis and cannot be used, therefore, as a means of identifying MVP."[26]

The definitive studies of Shah and Gramiak in 1970[27] firmly established the correlation, still indisputable at the time of this writing, between echocardiographic and auscultatory signs of MVP. Late or midsystolic prolapse, with its appropriate sign on echo, was associated with the auscultatory finding of midsystolic click and LSM, and a pansystolic prolapse correlated with a PSM whatever the cause. Thus my radiologist reports provided classic evidence that the pathology of my mitral valve had changed and correlated with the PSM which all doctors now heard on auscultation. Unfortunately, only Dr. Austin had listened to my heart at the time of my illness and heard the change in my murmur. Even if Austin had been telling the truth that my cardiomegaly had vanished, the PSP on echo was proof that the effects of the infection on the mitral valve were permanent since subsequent echoes did not show a return to a LSP and subsequent auscultatory examinations did not show a return to a LSM.

The appearance of "thickened" valves on my echo seemed to suggest IE. Dr. Adami's opinion, however, was that all prolapsed valves looked "thickened" on echo because they gave off more echoes than a normal valve. The thickening, he claimed, meant that there were multiple surface areas to give off echoes because of the bulging and ballooning of the valve. Pansystolic prolapse, he declared, simply meant my valve was giving off more echoes than most prolapsed valves. He insisted this was not a sign of more severe prolapse but of more extensive myxomatous degeneration. Of course, they are one and the same thing, that the more extensive the myxomatous degeneration, the more extensive the prolapse. But Dr. Adami could not see his own contradiction. He insisted that my past echocardiograms done at the time of my infection would have unequivocally shown vegetations that could not have been missed by either radiologist or cardiologist and that the present echocardiogram showed no sign of endocarditis. What I would never know was whether or not there had ever been evidence of vegetations on that TMSC echo that had so mysteriously disappeared.

"The prolapse is minimal," he announced at the end of his dissertation on echocardiographic signs.

The prolapse was minimal but the myxomatous degeneration was severe. Logic was useless when dealing with such a powerful person. But, I persisted fruitlessly, "Why couldn't this thickening of the valve and the increased echoes be signs of healed vegetations?"

"No," he repeated categorically, "they are signs of myxomatous degeneration."

When I insisted my previous echoes showed minimal or no prolapse which meant, according to his explanation, less surface area for sound to bounce off and that the PSP now meant more reflecting surfaces, he changed his story and said that all prolapsed valves looked like mine on echo.

Was Dr. Adami correct in his assertions? There is much evidence to suggest that he was not. At the time of my hospitalization, the echocardiogram had, and still does have at the time of this writing, serious limitations as a diagnostic tool. In 1973, a group of doctors from the Indiana University School of Medicine and the Krannert Institute of Cardiology in Indianapolis published the results of the first study of the echocardiographic visualization of the valvular vegetations of IE.[28] These doctors established the criteria for the interpretation of the echocardiographic pictures that represent vegetations. Normal valves without vegetations give off echoes that are "sharp and free of any thickening or shaggy echoes attached to the valves." However, these researchers found that valves with vegetations manifest "a non-uniform thickening in several areas of the valve" and that "in many areas the thickened valve has a shaggy appearance". The vegetations, however, appeared not to interfere with the movement of the valve. Most importantly, the location of the echocardiographic abnormalities correlated with the location of the vegetations at autopsy or surgery and clearly verified that what was seen on echo was, indeed, a foreign presence. Though the adjective, "fluffy", might replace "shaggy" in these interpretations, a fact which only points to the subjective nature of the descriptions, the criteria remained essentially the same at the time of my hospitalization and at the time of this writing and has remained the same in spite of improvements in the the equipment and techniques with the introduction of two-dimensional (2D) echocardiography which provides spatial information and a more accurate depiction of actual cardiac structures.[29]

In 1976, the same group of researchers from Indiana reported on the difficulties of identifying the vegetations of IE by means of echocardiography. Of 65 patients in their study who had clinically proven IE, vegetations were visualized on echo in only 22 or 34 percent. The remaining 43 or 66 percent of their patients had conclusive clinical and laboratory evidence of IE. The authors concluded that "Echocardiography therefore does not appear to be a sensitive method of detecting vegetations."[30]

Other studies confirmed the work of this group. A 1980 report from Duke University in North Carolina revealed that valvular vegetations were detected in only 54 percent of their patients with clinical and laboratory confirmation of IE, even with supposedly superior 2D echocardiography which is now uniformly used in 1989. A negative echocardiogram does not, therefore, rule out IE. Such observations led these doctors to warn that "decisions regarding clinical management (of patients with suspected IE) made solely on the basis of the presence or absence of vegetative lesions on echo are hazardous. Management of such patients must continue to be based on the clinical integration of multiple factors."[31]

In patients with MVP, the diagnosis of IE by echocardiography is even more difficult because the "machine" cannot distinguish between echoes from vegetations and echoes from myxomatous degeneration of the mitral valve. The same Indiana group that established the criteria for interpreting vegetations found that, in MVP patients with myxomatous degeneration of the mitral valve, "the appearance of the valve was different from those with vegetations in that the thickening was fairly uniform and the echoes did not appear shaggy." However, these writers warned, all patients with vegetations from IE do not have "shaggy" echoes and, hence, confusion arises.[32] After three years of further study of this subject, these researchers reached an even stronger conclusion on the insensitivity of echo. They found that one of their patients, who did not have IE, had "myxomatous degeneration . . . virtually indistinguishable by echo alone from bacterial vegetations."[33] Other workers, this group pointed out, have made the same observation in a patient with myxomatous degeneration of the aortic valve.

Other serious limitations of the echocardiogram in diagnosing IE were discovered by Chandraratna and Langevin from The University of Oklahoma Health Sciences Center in Oklahoma. They found that 40 percent of their MVP patients had "thick, shaggy echoes on the mitral leaflets which closely resembled those seen with valvular vegetations."[34] However, only one of their patients had bacterial endocarditis. The reverse could, therefore, be true in my case; the echoes of IE could have been mistaken for the echoes of myxomatous degeneration by TMSC's radiologist especially if he had not been asked by an unsuspecting doctor to look for the vegetations of IE. In considering all this, we have to remember that prolapsed valves deteriorate very slowly, over many years, and that rapid changes, as seen in my valve, pointed almost certainly to IE.

At the time of my hospitalization in April of 1982, many American researchers were pointing out the pitfalls even with the use of the superior 2D echo in confirming the presence of vegetations in MVP patients. At Stanford University School of Medicine in California, Martin, Meltzer and co-workers declared that "the studies of patients with mitral valve prolapse or myxomatous degeneration of the mitral leaflet, or both, may show excessive leaflet echoes uniformly distributed within the valve that may be difficult to distinguish from the "soft" echoes of vegetations."[35] The diagnosis would, therefore, depend entirely on the preference of the viewer.

Other problems were also pertinent to my case. Echocardiography, for instance, cannot distinguish between the fresh vegetations of active endocarditis and the healed ones of a "cured" infection.[36] Thus, the doctors I questioned could feel quite justified in saying that my echocardiograms, done after the infection, showed only the thickened or shaggy echoes of prolapse and not the signs of a past infection even though IE leaves the valves thickened in the same way that myxomatous degeneration does.[37] Both myxomatous degeneration and the fibrosis or calcification from the healed vegetations of IE result in an irregular, valvular surface that gives off more echoes. Furthermore, other startling studies show that there is no difference in the appearance of vegetations on echo before and after therapy. A group of researchers from the Mayo Clinic found no change in the echocardiograms of five patients before and after successful therapy.[38] Some researchers also say that the size and the intensity of the echoes actually increases after cure of the infection.[39]

According to research, the greater the valvular redundancy in prolapse, the greater the surfaces for the production of echoes. Obviously, too, valves that have less myxomatous tissue, or, in other words, minimally prolapsed valves such as mine were in the beginning, would give off less echoes. This raises the question, which I will deal with later, of whether IE per se causes the increased thickening of the valve or the accumulation of myxomatous tissue that replaces healthy tissue. Were the accentuated signs seen on my echo during this hospitalization in fact the signs of healed vegetations? It has also been noted in cases of IE that, after cure, the echoes become smaller but more reflective[40], once again strongly suggesting that my echo pictures could be showing the results of the bacterial infection of IE.

Another factor important in my case concerns the insensitivity of echocardiography in detecting valvular vegetations that are smaller than 3mm in size. This is true of both M-mode and 2D echocardiography.[41] Some researchers believe there is a direct relationship between the size of the vegetation on echo and the severity of the disease. In one study, 20 of 22 patients with detectable vegetations on echo either died or required valve replacement, but neither fate befell those with no vegetations on echo although they were proven to have the disease.[42] It could be argued, in my case, that vegetations may not have shown on my echo because they were too small. Oral antibiotics are known to reduce the size of the vegetations,[43] if they were, in fact, invisible on the February 26, 1980 echo, while they may have been present on the echo of November of 1979 at the time of my cardiac enlargement and prior to the administration of any oral antibiotics. However, recently when I was hospitalized for another bout of IE, a cardiologist, knowing nothing of my history, interpreted the thickened, shaggy echos as evidence first of fresh vegetations, then of healed lesions. Fibrotic, calcified vegetations remain on the valves for as long as sixteen years and have been observed at autopsy or surgery.[44]

Since Dr. Adami did nothing but refute medical facts in the matter of the echocardiography, I switched to the topic of the splenomegaly which was the cause of this hospitalization, but, here, his reasoning was just as foggy and misleading. "If you don't think my enlarged spleen is a leftover from a previous IE or indicative of a current low-grade, chronic infection, what do you think is causing the enlargement? Before 1979, splenomegaly had never been noted."

Dr. Adami replaced answer with cross-examination. "It was never noticed before then at any time, by anyone?" he repeated, rivetting his eyes on my face in such a manner as to shatter the falsehood he imagined secretly lurked inside me.

"I've never been told this before," I repeated. "I've had many examinations for university, for jobs . . ."

"You know," he said in his earlier velvety tones, "three percent of the population has unexplained splenomegaly from birth. I think you're one of those rare people."

"But," I countered with flagging spirits, "if I could be one of the rare individuals with unexplained, congenital enlargement of the spleen, why couldn't I have been one of the rare MVP people with IE?"

Dr. Adami smiled tightly and said, "I don't think you had endocarditis and you don't have it now."

At the time of that hospitalization, I had read very little about the spleen and, so, could not even challenge a conclusion so illogical as this. Subsequent research, after my discharge from hospital, disclosed that few authors of medical textbooks accept the idea of unexplained splenomegaly without any underlying disease. A 1980 textbook on radionuclide investigations of the spleen described a study of college freshmen in which the spleen was noted to be palpable in 2.9 percent of the students but that, by the end of a three year period, 70 percent of these spleens had become nonpalpable, which raised the question of whether these findings indicated "anatomic variants" or "disease"[45] such as mononucleosis. Of particular interest, the *Merck Manual of Diagnosis* gives no indication that such an "anatomic variant" exists without a "primary disorder" elsewhere in the body.[46]

It appeared that the more evidence pointed to a previous mild attack of IE, the more Dr. Adami vigorously denied such a possibility. Before his visit, Dr. Cabot had informed me of another abnormality in my heart. My echocardiogram showed changes in the tricuspid valve on the right side of the heart between the atrium and ventricle. The annulus or ring to which the tricuspid valve leaflets are anchored was said to be thickened. Naturally I was not expected to be upset by this finding any more than by what had happened to me in the past. To show alarm or anxiety, or even to question, would have confirmed Austin's hypothesis of "mental lability" and "pathological anxiety" in the opinion of these doctors. When I questioned Dr. Adami about this, he only offered me another superificial, unverifiable explanation designed to persuade me to accept the theory that I had never suffered IE. The tricuspid thickening, he said quickly, was an extension of the myxomatous process to the right side of the heart. Such an explanation could never be verified until surgery or autopsy. As I've already pointed out, myxomatous degeneration is an extremely slow process that increases with age. It does not happen in the short space of a year. At best the changes, if any, would be unnoticeable. This is, of course, the reason why so many prolapse patients' conditions remain unchanged for many years with nothing more than minimal regurgitation developing late in life. If Dr. Adami's opinion were correct, I should be as anxious about this underlying condition as about IE. Thoughts of the myxomatous process gobbling up my healthy heart tissue that fast were terrifying; it meant that I was aging internally at a frightening pace. On the strength of the evidence in the medical literature I had to reject his theory. I had come across few accounts of the involvement of the tricuspid valve or its annulus in the myxomatous process, and Dr. Cabot, himself, told me he doubted this theory. Also, usually the leaflets, not the annulus, are affected by the myxomatous process.

Research shows that valve ring abscesses are frequently missed on echo, especially M mode, though they are more likely to show up on 2D.[47] The nodes, which I suspect were vegetations, must have, however, been large enough to appear on echo. Although vegetations on the tricuspid valve ring may not show on echo, they have been found at surgery, even when the valve leaflets themselves, are free of vegetations.[48]

Dr. Adami's trump card in his fight to convince me nothing had happened to me in the past was startling. He denied that there was any uniform opinion in the medical literature on the use of antibiotic prophylaxis with dental manipulations! Dr. Warren and Dr. Tatler had not mentioned antibiotics with dental work. Both Cofman and Peter Austin had said it was a controversial subject. This was after Dr. Austin indicated in writing that I now required antibiotics. What were the real facts? Here, I was under supposedly serious investigation in hospital in April of 1982 and this was the kind of advice I was getting! Did the few opinions I collected, Hurst, Barlow, represent only a small, unconventional faction of the medical profession? As yet, I could not be certain. After some reflection, Adami conceded that I could use this protection, not because of medical necessity, but because of my "exaggerated" fears that I had suffered IE in the past. His opinion, he avowed, was based on the fact that endocarditis was so rare and that I had next to no chance of ever having had it or of acquiring it. He was using antibiotics as Peter Austin had and as Dr. Austin had used propranolol: as an anxiolytic medication.

From the moment Dr. Adami pronounced MVP a "benign syndrome", it was evident that he did not regard as significant or abnormal any of the complications I had endured. From the beginning of his visit, he wished to discuss my psychological health rather than my physical health and attempted several times to steer our discussion in the direction of a psychiatric investigation. His obstinate denial of all my legitimate concerns, his bizarre opposition to medical fact, left me bereft of any defense and filled me with a sense of monumental frustration.

To strip the patient of all defenses, to weaken him or her, is a genuine tactic of psychotherapy. A defenseless and, therefore, vulnerable, person is open to suggestion, to new learning and, inevitably, to the truths of others, whether they be false or not. It is a form of brainwashing. I learned subsequently that Dr. Adami was, in fact, a trained psychiatrist and had only gone into cardiology later in life. With his power and authority, he appeared determined to undermine and eradicate the knowledge I had gained from the medical literature to prevent me from further questioning of my past care.

The true nature of Dr. Adami's interview was ultimately revealed in his interrogation of my personal life. What was my family situation like? Was my relationship with my husband satisfactory? Was my sex life satisfying? What did I do with my time? What were my ambitions, my aspirations, my interests? When it came to describing my interests, writing novels and playing the piano, he pounced on these activities as highly "unconventional". It was inconceivable to him that I had given up a "lucrative" teaching career for such illusory goals. That the supply of high school English teachers had outstripped the demand was difficult for him to understand, operating as he did from the vantage point of guaranteed work that depends on the certainty of physical decay. When Dr, Adami's eyes fell on my piano scores, it was clear he believed he had caught the neurotic overachiever, redhanded. To be "studying music seriously at my age", as he put it, was "counter-productive". When I explained

I was preparing for my degree in piano, he began talking about the anxious MVP personality. In his view, I was taking on too much. He insisted on viewing my interests as prejudicial to my family and expressed considerable concern about whether or not my husband was freely supportive. His concluding advice seemed to be that I was putting undue stress upon myself, not to mention my family, and consequently, in his view, anxiety was affecting my health. It was the familiar doctor's attempt to find fault with the patient's way of life, in order to blame him or her for any illness. It seemed that anything a MVP patient did that was unusual was good evidence of neurosis. Only much later would I understand why many doctors automatically treated MVP patients as neurotic.

On the discharge notice, this psychiatrist, quasi-cardiologist, a term I might justifiably use as far as his consultation with me was concerned, offered his verdict that my head had caused my spleen to enlarge and, in the past, by inference, my heart, as well as changing my murmur, causing my fingers to club, nodules to appear on my tricuspid valve and my temperature to rise. The mind must certainly be very powerful, and I recommend that billions of dollars of research money be poured into studies on how the mind can cause an illness such as I experienced. Dr. Adami seemed to feel, the report stated, that much of the patient's "problem stemmed from her psychological reaction to these complaints," that is SOB, ankle swelling, splenomegaly, fatigue and all the events of the past. My despair, my frustration, that the truth would never be revealed and that I would never find the proper follow-up care for a MVP patient who had had genuine physical illness in the past wiped me out emotionally and spiritually.

Nothing was accomplished from this hospitalization, except that obvious abnormalities had accumulated. In addition to the thickening and nodules on the tricuspid valve, the laboratory reported urinary protein. Dr. Cabot insisted that this was normal and I simply had to accept his opinion at that time. One thing was certain. The confirmation of the splenomegaly indicated without doubt that the doctors at TMH must have misrepresented the facts or their radionuclide scan of my spleen had been done incorrectly, exposing me needlessly to radioactive materials.

Dr. Cabot forwarded Dr. Cory a copy of the Discharge Summary with instructions to him to carry on my care, checking my spleen monthly to see if it got any larger. As usual, this hospital summary was full of errors and, at times, I wondered whether I was, in fact the patient. Some errors in my medical history were disturbing such as "on January 7, 1980, the tooth was cracked". What did this mean? It implied that my tooth was functional up to this date and that someone or something had cracked it on that day when, in reality, this was the date of my periodontal surgery that resulted from the cracked tooth. Other errors were ludicrous, for instance, the statement that my cyanotic uncle had died of MVP in 1944. MVP was unheard of in that year, of course, and only emerged as a fully defined entity in the early sixties. In 1944, such a condition, whatever its name, would never have been considered as a cause of death. Nor was there any evidence that my uncle even had the same condition I had. And though the statement, "In February of 1980, she saw a cardiologist who diagnosed endocarditis", is closer to the truth than anything, no cardiologist diagnosed endocarditis at any point, and, so, this information does not belong in the record. But then the patient has no access to the medical record and has been granted no right in law to correct errors.

Dr. Cabot had sufficient courage to contradict Dr. Adami's explanation of the splenomegaly as a "congenital variant" and admit there was considerable evidence on physical and laboratory exam of a number of abnormalities. However, he seemed to lessen the significance of his findings by suggesting that my spleen be checked regularly, not so much because of an underlying organic disorder but because the patient, as he put it, is "so concerned about what all this means". But such a comment could also mean that Dr. Cabot was indifferent to the splenomegaly because he had ruled out any current infection and that, if anything, these signs were the "residua", as in the Libman cases, of a past infection and thus would eventually recede. Psychiatrist Adami's opinions carried a lot of weight, affecting, like Austin's, my credibility. Dr. Cabot stated "There is a question she thinks at that time (referring to the time of the dental abscess) of an enlarged heart." The word, "thinks", suggests that, in the absence of the concrete evidence in the x-rays, like Dr. Warren, Dr. Cabot was justified in doubting the cardiomegaly even though his x-ray of April, 1982 showed a "normal" sized heart rather than the "tiny", undersized heart I had prior to the infection and would suggest that my heart had increased in size rather than returned to the size before the infection.

To solve the mystery of the size of my heart, I tried to locate the x-ray which the internist in my home town had ordered when I first saw him, back in 1978, before my illness. My efforts to track down this x-ray were rebuffed with the wildest excuses. I first contacted a doctor who reported it was in the Radiology Department of the local hospital. Dr. Cory called but was told they no longer had the x-ray. A second call to this doctor gave me the name of the radiologist. He explained that some mysterious Dr. X, who was away for an extended period, had old records stored in the basement of his house. The six year time limit for keeping the film was not up. The radiologist said he would make some inquiries about getting a key and having someone look. It was a Robin Cook scenario. The radiologist called back and abruptly announced that there was no point in exploring Dr. X's basement files because my x-ray had been destroyed. Either Dr. X had come back from planet Y and checked his files in the short space of an hour or everyone was tipped off about my legal suit, and someone had been assigned, the radiologist, to convey the alibi to me. The question that arose in our minds was why, in a society that respects individual rights, are patients not permitted to purchase and store x-rays that are to be discarded. After all, the patient has submitted to the risk of radiation and the x-rays are ultimately of no use to anyone else but are of great value to the patient, if even to avoid duplication.

The situation was further complicated by a change in Dr. Cory's attitude.

When I questioned why my x-ray would be destroyed before the legal limitation period was up, he shouted at me, "Don't you complain to me about your missing x-rays!" Obviously, he was thinking of past events as well. "We've done all we can. We've gone to great lengths to help you." It seemed he defined one telephone call as going to great lengths. One explanation was that the x-ray had been forwarded to Dr. Austin long ago. I couldn't remember whether I had signed a requisition, but everything I had undergone proved that this was an insignificant formality anyway. My signature on films of "my body", which I was never allowed to see, was not worth the paper it was written on. The realization had stung me that I had no such rights at the time of the mysterious disappearance of my medical records. If the requisition with my signature had any legal effect, it would have been kept on permanent record as proof I had never released my records to a non-existent Dr. Korman. It would also have been proof of Dr. Austin's specific involvement in the disappearance since the requisition contained his name. For all the legal rights I had, Dr. Austin himself had probably signed a requisition asking for this x-ray long ago when he realized he had missed something at the time of my cardiac enlargement. This x-ray would have shown whether my heart had actually returned to its normal size, and Dr. Austin would not have wanted it around.

Some spokesman for the medical profession had surely got to Dr. Cory since he now refused to allow me to see any more letters or reports from other physicians. This was a stunning blow to me and altered our relationship. There was one final event in this fruitless search to get at the truth that appeared only to tighten the conspiracy of silence. Occasionally I saw a female physician in Toronto for pap smears and other female complaints. She had been my physician prior to my marriage. Dr. Cory's uncooperativeness sent me to her. I related my entire story, not leaving out any names of doctors or hospitals and with appropriate criticisms of my care. I also told her I had consulted a lawyer in order to retrieve my records which she cautioned I would have little luck getting. She was honest enough to admit that my murmur had changed dramatically since she had seen me before the infection and the spleen was definitely palpable. She repeated strongly that children were out of the question and insisted that I see a female cardiologist she knew for regular check-ups. Naturally we did not want to travel many miles for six monthly visits to see Dr. Cabot and welcomed the chance to have ongoing care in Toronto.

This female GP recommended a female cardiologist who had her office close to a Scarborough Hospital, and I was led to believe that she worked out of this hospital. While waiting in the cardiologist's office, I could clearly hear her conversing with another patient. What I learned was that she was attached to TMSC. This was shocking and disappointing to me. When she finally examined me, her behaviour was very curious. After insisting I had never had endocarditis in the past, she said my murmur was insignificant, and, contradicting the GP, said pregnancy in no way posed a risk. Furthermore, my spleen was not enlarged. I insisted the ultra sound had shown an enlarged spleen. She gave another angry, careless check and threw her hands up in the air in a gesture of bored impatience. Her reaction was not that of someone learning a person's history for the first time and carefully taking note but of someone who has heard it all before and is both angry and anxious when confronted with the live specimen, protective of her colleagues and herself and unwilling to get involved.

"Oh all right!" she exclaimed haughtily, "it is enlarged! So what! What do you want me to do about it! It doesn't mean conclusively that you've had endocarditis."

Clearly, she was a step ahead of me, already anticipating what it was I wanted to prove. I could not return to her because of my litigation against TMSC which, if she did not know, would soon. She asked me for my records from TMH and my recent hospital investigation. A few days later, to my astonishment, I received a letter in which she once again asked for my records and even enclosed the requisition forms for me to sign! This struck us as very unorthodox and suggested she was a little too eager to get her hands on my medical records.

There was another piece of information enclosed which shocked both my husband and myself. After all my efforts to get a definite opinion about the use of antibiotics with dental work for MVP patients, this doctor was sending me a photocopy of the American Heart Association recommendations which spelled out the antibiotic prophylaxis regimen with dental and other procedures for MVP patients! This was incredible and could only point to the fact that she was well aware of my case. Confidentiality was just another of those pieces of rhetoric that floated out of the mouths of doctors.

As well, she enclosed a copy of a card I was to carry indicating the patient required protection from bacterial endocarditis. Every other cardiologist, except the American doctor and Cabot, had tried to convince me of the controversial nature of this issue. We could only conclude that this cardiologist was familiar with my case and my malpractice suit and was protecting herself, or that TMSC had warned all its doctors of the "new" ruling about MVP and IE and the necessity for antibiotics in these patients. This doctor-patient relationship spelled danger and, so, we opted for travelling to see Dr. Cabot who manifested some interest in my wellbeing.

11

Oracle at Delphi

Dr. Will's last gift to the Foundation was his own home, which as Mayo Foundation House has become a centre for the fellows' activities, both social and professional . . . young doctors meet with their teacher to discuss medical problems . . . the evening starts off with a formal paper by one of the fellows who has been making a special study of the topic. Then a staff member from the Section on Cardiology talks about the things a bad heart can do to wreck a kidney operation . . . after a while the head of the postmortem service reports cases that have come to his division because some risk was overlooked in a seemingly simple operation. The surgeon may be operating for nothing more than an ingrowing toenail, he says, but if he has failed to take into account a *leaky heart* and the patient dies during the operation, the death is charged to the ingrowing toenail because that's the only way to keep the mortality figures straight.

> Helen Clapesattle: *The Doctors Mayo* (Minneapolis: University of Minnesota Press, 1941), pp. 379-80.

For many years diagnosis by use of the proctoscope . . . was one of the incidental duties of the urologists. Then one day Dr. Will remarked casually to young Dr. Louis A. Buie that there was a big opportunity waiting for someone enterprising enough to concentrate on proctology. Because no one liked the idea of spending his days examining and treating rectums, a great many persons were suffering from uncorrected deformities or diseases of that part of the body and they would seek relief if it were available. Dr. Buie took the hint and within a few years he was doing so much work in this field that a separate section on proctology was formed with him as head. By the end of the 1930's his section was one of the busiest at the clinic — another demonstration of Dr. Will's genius for seeking opportunities.

> *The Doctors Mayo*, p. 217.

The reader might well ask why I did not give up in defeat, why I persisted in asking the sphinx to solve its own riddle. My last hospitalization provided me with more irregularities and more evidence of past IE, yet less explanation. I strongly believed in preventative medicine and only vaguely understood that my febrile illness in association with an endodontal infection, if it had been investigated right from the beginning, might have provided some valuable clues to the prevention of deterioration in the MVP syndrome. But, from the start of my illness, there had been indifference. I was never able to get answers, yet I would learn later that there were answers to my simple questions in the medical literature.

And what doctors suggested, in order to protect their colleagues and halt snooping into their business, was not, in reality, a neurotic obsession with my heart or my health but an obsession with truth and with the desire to pave the way for a more honest, open relationship between the physician and the patient. And though I actually considered seeing a psychiatrist, I did not because I realized that my feelings were not so much anger from what had happened to me but anger that I did not have access to personal health information. I knew a psychiatrist would try to teach me acceptance and submission rather than rejection and revolt. I believed that something had happened to me in a subtle, insidious way and that the information about me would be of benefit to others with MVP.

I wrote some letters to other U.S. medical centres and doctors who were responsible for the articles I had read in the medical literature. My aim was to talk with them about MVP. Understandably, I could not find a doctor who was prepared to answer my questions without examining me, though, unlike the Canadian doctors I had seen, all agreed that my medical history was suspicious of IE. Eventually, after a year, I obtained an appointment at the famous Mayo Clinic in July of 1983. My first choice had been the Stanford, California Medical Centre because MVP patients with IE had been studied there. However this was too far to travel. In one of their studies, there were patients whose murmurs changed during IE, from a LSM to a PSM, as mine had. Nor had they required immediate valve replacement because of heart failure.[1]

The Mayo Clinic naturally asked for my x-rays, echoes and other documents from the time of my illness. Since I couldn't oblige, I had to settle for my most recent tests. I now wanted clarification of the cause of the splenomegaly, the tricuspid valve changes and my current symptoms as well as the apparently permanent damage to my mitral valve. However, when I tried to collect these test results, the liver spleen scan, the print-outs of the echoes of the mitral and tricuspid valves, chest x-rays, lab reports, Dr. Cabot refused me permission and said that they were unnecessary for another opinion. This meant, of course, that my vanishing records were also unimportant. My conversation with him was a scenario straight out of a Kafka drama. The documents I was asking for were not the property of Dr. Cabot but of the hospital. A patient should not have to go through the treating doctor to obtain them. But the truth of the matter is that all doctors make it their business to know where a patients' records are going when that patient is looking for another opinion. Dr. Cabot's explanation was that I had to check with the appropriate departments, that he did not control these records. This was true, but the departments, of course, deferred to him, the treating physician, before releasing any documents to the patient. It was the same sequence that had taken place with Dr. Austin and Dr. Cofman.

When I insisted on my right to take these documents to someone else, Dr. Cabot suddenly claimed there was no permanent record of any of my tests. When he could not convince me, he threatened that, in the future, patient records would not be transferable. Though this sounded like the ultimatum of a military tribunal whose object is to crush freedom of information, it was a threat that was well within his power and the power of the entire medical establishment to fulfill.

In a final desperate attempt to stop me from investigating, Dr. Cabot asserted that I didn't have MVP. That was the decision, he said, of a senior resident in cardiology. When I protested, asking what it was I had, he modified his story to borderline prolapse and then hung up curtly, leaving me with waves of frustration and shock that supposedly responsible, professional people could behave in this way. A sickening sense of powerlessness engulfed me. In our youth, we imagine, like Kino, in Steinbeck's novel, *The Pearl*, that we can move mountains but, as we grow older, we realize that mountains can be moved only at certain times and only by the Atlases of the world who hold them up.

A short while later, Dr. Cabot called me back and, in a daze, I heard him recite the documents I could pick up from his office which included everything I'd asked for except, curiously, the echo print-out showing the tricuspid nodules, and I wondered if this was because the sudden appearance of tricuspid changes, could not, unlike the spleen enlargement, be as easily attributed to something other than IE.

We arrived in Rochester, Minnesota just as the sun was setting, and long, dark shadows had fallen over the city. Rochester is small, only 60,000 permanent residents which, as the Patients' Guide to The Mayo Clinic proudly claims, swells to several hundred thousand with the influx of the sick. The land is flat, the city rising like an oasis in the middle of nowhere. The closest big cities are Minneapolis, 80 miles northwest, and Chicago, 275 miles southeast. The Mayo Clinic, lifeblood of the city, employs several hundred medical and surgical specialists and, along with the St. Mary's Hospital and the Rochester Methodist Hospital, quite conceivably provides the bulk of employment for its inhabitants. Recognizable commercial enterprises, like Libby's corn company, are distinctly anomalistic in this modern mecca. The Mayo Clinic affects everything, from special rates in hotels, motels, restaurants to even retail shops. And the sick person, like the tourist, is fair game for every sales strategy in the book. Without the clinic, Rochester, like some Northern Canadian mining town divested of its gold, might well descend to the level of a ghost town.

Rochester, dependent for its survival and its prosperity on the singular industry of the Clinic, reminded us somehow of another equally famous city, Las Vegas, Nevada, paralleling in wantonness the virtues of Rochester. The population of Las Vegas, similar to that of Rochester, also swells to an enormous size with the influx not of the unfortunate sick but with gamblers. The survival, the cashflow, of these twin monoliths is inextricably bound up with the psychology of gambling. The health gamble replaces the financial gamble. The cat scans, echocardiograms, stethoscopes, proctoscopes and scalpels are the slot machines, and the diagnosis of the problem and, therefore, the cure, the jack pot. A similar desperation propels the pilgrim to either shrine to pray for a miraculous cure of his physical disease or his financial ills.

Centres like Mayo are the Delphis of modern western civilization, their doctors, the Apollos. They are viewed as the convergence of the classic and Christian myths. The simple homilies of simple folk bear this out. "We didn't know what was wrong with Harry. We went to dozens of doctors in Wisconsin. None of them could find the problem. If we're gonna find it and cure it, it's gonna be right here." The cure is implicit in the act of diagnosing the malady. A problem identified is a problem banished. We live in a society that relies on Mr. Fix-it. The handyman advertises that "no job is too big or too small" for his services. After all, Jesus was a carpenter and, in his Apollo-God capacity, the doctor is the "supreme carpenter". Modern medicine thus caters to the deluded belief that fixing the problem is preferable to preventing it.

The omnipresent carnival atmosphere of Vegas mingled with the religious fervor of Mayo from the moment we stepped inside the revolving doors of the Clinic at 7:30 a.m. and threaded our way through the swarming crowds to the Admissions desk. There were few signs of illness. It was like registering at a hotel or spa rather than a medical centre or waiting in a ticket line-up at a train station or an airport where people inched ahead, kicking their luggage before them. Two lines stretched out, one for those with and one, three times as long, for those without appointment. In an auditorium with row upon row of chairs, we waited for the prestigious plastic Mayo card which solidifies membership in this exalted community and encourages the patient to drop in at any time as if the Clinic were some exclusive, local professional club.

After a two hour wait, we proceeded to the appropriate department, mine Internal Medicine, for the book of appointments. This was an all day wait. The excuse was the "broken computer". Even Delphi is subject to the tyrannical antics of technology. When our name was called, we started up from our doze, praying vainly that the wait was all over. But it was only time for the blood test. We were directed to the proper floor. This assembly line procedure takes five minutes, but the wait takes at least two hours. Masses of people, snoring, knitting, reading, eating were stuffed into a huge waiting room with domed glass ceilings through which the hot sun poured down on a massive, potted jungle that reminded me faintly of the promenades of Eaton's Centre in Toronto. There were at least a half dozen laboratories doing the blood tests.

Once done, we returned to the Internal Medicine floor and waited until late afternoon when beaming smiles announced the computer was fixed. More waiting. Then the presentation of the precious book of appointments. When I received this package, looking like a passport, I was struck with the finality of being rubber stamped on the forehead like Cain or branded on the rump like a cow. The clerk read the appointments to us and carefully interpreted the instructions as if they were the occult symbols of a sorcerer. My initial appointment was with the Consultant in Internal Medicine, the Clinic physician assigned to my case who arranges the tests he feels necessary. First, I was bewildered that he was an internist, like Dr. Cabot, rather than a cardiologist. This visit was followed by an ultrasound scan of the spleen and an electro-cardiogram. Two tests, which I had never had before, stood out as death sentences, a proctoscopy and a barium enema x-ray. The clerk delicately explained that these tests meant castor oil, cramps and enemas in preparation for the tubes that would invade the body. When she was instructing me where to purchase the enema bag and the castor oil which she was pleased to say tasted like cherries, I found my voice. A timid, bewildered protest was bubbling up inside me. Why was I scheduled for such an examination? She didn't know, of course. I quickly remembered that I had listed diarrhea as one of my symptoms but was completely bewildered as to why this would call for such an invasive test. To my shocked dismay, apart from the electrocardiogram, there was no consultation with a cardiologist and no echocardiogram listed anywhere in the booklet.

"Your Consultant didn't think such tests were necessary," the clerk said. "But, I'm here about my heart!" I emphasized impatiently. We hadn't driven 1500 miles for proctoscopies and barium enemas which I supposed could have been done just as well at home. I repeated rather methodically why I had come. It seemed that the causal connection between my past events and present condition was being ignored in favour of investigating some other imagined disease, such as cancer of the colon or inflammatory bowel disease which in no way related to my medical history. "Well you'll have to wait until you see your Consultant," the clerk said in a resigned voice. "But I wouldn't want to stay for a whole week unless I can have a consultation with a cardiologist," I replied emphatically. "Well, just a minute," she said all flustered and then went off to inquire. I could see it was not her problem and I felt badly that I had upset her. I glanced at my husband, adrift among the throngs of slumped, inert forms imprisoned in their rows of identical chairs. He sat opposite the huge mural depicting the illustrious achievements of medicine and Mayo. I'd heard so much talk of unnecessary tests that I began to doubt the motivation of the gigantic industry of the medical profession.

The clerk returned and said, "Well you were supposed to have a heart x-ray. Everybody has a heart x-ray. I don't know why it's not in here. It's supposed to be this afternoon at 4:00."

"But I don't need a heart x-ray. I had one barely three months ago." I reminded her that I had submitted my two x-rays from April of '82 and '83 for the internist's opinion. "I don't think I should have another heart x-ray so soon. Hasn't the Consultant looked at them?" I asked.

"I'm sure he did. He wouldn't order another so soon if he thought it dangerous or unnecessary."

Naturally I wondered if there was something wrong with my x-ray that Dr. Cabot had missed. After all, he was unable to give me a reason for the enlarged spleen. She was waiting with her pencil raised to mark the heart x-ray at 4:00 p.m. that afternoon, and I felt I could do nothing but submit.

My instructions were to ask the Consultant about an appointment with a cardiologist and the echocardiogram. If he felt they were important, the clerk said, he would arrange them, but, she warned, everything had been arranged months in advance and there was little hope of change.

I slunk away with a feeling of frustration and the impression that cardiologists had little time for MVP patients. The suspicion grew that I would not get answers to my questions here. What I really wanted to know was the reason why I had classic signs, described by Libman, of a previous IE and why I had symptoms related to further deterioration in my mitral murmur. But I had arranged this visit myself. I had not been recommended by any doctor in Canada. There are few doctors in Canada or the U.S. who would not regard this as unorthodox and few who would approve. Such independence can only mean that the patient is dissatisfied and is likely attempting to gather evidence surreptitiously for use in a malpractice action, especially if that patient refuses to give the names of other doctors and asks that all results of tests and consultations be forwarded to him or her personally. Such unorthodox procedures usually result in as little information as possible, but, at that time, I was still too innocent to realize this.

In arranging these appointments, little or no consideration, it seemed, had been given to the patient's time or pocket book, and it appeared that the cardiology consultation and examination would be held over to the following week. Like everyone else, we crept about only mildly protesting, wondering what to do in between appointments to kill the boredom. There's the pool at the hotel but a glance at the sleek, bronzed creatures on the sun circuit makes one feel whiter and more unhealthy than ever. There are the movies, the shops, the restaurants that lure the Mayo pilgrims into buying or eating out of boredom.

And there were the most famous attractions, the mansions of the founding fathers of the Clinic, the Brothers Mayo and their colleague, Plummer, after whom only a mere building is named. Dr. Plummer's mansion, "Rochester's only castle", as the Mayo guide brochure boasts, dominates the entrance to Rochester and is the first thing the visitor sees when approaching the city. The huge chimneys of this mysterious structure soar up out of the secretive foliage offering a tantalyzing glimpse of unbelievable wealth. This huge colossus bestrides one of two singular hills of this flat city. In the quaintness of its design, the English Tudor Country House with its rose garden, the architect had attempted to save his Gothic monstrosity from the vulgarity of that peculiar American union of capitalism and medicine by a colonialistic condescension to the superiority of the tastes of the British aristocracy. But Dr. Plummer's rose garden is distractedly American in its Brobdingnagian extravagance. A medieval tower glowers over the rose garden and the mansion perched high up on its plateau with a spectacular view as from a peak in the Andes. This awesome crenellated fortress is in no way attached to the house. Its "raison d'etre" is only reluctantly revealed upon questioning the guide. The tower, it seems, defended the doctor's roses from the forces of nature. This structure was built, she explains, for the sole purpose of watering the doctor's roses in an ecologically threatened area. This tower stands as a kind of challenge to the humble claims of the Mayo Brochure that "no financial benefit shall accrue to any staff member, officer or employee beyond a reasonable compensation."

One can't overlook the entrepreneurial spirit that went into the building of the Mayo Clinic when one hears the frequent Mayo visitor repeat that the long wait for appointments is related to the doctors' interest in the hotels. History might corroborate the truth of such a statement in that "this big business plant" had, indeed, in the past, established an intricate maze of hotels, The Kahler Corporation, with subway tunnel that connected them to "the Clinic".[2]

Mayowood dominates the second hill, the power of medibusiness looking down upon the frailty of humanity. This was the home of Charles Horace, son of William Worrall Mayo. The father and his sons were responsible for one of the first private group medical practices in the United States, one which became an excellent example of the profit of wedding medical science and free enterprise in the early 1900's. Like the Plummer home, this thirty-eight room mansion was a showplace for the French, Spanish, English and American antiques Charles Mayo had collected, symbols of the extraordinary wealth that could be had from the business of treating the sick. Cowering beneath the ostentatious Plummer mansion is the lowly Ramada Inn where we stayed, its non-descript modernism representing the downward slide into he commercialism of sickness.

At 10:30 a.m. the next morning I was again face to face with one of the "exalted authors" of the medical literature I had read. My Consultant was a soft spoken, well-bred, relaxed individual who appeared not to react with any degree of hostility or disapproval to my questions. After an internal examination, a standard that goes with the visit, he began taking my medical history. He first glanced at Dr. Cabot's two x-rays and said, as I expected him to, that my heart was normal in size. It seemed pointless to raise the issue of the tiny, smaller than normal heart prior to 1979.

We discussed the question of the cardiac enlargement occurring simultaneously with the echocardiographic documentation of holosystolic prolapse and Dr. Austin's clinical observation of increased regurgitation all in the presence of a severely abscessed tooth. The Consultant expressed regret that he did not have the chest films and the echo print-outs of those events. In fact, he asked if it were at all possible to telephone my home and have someone forward the radiologists' reports on these films and echoes to him. I had not brought them because I now believed it would make little difference to what a doctor would say about my past events. Later, when I was home, I sent him the five radiologist's reports from 1978, 1979, 1980, but, as I guessed, without the films and echoes, he was unable to say what had been the cause of the change in cardiac size and the change in murmur.

However, at our meeting the internist confirmed that the change in my murmur at the time of my fever and oral infection would have correlated with the change in the echocardiogram from the late systolic buckling or dipping to the pansystolic sagging and that this change represented a permanent change in my valve, not a transient finding that would reverse itself as Dr. Tatler had said. This seemed to be a step in the direction of some positive answers that I had wanted all along. However, it would become clearer, in the course of our discussions, that he would offer no criticism of my past care.

The splenomegaly, he conceded, could be a leftover from a previous infection. He could never state, he said, with 100 percent certainty, that I had never suffered IE. His opinion then confirmed Dr. Hall's at TMH. The internist repeated that having the films and hospital records from the time of my illness would help to establish a past IE. This was both welcome and unwelcome news that brought a renewed sense of impotence and frustration that I had not had control over these documents to prevent their loss which robbed me of the certainty of knowing whether or not I had suffered a life-threatening disease that would ultimately limit my lifespan, predispose me to repeated episodes or relapses in the future and which could be responsible for my present health. And, most important, the loss of this medical history would make it very difficult, even eight years later, when I once again had classic signs of IE, to convince a doctor that I should be tested for this disease.

I told the Consultant of my disappointment that my specific cardiac complaints were not being addressed. "Well," he hesitated,"I guess we could arrange something. But your appointments are already booked. You might have to wait until Monday." My hopes sank. There were hours in between appointments. After seeing the Consultant there was nothing until the chest x-ray at 4:00 p.m. On Wednesday, there was only an electrocardiogram at 8:00 a.m. On Thursday there were the proctoscopy at 8:00 and the barium at 10:00 and nothing that afternoon or on Friday. I showed him my appointment booklet.

Eventually we did get an appointment with a cardiologist after a wait from 11:00 a.m. until 4:00 p.m. for the return of my booklet while the clerks again struggled with their downed computer. All we could do was philosophize on the brilliance of this mechanical appendage of the human brain. We went out of the waiting room so that I could have the chest x-ray, came back and waited again until almost six o'clock when at last they announced victoriously that they had won their battle with the stubborn computer and I now had my Friday appointments, an echocardiogram and a visit with the cardiologist. We stumbled out, sadly convinced of the power of the corporate machine.

The vacant hours were filled up with some pool dipping, visits to the doctors' houses, the Mayo Medical Science Museum and the Mayo Memorial Park. This park near the Mayo Civic Auditorium is just one of the many impressive tributes to the Brothers Mayo. The Mayo brothers who had, themselves, contributed financially to the establishment of this park, assured their own fame on an even more exalted level. A statue of Dr. William Worrall Mayo with the inscription A Man of Hope and Forward Looking Mind dominates the park. There's an expression in the medical literature that mitral regurgitation begets mitral regurgitation. The same could be said of success, wealth and fame. For the Mayo brothers, it would not have been difficult to be hopeful and forward looking. Equally imposing are the statues of the two sons in their surgical gowns. Beneath their raised dais is a shrine shaped like an amphitheatre, as if in anticipation of the pilgrimage of hundreds of thousands of people to this Holy Place. All that is missing to complete the evocation of the truly spiritual power of these servants of the Lord is the familiar collage of crutches, braces, wheelchairs, canes and other appliances the disabled in their miraculous recoveries leave behind as testimonies at the shrines of Lourdes, Guadelupe or Ste. Anne de Beaupré.

When the dreaded hour came for the proctoscopy and the barium enema x-ray, I waited with the young and the old, with the anxiety-ridden and the indifferent. Two older women, who, with the great cancer scare, talked about the necessity of having their colons checked as regularly as their hearts chatted as though they were at their hairdressers or waiting for a round of golf. One knitted and reminded me of her literary sister, Mme. Dafarge, impassive, "pathologically calm", before the impending horror.

A nurse delicately ushered me into the examining room where I was confronted with a big, pudgy man who was wiping his instrument, the proctoscope. Words made up of borrowed foreign parts, like "procto" from the Latin for rectum, always have a comforting, euphemistic effect. I had time only for a swift glance at this long tube which he waved like Circe's wand that changed men into swine and, then, he directed me to kneel on a contraption oddly resembling a priedieu. Then the dress was lifted, the nakedness revealed, and all the humiliation that human flesh is heir to having annihilated the sparks of humanity, I folded my hands on the shelf. Unable to conjure up any prayers, I contented myself with the soothing words of Isaiah that all mankind is grass and their glory like the flower of the field while the beatified faces of the Mayo Brothers in a picture on the wall grinned down upon me in malicious approval of my mortification.

Then came the painful barium that snaked its way through the large intestine and the rush to the john with the pinky, white liquid, looking as innocent as an icecream soda, gushing out. Little did I know that this intensive pain which others told me they did not feel, was hardly normal and likely was the reason for what I was soon to discover once I returned to Canada.

The Friday echo accomplished I reported for my examination with the cardiologist. This time, I insisted on the presence of my husband, even though the intimidating "barriers" in the Mayo set-up had discouraged me on my first visit with the Consultant. The surprised doctor reluctantly agreed. After his examination, I asked if he would describe my murmur as pansystolic. "Yes, I guess I would have to say that. It's a long murmur."

His opinion now verified the opinions of many other doctors I had seen, and I thought with dismay of Dr. Cabot's protestations that I did not have MVP. "I had a much shorter murmur, late systolic, before my illness. It was very faint and could not be heard all the time." Once again, I was tailoring my questions as if I were cross-examining him or the ghost of Dr. Austin.

And I knew as I asked my questions that the cardiologist would suspect I was up to no good. "I didn't examine you then so I can't comment. Your echo showed virtually no prolapse."

Again, there was the confusion. "Oh," I could only repeat numbly. I would never know if this were true or not.

"But I don't regard that as definitive."

"Why not?"

"Lots of reasons — technician's error, inadequacies of the echocardiographic equipment. What I hear with the stethoscope is the most important."

"Could the infection from the dental work in 1979 and 1980 have caused this change which was documented at the time."

"It could have," he responded. "I can't rule out that you never had endocarditis, but you seem to be relatively healthy now."

"What about the fatigue and the SOB with activities I accomplished easily before."

"I can't really say at this time. According to ultrasound, your spleen is still enlarged."

I wanted to say but that's what I came for, to find the cause of these symptoms, not for proctoscopies and barium enema x-rays which, of course, were normal. Nor did I need more spleen ultrasounds or heart x-rays. But I only asked, "Could the splenomegaly be left over from an infection?"

"That's possible. I would recommend a MUGA test with exercise. We could not do it today of course. This would show how your heart is functioning as a result of whatever process was going on." My husband and I looked at each other. We could not afford to stay longer. "I could have this done just as well in Canada," I said hastily.

Again I wanted to protest that this should have been done instead of the proctoscopy and barium enema but I didn't. "What is your opinion of the tricuspid changes?"

"I don't know. Our technician didn't see them this time."

But then the technician hadn't pick up the prolapse I said to myself. I was disappointed not to have some clarification of this. We then discussed a blood abnormality which had not been found in Canada but which would, with further reading, become important in the collection of signs of IE. My second blood test confirmed a "monoclonal gammopathy". I didn't know what that meant. The Consultant in Cardiology explained that this was an antibody found in my blood serum, that is the amber coloured liquid which remains after the red blood cells have been allowed to clot and shrink. Serum is composed of a multitude of properties including the immunoglobulins or antibodies, like the monoclonal immunoglobulin found, which defend against disease. The cardiologist confirmed that this antibody as well as the splenomegaly could be lingering signs, what Libman had called the "residua" of a subacute bacterial infection, but he said he would never know for sure.

Our interview ended, as all the others, with no authoritative confirmation that cause and effect were linked but with increased suspicion that they were.

As we left, the cardiologist threw out a parting shot which he had obviously been saving for the end of our discussion. It was a warning on behalf of the medical authorities to keep my place in the power structure and refrain from challenging the strongest and most united collective mentality. "You shouldn't read the literature," he said not unpleasantly. "It doesn't do you any good. For the good of your health, I would suggest you stop reading."

I made no response to this statement which surprised me though it should not have in view of its consistency with the opinions of other doctors I had met. Unfortunately it had been made all too clear to me in the past that if I had read the literature and known of the dangers of endodontal infection and periodontal surgery without antibiotics and if I had known what endocarditis was, I would not be in the position I was now in and I would certainly not have let the dentists deceive me for a whole year about an abscessed tooth.

At my closing visit with the Consultant in Internal Medicine, we discussed the monoclonal antibody, immunoglobulin G. This antibody, he said, was found in chronic infections and was likely connected to the enlarged spleen, and both could be left over from a significant bacterial infection. The monoclonal antibody should be checked every six months he added. This curious finding was linked ironically to the disease, "myeloma", a musical sounding word that is the name of a deadly disease, bone marrow cancer. Why had the word, myeloma, appeared on my blood test card I asked?

"It's just a routine test, an incidental finding. It may mean nothing. There's certainly no clinical signs of myeloma."

However, this immunoglobulin abnormality would show up for some years after along with other immunoglobulin abnormalities and raised the interesting question of whether certain kinds of cancers could be precipitated by a serious bacterial infection years after the event. Like the cardiologist, the internist stressed the need for antibiotic prophylaxis but curiously only with dental extractions and this was confirmed in a written report which I received later. However, at the time of my visit to the Mayo Clinic, coverage was recommended for any procedure that draws blood and, in particular, had been recommended for barium enema x-rays.

When it was all over, we walked down to the collection bureau for our bill, a whopping $1263.10. We knew it would be a lot but not quite that much. This was for three doctor visits, echocardiogram, electrocardiogram, ultrasound of spleen, chest x-ray, proctoscopy, barium enema x-ray, laboratory work and visit to a dentist. The cost of medical consultation, electrocardiogram, phonocardiogram, chest x-ray and echocardiogram on my previous visit to the U.S. was only $237.00, less than the cost of the $250.00 echo alone at Mayo.

We came away from the Mayo Clinic with only one piece of information that was significant, the presence of the IgG immunoglobulin which later research would tell us was found in cases of IE and could be a leftover from such an infection. But we had learned nothing about the cause of the tricuspid nodules and the enlarged spleen, and, in its personal report to me which constituted the medical record, The Mayo Clinic described my murmur in completely meaningless terms as a "systolic murmur". Such a general opinion in no way substantiated my claim that my murmur had deteriorated as a result of any previous infection that had not been prevented or treated properly.

I also came away with a problem. Because of crippling back pain on the way home, we stopped off in the emergency department of a Windsor Hospital. I was given a shot of Demerol and, unfortunately, x-rayed again. The emergency doctor, on looking at my x-ray, asked if I had recently had a barium enema x-ray. I filled him in on the details. It seems either too much barium, which is used as an opaque contrast medium for roentgenographic studies of the gastro-intestinal tract, had been injected or too much force had been used, resulting in barium being displaced into my appendix. The barium cannot be rejected naturally by the body. Though supposedly an inert substance, this mineral can be dangerous. The authors of *The Pharmaceutical Basis of Therapeutics* warn that "although the insoluble barium sulphate is not normally absorbed by the body, it can produce local "granulomatous reactions" (lesions or scar tissue), for example, granulomas of the rectum. In fact, proof of this is found in a study done in 1962 which these authors cite. It was observed that, over long periods of time, men who worked at mining, sorting, grinding and bagging ore barytes (barium sulphate) have developed "barytosis", a granulomatous disease of the lungs or a form of cancer.[3] Later, Dr. Cabot would tell me that the barium could not be removed from the appendix and that it was a "wait and see situation" which, of course, only increased our anxiety.

In the entranceway to the Mayo Clinic, there is a very famous work of art, the Mestrovic statue of Man and Freedom. Picture a figure, suspended from the wall, the muscles of the chest pushed upward and the torso leaning forward with arms outstretched as if to take flight, hands shaped to hold nothing but the illusive dignity of air, the face turned up towards the heavens in a gesture of supplication. The sculptor was a modest man of humble origin, a shepherd in his Greek childhood, whose great art has been used to symbolize what some might consider an even greater art, medical science. The posture of this figure implies that freedom is defined as the liberation from disease. The dark, naked figure with bent knees and raised arms against the stark white background is unmistakably intended for comparison with the crucified Christ. How fitting that a shepherd should have created it! Its subliminal message is that another kind of salvation exists, through the gods of medicine and their miracles. But this statue representing the act of "striving for freedom", as the Mayo Brochure sumptuously describes it, symbolized something else for us. The striving for truth, for access to personal health information in the face of insurmountable barriers was a kind of crucifixion, and any patient, any individual, who has been deprived of precious moments of health, of life, who has been victimized by any powerful group in society is, indeed, a crucified soul.

On our way back to Canada, prior to my back problem, we had stopped at Spring Green, Wisconsin to see Christopher Marlowe's Tamburlaine The Great, the "scourge and wrath of God" who hung the slaughtered corpses of the Virgins of Damascus upon the walls and justified his evil deeds with the belief "That virtue solely is the sum of glory" which, it seemed to me, was a suitable motto for the Mayo Clinic. It was here that we saw the mind-boggling phenomenon, referred to in the tourist brochures as The House on the Rock. Built by an architect, Alex Jordan, on top of a 400 foot rock, this house, incorporating the stone as part of its walls was intended to unite man and nature, to wed the author's own stone ceramics to the very elements out of which they were fashioned.

But, this truly unique idea of a house growing out of a rock has slid inexorably downward into commercialism. What began as small, original, a journey into the spirit of man and his environment, has expanded, with the profit motive, into the huge, the common and the vulgar. Now a fortune-hunter's tourist trap, it attracts more and more people by its ever-increasing quantities of objects that dwarf the original house and display of ceramics. The colossal has become the sole measure of value, and hugeness has become tedious. Buildings have been erected all around the original monolith to hold gigantic, pneumatic instruments that pour forth the same ear shattering decibels of sound, and thousands of dolls' faces wear the same plastic look of assembly line brush and paint bucket. The sheer opulence and fakery of bombastic papier mâché cannons, gigantic calliopes and a carousel which boasts to be the biggest in the world, simply explode into meaninglessness when one lands in the midst of customized diesel and hydraulic behemoths, wheels, drums, kettles, pistons, all with no apparent function except to be big. Their shapes and outlines escape the deciphering talents of the small, intricate lens of the human eye. Though the brochure says real trees continue to grow inside the house and pierce the roof, close inspection reveals these trees are, in reality, dead, their tops cut flush with the ceilings. And beneath the mania for collecting objects is the mania for collecting money, $20,000 on a weekend. The image of the artist at work building his home, "disdaining to delay for the installation of technical machinery" and, consequently carrying "the needed stone and mortar in baskets upon his back, climbing the most difficult slopes by ladder, then climbing unaided the rest of the way"[4] dissolves into the most ephemeral of fantasies when one steps into the numbing bizarrities of this mutation of the artistic spirit. Somehow, such a gigantic commercial enterprise seemed a fitting conclusion to our Mayo visit, a lesson that size is not all. We were reminded of the elaborate scale upon which Mayowood was built as the brochure states: "the poured reinforced concrete construction necessitated the bringing to Rochester from Chicago one of the largest concrete mixers ever seen in this area."[5] Such achievements, like that of Mayowood and the Plummer castle do not represent the striving after freedom depicted in the Mestrovic sculpture but the striving after hugeness, after power, after wealth, which in turn is the impulse of the medicrats and the whole medibusiness of health care.

PART TWO:

THE CRY OF THE HEART FOR HELP

12

The Cat and the Pigeons

He has become really formidable; whenever any proposition is brought up, he will argue to the bitter end for the opposite side. He is firm in dispute, obstinate as a mule, he never alters his opinion, and he follows a line of reasoning to the last example, he accepts without question the opinions of the great ancients, and he has always refused to listen for a moment to the arguments and experiments concerning the alleged discoveries of our own time with regard to the circulation of the blood and similar nonsense.

Jean-Baptiste Molière: *Le Malade Imaginaire*, Act II

MVP is a classic example of a vastly misunderstood disease. If lay people were to read the medical literature, they would find that many diseases, which the medical profession presents to the public as hot discoveries, have, in fact, lengthy histories. The first references to the syndrome now known as MVP go back as far as the American Civil War. An examination of the history of this disease shows how it came to be regarded as benign, nothing more than an auscultatory curiosity, and why the majority of doctors even today still ignore its risks.

Heart Sounds

MVP is identified by an abnormal sound in the heart which doctors call a click. It is heard with a stethoscope which is the best way of detecting MVP according to most researchers.[1] Commonly, there is a murmur as well. These auditory phenomena, the click and the murmur, are confined to systole, the contraction or pumping interval of the cardiac cycle, as opposed to diastole which is the filling interval. When we press an ear to the chest wall, we hear, in the normal heart, two distinct sounds which doctors name quite logically as S_1 and S_2 or in lay language, "lubb" and "dup". The interval between S_1 and S_2 is systole and between S_2 and S_1 diastole.

For the doctor's clinical or auscultatory purposes S_1 is associated with the synchronous closure of the mitral and tricuspid valves[2] in the left and right sides of the heart, though these two valves do not, in fact, close simultaneously.

The sounds are, in reality, produced by vibrations caused by the movement of blood during systole when the ventricles forcibly contract to push the blood through the aortic valve into the aorta for distribution to the entire body and through the pulmonary valve into the lungs. At the commencement of systole, there is an acceleration of the blood flow followed by an abrupt, brief deceleration which causes tensing of the parts of the heart involved in ventricular systole, i.e. the atrioventricular valves, papillary muscles, chordae tendinae, valve leaflets and valve rings.[3]

The second heart sound, S_2, concerns the mechanism of diastole. Likewise, the doctors say this sound is actually caused, not by the synchronous closure of the aortic and pulmonary valves after the oxygenated blood has entered the aorta and the deoxygenated blood has entered the pulmonary artery and the lungs, but by the vibrations set up by the abrupt deceleration of the blood in the tubular vessels and their walls and the valve leaflets.[4] Apart from these two normal sounds, S_1 and S_2, almost all other sounds are abnormal and associated with disease.

Da Costa and The Non-Disease Theory

Extra systolic sounds, occurring in the systolic interval between S_1 and S_2, and the symptoms associated with them, were first recorded in the 1860s by a Northern American army physician, Dr. J. M. Da Costa, during the American Civil War.[5] Had it not been for this great American conflict, Da Costa may not have had the right setting to study this phenomenon. A war favoured him with ideal, experimental conditions in which large numbers of men were subjected, uniformly, to maximum psychological and biological stress.

Da Costa's observations and conclusions were based on three hundred cases of soldiers who were found to have abnormal heart sounds in systole and a set of symptoms that emerged, for the first time, when the men were engaged in a war. Da Costa provided a description of the typical soldier with cardiac symptoms who came to his attention:

> A man who had been for some months or longer in active service, would be seized with diarrhoea, annoying, yet not severe enough to keep him out of the field; or attacked with diarrhoea, or fever, he rejoined, after a short stay in hospital, his command and again underwent the exertions of a soldier's life. He soon noticed that he could not bear them as formerly; he got out of breath, could not keep up with his comrades, was annoyed with dizziness and palpitation, and with pain in the chest; his accoutrements oppressed him . . . it was decided he was unfit for duty, and he was sent to a hospital, where his persistently quick acting heart confirmed his story, though he looked like a man in sound condition . . . the irritability of the heart remained, and only very slowly did the excited organ return to its normal condition.[6]

The chief symptoms of which the soldiers complained, palpitations, dizziness, chest pain and dyspnea or shortness of breath, are among those modern researchers attribute to prolapse of the mitral valve. As well as symptoms, Da Costa described certain clinical findings, extra systolic sounds, heard with the stethoscope, that modern medicine now realizes are part of the picture of MVP, such as "double beats and intermissions" and what Da Costa called a "curiously broken" sound "like the motion of an only slightly elastic or cartilaginous substance"[7] that seemed to duplicate the first heart sound. He was, in fact, hearing the "click" of MVP.

Da Costa also recorded the sound of the systolic murmur. At that time, doctors believed that only the murmur, which began with S_1 and ended with S_2, or replaced those normal heart sounds, was a regurgitant murmur indicating organic valvular disease. And, even then, this sound was considered grave only if cardiac enlargement was present. This type of murmur, which began with S_1 and ended with S_2, is referred to as a pansystolic murmur (PSM). This was the kind of murmur I developed as a result of my IE. Da Costa found the PSM to be uncommon just as it is considered to be in MVP patients today.[8] Far more common was the mid to late systolic murmur which was heard best with the stethoscope placed over the apex of the heart. Da Costa's description of a blowing, inconstant murmur matches the descriptions of the mid to late systolic murmur of MVP today.[9]

Da Costa was puzzled by this curious extra sound in systole. Was it associated with regurgitation of blood backwards into the atrium and thus valvular disease? Da Costa published an article in 1871 which was the fruit of an even earlier work, the *Medical Diagnosis* of 1864. The terms he used, "irritable heart" and "functional disorder of the heart", to describe what he found, conveyed his opinion that organic disease of the heart was not present, despite his references to the "valvular" nature of these extra sounds.[10]

Da Costa boasts that his observations made him famous "within and without the walls of the hospital".[11] The institution he referred to was the Pennsylvania Military Hospital where he had been appointed visiting physician in 1862 and where he was sent all cases of this "peculiar functional disorder of the heart". The term, "irritable heart", which he coined even spread abroad and was used in a report published in the prestigious *British Medical Journal*.[12]

Da Costa believed the disorder was extremely common, likely found in soldiers of every war, including Napoleon's, and evidence of its existence, he said, existed in the *British Blue Book of the Crimean War of 1854-56*. As well, he had observed the disorder in civilians and recommended that it should be "equally interesting to the civil practitioner on account of some obscure or doubtful points of pathology"[13] In other words, he saw something in the pathological specimens which could not be dismissed outrightly as without disease. But no conclusion appears to have been made regarding the presence or absence of disease.

Because of the prevalence of this disorder, Da Costa issued a warning to physicians not to confuse the extra systolic sounds with valvular disease such as that known to underlie the regurgitant, pansystolic murmur with cardiac enlargement and evidence of rheumatic heart disease. His purpose was to avoid alarming patients. To that end, if, in these cases, edema was found, ordinarily pathognomonic for heart disease, he advised it should be dismissed as "transitory" and "limited to the lower extremities".[14] Da Costa thus laid the foundations for the modern approach to MVP. "Non primum nocere", first do no harm, the physician's oath, might better be called "non primum terrere", first do not frighten.

But, curiously, earlier in his studies, Da Costa had believed that the "irritable heart" did, in fact, become a diseased heart. And he had evidence for this opinion. Of his two hundred cases, twenty-eight had developed hypertrophied hearts while a further 36 hearts were possibly enlarged. But, unfortunately for individuals with MVP today, Da Costa doubted his own evidence of the seriousness of this condition. When asked, "What becomes of these kinds of hearts?", he answered that the hypertrophy was naturally arrested and the heart returned to a perfectly normal condition.[15] My cardiologist, Dr. Austin, came to the same conclusion made over one hundred years ago, that, during an insignificant oral infection, my heart enlarged with no apparent reason and then miraculously returned to its normal size without any treatment.

Cuffer and Barbillion: Disease vs. Non-Disease

It was in France, however, that the extra systolic sounds were viewed with seriousness. The French, like Da Costa, observed the same signs and symptoms in the civilian population, and, in 1887, two Parisian physicians, Cuffer and Barbillion, were the first to report the observations Da Costa had made in America. However, they called the extra sound a "systolic gallop" or "le bruit de galop mésosystolique" in an article they published in the well known Paris Medical Journal, *Archives Générales de Médecine*.[16]

By giving the new phenomenon the name "gallop", they drew attention to its seriousness. The gallop sound was well defined at this time. In fact, it was also a Parisian, a Professor Bouillaud, who, in 1835, first described and named the gallop sound which he said resembled the hoof beats of a galloping horse.[17] The word, "gallop" has a particular significance to medical people. The "gallop" was a name given to an extra sound heard, not in systole, but in diastole. It was associated with a combination of cardiac and renal disease. Cuffer and Barbillion found it, as did Da Costa, in cases of typhoid fever. The diastolic gallop was always considered grave. It was believed the patient usually died within ten to fifteen months of its diagnosis.[18] It was regarded as the patient's death knell, imagistically rendered by Obrastzow in 1905 as "the cry of the heart for help".[19]

The two Parisian physicians naturally discussed whether or not the sound they called "the systolic gallop" had the same grave prognosis as the gallop in diastole. They felt it might have because this extra systolic sound had certain features in common with the diastolic gallop. Both sounds they described as more tactile than auditory. Cuffer and Barbillion, translating the extra systolic sound accoustically as "vou tou-ta"[20], or in English "lub-click-dub", described it as "sourd, et affectant le tact plutôt que l'ouïe" because it was accompanied by a visible and palpable sensation of a slight elevation in the chest wall.[21] This was exactly the way the diastolic gallop behaved. Though Da Costa never used the term "gallop" when describing the extra systolic sound, he referred to the physical sensation as a jerky cardiac impulse or a palpable sensation when he placed his hand over the patient's heart.[22]

Cuffer and Barbillion, unlike Da Costa, claimed the extra systolic sounds signified cardiac disease. If the "gallop rhythm", according to Cuffer and Barbillion, was closest to the first heart sound, the prognosis was more favorable; if closer to the second, serious, and an indication of dilatation of the heart.[23] Their opinions were extraordinary for their time. The "systolic gallop" was a controversial subject in Paris, and the prevailing theory among physicians was that the extra sound was insignificant, that it came from outside the heart rather than inside and that it was caused from pleural pericardial adhesions or scar tissue which annealed the pericardial sac to the lung as a result of an infection such as pericarditis. Cuffer and Barbillion stuck to their guns and concluded that "nous pouvons . . . éliminer toute arrière pensée de . . . bruits extracardiaques."[24] To these two physicians, the sound was purely cardiac and could indicate an invisible lesion somewhere inside the heart. This "bruit cardiaque pur", they warned, should not be carelessly dismissed but should "éveiller la sollicitude du médecin, précisément à cause de la possibilité d'une lésion du myocarde plus intime et plus profond qu'on ne pourrait le supposer."[25] This warning would not be heeded until eighty years later. Their hypothesis that the sounds were caused by a myocardium weakened by disease, possibly a chronic myocarditis,[26] that is an inflammation of the heart muscle, is now being investigated in our time.

Modern researchers say that the "gallop" sound is strictly a diastolic event and that, in the older literature, the term, systolic gallop, was indiscriminately used for all extra sounds in systole. But, even the earlier writers recognized the inaccuracy of the application. In 1933, Wolferth and Margolies suggested abandoning usage of the term altogether chiefly because of the connotation of grave illness,[27] and Harvey repeated this advice in his 1949 textbook on auscultation.[28] Much later, in Hurst's text, *The Heart*, it was pointed out that the older researchers were describing the "systolic click" of MVP and the term, "gallop", the writers advised, should be discarded.[29]

The modern researchers came to this conclusion because Cuffer and Barbillion's description of the mid-systolic gallop sound matched that of the modern MVP click. The sound was found, the French doctors said, in thin people and was often accompanied by a murmur. They reported that the click increased or diminished in intensity and sometimes disappeared altogether, only to be heard several days later: "Il est difficile d'apprécier les conditions qui peuvent modifier ce bruit de galop, de reconnaître sous quelle influence il augmente ou diminue d'intensité, et de savoir pourquoi il disparaît parfois très rapidement pour se montrer de nouveau quelques heures ou quelques jours après. Il est certain que ce bruit est passager et capricieux."[30] Doctors today are equally perplexed as these two 19thC Parisians were when faced with a sound that changed in intensity and even disappeared. In proclaiming, contrary to contemporary medical opinion of the day, that disease underlay these fickle sounds, Cuffer and Barbillion sparked the controversy that would rage right into our own time over the nature of these findings.

Gallavardin and The Pleural-Pericardial Adhesion Theory

The popular theory of the non-disease origin of the sounds took root with the declarations of another French physician, Gallavardin. In 1913, he wrote in the *Lyons Médical Journal* that "le claquement mésosystolique", a term that really translates into the modern "mid-systolic click", or "le pseudo-dédoublement du deuxième bruit", a term more closely approximating that of Da Costa, was extra-cardiac and caused by pleural pericardial adhesions from a transitory pericarditis or some other illness such as typhoid fever.[31] What was astounding was that Gallavardin had little proof. His opinions were based on autopsies of three of his patients in whom he had found strands of pleuro-pericardial adhesions.[32] There was no evidence that he cut open the hearts of these patients, for surely he would have found the typical pathological features of prolapsed mitral valves.

Gallavardin's influence was great. The theory of the extra-cardiac nature of the abnormal systolic sounds spread. Other prominent writers, like Lian and Deparis, as late as 1933, were concluding, without proof of autopsy examinations, that the clicking sounds in fifty of their patients were caused from pleural-pericardial adhesions, simply on the strength of Gallavardin's three autopsied cases.[33] For the next fifty years, those three autopsied cases of Gallavardin would be used as evidence of the extra-cardiac theory. Furthermore, six of Cuffer and Barbillion's patients with the extra systolic click had died of diseases such as typhoid, tuberculosis and kyphosis, which is tuberculosis of the spine, and none had primary cardiac or renal involvement.[34] These cases then also became evidence of the extra-cardiac theory to explain the systolic click.

Griffith and Hall: Mitral Regurgitation and The Disease Theory

Around the turn of the century, a drop of wisdom was injected into the debate when two American doctors, Griffith in 1892[35] and Hall in 1903[36], without mentioning clicks or gallops, reported on the peculiarity of the mid to late systolic murmur. Like Da Costa, they stressed its frequency in the general population. Once again, the diastolic sounds, the gallop and murmur, associated with stenosed or narrowed valves resulting from rheumatic fever, became the yardstick for evaluating the seriousness of the systolic sounds. Griffith and Hall were as puzzled as Da Costa by the mid to late systolic murmur. They wondered how it could signify regurgitation of blood since it did not behave typically like a regurgitant murmur, that is, occupy all of systole. These two physicians, overlooked, rarely quoted in the old literature, made the most imaginative and most correct contribution to the history of MVP. Though their explanations differed, both were convinced that this peculiarly-timed murmur, like the longer pansystolic murmur, indeed, signified a leaky mitral valve with retrograde flow of blood into the left atrium. Symptoms which Da Costa had dismissed as transitory, such as edema of the lower extremities, as well as shortness of breath and rhythm disturbances, helped to shape Griffith's and Hall's opinions. Griffith proposed that the vibrations heard earlier in systole indicated regurgitation but were simply inaudible. "It seems", he stated, "much more probable, however, that cases such as those reported are instances of mitral regurgitation of much greater degree than the murmur alone would indicate . . . the regurgitation . . . probably lasted through all, or nearly all of the systolic period, but usually became audible for unknown reasons, only towards the middle or latter portion of it."[37]

Griffith was unable to refute the contemporary theory of cardiac hemo-dynamics, that a valve could not leak near the end of systole because the pressure of the blood in the ventricle is at its lowest at the end of that period of the cardiac cycle. While Griffith tailored his hypothesis to accepted opinions, Hall was more daring. He advanced an idea that is current with today's more scientific explanations of blood hemodynamics. For Hall what could not be heard was not there. Without benefit of modern cineangiographic studies, Hall conceived that regurgitation could occur "only" in the last half of systole and that the valve could be incompetent "only" at that time. And contrary to the weighty opinions of Gallavardin and others influenced by him, Hall insisted there was underlying valvular disease that caused the incompetency. To explain the leakage in late systole, Hall hypothesized that disease of the papillary muscle, which supports a portion of the mitral valve, could be responsible for its improper closing. This was a startling supposition for 1903. Modern researchers have suggested that the clicks and chest pain in MVP could be caused by ischemic disease of the papillary muscle.[38] Ischemia (iss-kee-mee-uh), the noun, and ischemic, the adjective, come from the Greek word, ischaimos, which means the stopping of the blood supply in an area and hence oxygen, thus creating a local anemia.

The extra-cardiac, pleural-pericardial adhesion theory of Gallavardin's school of thinkers so dominated the first half of the 20thC that little attention was paid to the theories of Griffith and Hall. In fact, the murmur, accompanying the "gallop" sound, was rarely mentioned. Thayer, 1926,[39] Wolferth and Margolies, 1933[40], Thompson and Levine, 1935[41], Johnston, 1938[42] and Luisada, 1949[43], devote much discussion to the systolic "gallop rhythm" or "click" but pass over the murmur without remarking on its connection with these other sounds or referring to Hall's or Griffith's work. However, from another point of view, the observations of these writers may mean that many more people had clicks than murmurs, an observation born out by modern studies.

The gallop sound or what we now call the click, curiously varying from one systolic cycle to the next, from early to late systole, fascinated and puzzled the earlier researchers as it has the modern. But, if they had paused to reflect on the murmur, as Hall and Griffith had done, they might not have adopted Gallavardin's extra-cardiac theory so unquestioningly to explain extra systolic sounds. Six years before the introduction of life-saving antibiotics, in 1938, Johnston summed up the opinion of the day, relying upon Gallavardin's three autopsied cases, done at the turn of the century, as proof.

> All evidence both from their clinical characteristics and from the measurements showing the great variability with which the clicks appear in systole indicates that they arise outside of the cavities of the heart and are not dependent upon intraventricular or intra-aortic pressure changes as are the heart sounds and murmurs. It is also apparent that they are in some way produced by the motion of the heart . . . we thus return by a somewhat round about process of exclusion to the theory that the clicks are due to pleuropericardial adhesions, or to some anomaly of these structures which allows vibrations to be produced in systole. None of our cases have come to autopsy and the only direct evidence supporting the theory is found in the three autopsied cases of Gallavardin.[44]

Johnston, like others, only briefly mentioned the late systolic murmur and placed it in the same category as normal heart sounds. Gradually, without any of the imaginative thought of Griffith or Hall, the opinion would take hold that the murmur, as well as the click or gallop, was, by association, extra-cardiac and thus of "no unfavorable influence upon the subsequent course of the patient's life."[45]

Sir Thomas Lewis and Soldier's Heart

The French theory passed into the English domain and, when the giants of the first half of the 20thC, Lewis, MacKenzie and Evans, got hold of it, there was no turning back. The ideas of Hall and Griffith slipped quietly into oblivion. The opinions of the British physician, Sir Thomas Lewis, carried enormous weight. The reason was, once again, the social phenomenon of war. During World War I, Lewis was a medical officer as Da Costa had been in the American Civil War. War had that unique potential to rapidly produce a set of symptoms and clinical signs, which probably had remained quiescent in civilian life, that could easily be attributed to a psychological cause. Shortly before the conclusion of the war, Lewis published a book, *The Soldier's Heart and The Effort Syndrome*, which established the criteria for distinguishing between organic and inorganic heart disease. The book's purpose was to assist military physicians in choosing men for active duty. Lewis was convinced the systolic murmur had been responsible for the unnecessary discharge of soldiers from the army as permanently unfit. To Lewis this was a supposed cardiac illness. Disturbances in the cardiovascular system, he said, had numbered one for every four cases of wound.[46] Since the war had a huge appetite for manpower, this was clearly disastrous to the nation's defence.

Lewis and Da Costa had observed the same symptoms produced under the same conditions of maximum psychological and physiological stress. Lewis chose to believe that Da Costa had fostered the idea that "irritable" heart lead to permanent cardiac enlargement[47] when, in fact, Da Costa had debated the issue and discredited the condition, concluding that the hypertrophy was transitory as was the edema. Lewis appears to have deliberately misrepresented Da Costa's views in order to emphasize all the more forcibly his own theory that what both were describing was a set of symptoms and not a disease.

Although he described a number of murmurs, Lewis, in reality, was talking about different aspects of the same systolic murmur. One of the murmurs, which he found most common in both soldiers and civilians, he called the "cardiorespiratory murmur."[48] Doctors, as late as 1968, equated this murmur with the extra-cardiac murmur of Gallavardin and, hence, with the late systolic murmur of MVP. In that year, 1968, Caceres described the cardiorespiratory murmur at great length; it was innocent, often introduced by a click and found generally in patients with pectus excavatum or the indented sternum found in both MVP and Marfan's disease.[49]

Lewis associated this murmur with rapid heart beat and described it as best heard at the apex as a short, high-pitched, blowing sound, the last word being the one Da Costa had favoured. Lewis dismissed this murmur as no more than a breath sound, "the natural accompaniment of the over-reacting heart."[50] Other murmurs he described were clearly linked with pericarditis as Gallavardin had observed. In these cases, Lewis considered the extracardiac sound to be produced by "roughening of the pericardium or pleura", that is the serus membrane covering the lung.[51]

Like Da Costa, Cuffer and Barbillion, Lewis observed that the systolic murmurs varied in length and intensity according to different examination postures.[52] This was one of the important clues that modern researchers would use to link MVP with many of these earlier murmurs. In the controversy over their significance, Lewis unequivocally stated that these sounds likely came from outside the heart and, therefore, had little prognostic significance. As a matter of course, he did not mention Griffith and Hall.

But Lewis was not content with an attack on the seriousness of the systolic murmur. He attacked the whole traditional concept that the sound of a murmur, heard with the ear or the stethoscope, meant that there was a leaky mitral valve, and he was, evidently, the first to do this. "There are no symptoms to be attributed usefully to mitral regurgitation," he said. "The only sign that can be named is a systolic murmur."[53] Even the pansystolic murmur, established as the hallmark of regurgitation, is unverifiable in Lewis' view, unless there is a history of rheumatic heart disease and probably a diastolic murmur as well. He says that pathological evidence cannot be found in the valves at autopsy and though he described a stretched, relaxed or "wide" mitral ring,[54] an observation made in cases of MVP[55] today, any thought that this could cause leaking, Lewis dismissed because of the absence, as far as his ears were concerned, of a murmur in life in many of his cases. And though he described "crumpling" of the mitral valve at its edges, a description that also closely resembles that of modern pathological observations, he did not regard this as an indication of valvular disease since many men, he vowed, carry this into old age.[56]

Lewis concluded that the systolic murmur only meant regurgitation in cases of obvious bacterial infection, or IE, with cardiac enlargement, or in the elderly. Age per se means a dilated heart, he declared imperiously, and, thus, blood must be leaking during systole from ventricle to atrium.

> Confidence in the value of a diagnosis of mitral regurgitation is reduced not only by frequent doubts as to whether regurgitation actually exists or not, but by our total inability to state its degree if it is there. There may be some grounds, though they remain inadequate, for claiming that harshness, thrill, (a fine vibration felt when the hand is placed over the heart) audibility over a wide area, or other characteristics, mark the murmur of mitral regurgitation; no claim has yet been made that particular qualities betray the slight or the large leak. Assuredly if the diagnosis of regurgitation, qua regurgitation, matters, it matters according to its degree. Briefly, the diagnosis of mitral regurgitation has a very limited importance, it may be useful as an early indication of muscular failure in acute infectious disease and occasionally in old age."[57]

Lewis warns emphatically that the mitral murmur "should not be allowed to modify prognosis or treatment" and "to regard any distinct systolic apical murmur as meaning a diseased valve is indefensible."[58] Indefensible! These are strong words that have influenced medical opinion for well over half of the 20thC with disastrous repercussions for many unfortunate people.

There is particular tragic irony in Lewis' casual remark that it is the degree of regurgitation that matters. It was precisely this that mattered at the time of my illness, that signified that I, in fact, had an IE which was ignored by every doctor and dentist who saw me. For Lewis seeing was believing. Proof of regurgitation would have to await the advent of cineangiography when the leakage could be quantitated and correlated with the auscultatory features of MVP. But, even today, despite the observations made with angiographic studies, my internist argues that there is no proof that the PSM denotes a larger leak than the LSM. Lewis' opinion, indicative of his cautiousness, on behalf of the war effort, and his lack of imagination did not alter in the twenty year period in which his book, *The Soldier's Heart and the Effort Syndrome* saw two printings.

James MacKenzie and the Escape Mechanism Theory

James MacKenzie, who with Lewis founded the medical journal, *Heart*, topped his contemporary by concocting what must be one of the wildest hypotheses in medical history. To crush the idea that mitral regurgitation had any importance whatsoever, MacKenzie proposed the "escape mechanism" theory. In his 1913 textbook, *Diseases of the Heart*, Mackenzie explained how regurgitation could be beneficial to the healthy, excellent function of the heart.

"If we consider how little we know of the causation of murmurs, it will be realized how little justification we have for treating them as abnormalities. Even if they were due to regurgitation, it is quite conceivable that the regurgitation might be an essential to a good functioning heart."[59]

In effort, MacKenzie explained with allusion to Lewis, the heart is over distended with more blood and cannot contract as strongly or forcefully as it should. This blood must remain in the ventricle. Leakage back into the storage chamber of the atrium would offer a natural escape device for some of the extra blood to relieve the chamber of over distension, thus preventing eventual hypertrophy of that organ from repetition of the same set of events over time. MacKenzie, of course, completely overlooked enlargement of the left atrium and the effects on the body of an inadequate supply of blood. This design created by God or Mother Nature must be accepted, he insisted, because "the fear of regurgitation has attained the dimensions of a bogy in the medical mind" and ought to be laid to rest.[60] Lewis had advocated dismissing regurgitation because he felt it could not be known whether it was there or not, and MacKenzie advised accepting it as part of our physiology designed by the Creator.

The Cat and The Pigeons

One year before the introduction of lifesaving antibiotics that could have been used from the beginning to prevent IE in patients with late systolic murmurs, the controversy reached its zenith, exploding in the pages of the distinguished *British Medical Journal*. In a 1943 article, William Evans, using the same arguments as Lewis, that regurgitation could not be proven scientifically, boldly pronounced that the term, mitral incompetence, ought to be struck from the medical vocabulary. Fifty years and more of time, effort and expense would simply be cast aside in the typical cyclical journey of medical research. "It is time," Evans said, in discussing regurgitant murmurs, "to be rid of the term; if preserved it will continue to frustrate the proper management of patients presenting them. The time is overdue to unify our views on the commonest of them all, the systolic murmur in the mitral area."[61]

Evans, like researchers today, bolstered his confidence in his own claims by reliance on technology. "Electrocardiography and cardioscopy" (x-ray of the heart) will prove definitively, he said, whether there is disease of the heart by identifying accurately the second gold standard after stenosis, that of hypertrophy, alterations in the size and shape of the heart. The absence of these two features, stenosis and hypertrophy of the heart muscle, would confirm that all "queer" sounds in systole are totally insignificant. The idea that the heart must be "large" before a diagnosis of disease or failure can be made persists today, confusing the picture in cases such as mine, and likely that of many other patients with MVP, where the heart is smaller than normal to begin with and thus when it enlarges remains within generally accepted measurements. Evans had influence, but his attempts to explain why systolic murmurs should be dismissed were unsound. In discussing these, he said that he found them frequently in people with "conspicuous depression of the sternum",[62] or, in other words, the flat chest or "slick chick of Dr. Warren, or the "pectus excavatum" of the full-blown Marfan's patient. In one of the most confused and contradictory pieces of writing in the medical literature, Evans claimed that "when the murmur is decidedly louder in the upright posture it is the innocent kind" and in "instances in which a trivial systolic murmur becomes louder in the reclining posture . . . the innocent nature of the murmur can be presumed."[63]

Several of Evans' colleagues responded with dismay or scorn. C. H. Ross Carmichael, for instance, said he discussed the article with his colleagues and found all of them as confused as himself by Evans' "foggy" reasoning and "hazy" theories.[64] And Dr. Gaskell, another colleague, said that the befuddled logic of Evans prompted him to write that "at first I thought that, after forty years of continuous auscultation of hearts and trying to estimate the significance of abnormal noises, especially while on medical boards, the complete fogging induced in my mind by his article was the result of my own senility, though I was not conscious of any mental deterioration."[65] The inference is that Evans' own opinions reflect senility. It is unfortunate that the frankness, the criticism, the checks and balances, manifested in these debates expressed in the medical literature of the forties, are virtually absent from the medical literature today.

Gaskell also recognized the true nature of Evans' article. As he meta-phorically stated it, this article "put the cat among the pigeons".[66] The purpose of Evans, the cat, is to scare off the pigeons who believe that extra systolic sounds mean mitral incompetence. Doctors, in 1980, in my own case, were actually using the foggy arguments of Evans when they insisted that, though my murmur had become louder and longer in the upright position, it was still innocent or benign just as it was before the infection.

It can only be called tragic that this thin vein of truth running through the older medical literature was not dug out and given prominence. Gaskell reasoned, as did Griffith and Hall, that:

> all noises or sounds must be the result of some physical phenomenon: nobody at least can dispute that. Surely stenosis or no stenosis, there must be regurgitation of blood back through the mitral orifice. What else could cause the sound we hear? The blood is already in the ventricle before we hear it, the ventricle contracts, and unless the sound is caused by regurgitation back through the valve it must be caused by something else, and is, therefore, not a mitral murmur. If it is caused by back-rush through a damaged valve, then the valve is incompetent or leaky and there must be such a thing as mitral incompetence. You cannot have it both ways.[67]

Paul White and Papillary Muscle Dysfunction

Disease or no disease, regurgitation or no regurgitation. This was the question. Other writers of the first half of the century challenged the non-disease theory with sound explanations that proved to be verifiable today. In 1931, Paul White, taking up an observation that Lewis had made from autopsies of soldiers' hearts but had discarded and that has since been verified by modern pathological examinations, suggested that extra systolic sounds, clicks and apical murmurs, could be accompanied by regurgitation and dilatation of the heart due to stretching of the mitral valve ring and downward displacement of the papillary muscle.[68] In other words, an unknown disease, which doctors of the seventies and eighties would investigate, was weakening the valvular tissue. White also pointed out that abnormal chordae, which are elongated or stretched, a pathologically proven feature of MVP, could also cause the valve leaflets to close improperly.[69] It might be remembered that Hall had also pointed at the papillary muscle as the causative factor and that both Griffith and Lewis described stretching of parts of the valvular apparatus, in particular valve rings.

The Revival of the Extra Cardiac Theory in the 20th Century

As late as 1958, modern, supposedly sophisticated "pigeons" were falling prey to the cat. Aubrey Leatham, who would later call all the attention MVP received a "fiasco",[70] was still hammering away at the extracardiac theory of 1913. In a paper, which summarized auscultatory signs, he redefined the extra systolic sounds of Gallavardin and reconfirmed the position that they do not come from within the heart and thus are unrelated to disease of the valves. His opinion comes almost one hundred years after Da Costa first drew attention to the peculiar disorder which he called "Irritable Heart".

> Extracardiac sounds occur about mid or late systole, after ejection at a time when . . . no valve movements are taking place . . . thus timing of these sounds strongly suggests that they are not intracardiac and this is supported by their tendency to great variation within the phase of respiration and with posture. They are entirely innocent and may be frequently pericardial in origin.[71]

Leatham fell, like all the others, into two traps. He could not believe a valve would leak in late systole because of the accepted notion of the hemodynamics of cardiac function and, like Evans and the much earlier writers, the variability in intensity of the murmur with respiration and position of the patient could only point to the insignificance of the sounds. By 1980 Leatham had written a paper which showed he had finally abandoned Gallavardin's theory.

Pathological Evidence of Disease

The turning point in the whole debate over extra systolic sounds came when Dr. J.V.O. Reid of the University of Natal in Durban, South Africa revived White's neglected theory of the chordal origin for the clicks. His 1961[72] study revealed that the hearts of five of his patients with murmurs had, at autopsy, definite pathological abnormalities. Hence the value of autopsy to research. Like Hall, Reid implicated the papillary muscle. He explained that either a diseased papillary muscle was improperly contracting or the chordae that hold the valve in place, being too long because they were stretched, would slacken in mid-systole preventing the leaflets from coming together securely. This would happen once the pressure in the ventricle declined and the heart became smaller. Such a theory would not have to take into account the longstanding hemodynamic concepts which Leatham and others could not overcome, that the leak should occur when the pressure in the ventricle is at its greatest at or near the beginning of systole at the moment blood is forced out of the ventricle.

Reid coined the word, "chordal snap"[73], to describe how the elongated chordae could, at the time of highest pressure in the ventricle, be snapped taut, with expansion of the heart filled with blood, producing the sound of a click. Like his predecessors, Reid realized that pathological change in any of the parts of the heart necessary to complete successful systole could "predispose to the occurrence of a mid-systolic click and be found especially in cases where there is a murmur."[74]

The squabble of the cats and pigeons would temporarily grind to a halt in the sixties when the pigeons would bring forward incontrovertible evidence which the cats, still clinging to their old ways, could no longer attack and kill. The pigeons, for a time, were not to be frightened off by the louder cries of the cats. But some cats, like Austin, would remain unconvinced, resulting in tragedy for their patients.

13

Witwatersrand:
The Gold Under the Reef

There is clinical evidence consistent with mitral valve prolapse in the form of a non-ejection click at the apex. This diagnosis has been established on a number of occasions and historically, there is echocardiographic evidence which supports this. I do not believe, however, that the murmur is mitral regurgitant . . .

Personal communication from a cardiologist to my general physician,
August 3, 1983.

The Late Systolic Murmur

Witwatersrand means white waters reef and is the name of the university in South Africa where Dr. John Barlow is Chief of the Cardiovascular Division. Prior to my illness, when I was searching for information on MVP, Barlow's name was one of the first I came across. In 1965, a cardiology convention was held on the subject of late systolic murmurs and non-ejection clicks or MVP at Witwatersrand. Dr. Barlow was asked to speak and, on introducing him, Dr. Bernard Tabatznik drew attention to the metaphorical implication of the name, Witwatersrand; it is under this reef with the beautiful-sounding name that the gold lies. Barlow, who is also associated with the Johannesburg Hospital, was born in Capetown and obtained his medical education in Johannesburg and London. Like W. Proctor Harvey, Barlow has maintained a keen interest in auscultation of the heart throughout his professional life. His expertise in this area has been captured on recordings that are used to assist medical students all over the world in learning how to listen to heart sounds. In the words of his colleague, Tabatznik, Dr. Barlow is "unique", "controversial", "iconoclastic" and this is likely why he could, unlike his contemporaries, come to some startling conclusions about the hotly debated extra systolic sounds.[1] The controversy he stirred up regarding MVP set, as Gaskell had put it, the pigeon among the cats.

In October of 1963, Barlow published an immensely significant paper on MVP in the *American Heart Journal.* In it, he demonstrated indisputably that the murmur heard in late systole was, like the traditional PSM, caused by the regurgitation of blood backwards through a mitral valve that was incompetent only late in systole.[2] This was, indeed, the gold under the white reef, the precious knowledge that could save patients from deterioration of their valves and, ultimately, from death. Barlow's work demolished, forever, the doubts that extra systolic sounds, clicks and murmurs, came from inside the heart and indicated valvular disease and regurgitation. Barlow was able to confirm unequivocally that blood leaked into the atrium in late systole by means of cineangiography, specifically catheterization of the left ventricle. This invasive test involves the insertion of a long, slender and flexible tube, called a catheter, via the femoral artery in the groin, threading it, retrograde, against the blood flow, up the aorta, across the aortic valve and into the left ventricle. A radiographic contrast material, or dye, is then injected which permits high speed x-ray motion pictures or ventriculograms. The severity of regurgitation, the presence of congenital or acquired valvular lesions, the pressure in the left ventricle and its motion, the volume of blood in the heart at the end of systole and diastole and the ejection fraction, which is the percentage of blood pumped out of the ventricle with each systole are among the determinants of the heart's pumping function that can be measured.

However despite modern medical technology that permits visualization of the mysterious workings of the heart, without imagination, Barlow would never have undertaken such a quest to prove the existence of mitral regurgitation in late systole. Barlow not only proved this but also attempted to quantitate the leakage and correlate it with clinical signs, the systolic sounds heard on auscultation. He found that "the amount of dye which entered the left atrium was surprisingly large in the patients with pansystolic murmurs, whereas, in those with murmurs confined to late systole, a small jet was seen with each ventricular systole."[3] Barlow and co-workers also found that, in 25 patients with no clinical signs of mitral regurgitation, i.e. the sound of a murmur, there was no blood forced back into the left atrium. In a later paper, published in 1984, which Dr. Barlow sent to me, he stated that "patients with holosystolic murmurs have relatively marked MVP."[4] Barlow's studies provided additional proof for me that my mysterious "infection", which was accompanied by a change in my murmur from late systolic to pansystolic, meant that the leak in my valve was more severe. My symptoms of SOB with exercise and increased fatigue had, therefore, some explanation.

After Barlow's observations organic disease of the mitral valve could no longer be denied in the presence of extra systolic signs of a murmur, despite the absence of the traditional markers of heart disease: cardiac enlargement and deformities of any part of the heart's structure. Like Da Costa, Lewis and McKenzie before him, Barlow emphasized the frequency of clicks and late systolic murmurs in the general population and said this was the cause of the presumed innocency of these sounds.

The Systolic Click

By the same hypothesis, which earlier researchers used to show that murmurs, like clicks, were extracardiac, Barlow suggested that, by association, the clicks, like the murmurs, are intracardiac. He drew upon the ideas of Reid, who was at the same hospital, that the clicks come from within the heart and are caused by disease of the chordae of the mitral valve. Pathological studies support this opinion. One of Barlow's female patients, who was known to have an isolated mid-systolic click in life, was found at autopsy to have a single, fibrosed mitral valve chorda, the cause of which, either rheumatic heart disease (RHD) or IE, was unknown. Another female patient who had a click in life and died of uremia had no abnormality of the heart except for pleural pericardial adhesions of the sort Gallavardin had described.[5] It might be asked, however, whether histological examination of the valvular tissues would have shown the presence of excessive mucopolysaccharides and thus the existence of MVP, or, taking into account the studies of Libman, if this woman's uremia had resulted from a remote episode of IE with kidney involvement.

Though this second case might seem to confirm Gallavardin's theory that clicks came from outside the heart, Barlow argued convincingly that the co-existence of clicks and murmurs in six of his other patients made it extremely unlikely that the clicks were extracardiac since he had now proven that late systolic murmurs were caused by mitral regurgitation. Barlow's belief that the clicks as well as the murmurs were intracardiac was verified a few years later, in 1966, when Criley et al, using the same cineangiographic techniques as Barlow had used, confirmed that the click came from within the heart and occurred at the point of maximal prolapse of the leaflets into the left atrium.[6]

Innocent Murmurs

Barlow's contemporaries in the United States, like McKusick and Humphries, at the famous Johns Hopkins School of Medicine in Baltimore, were, in 1962, still clinging to Gallavardin's extracardiac theory of pleural pericardial adhesions to explain mid-systolic clicks and LSMs. They claimed that the late systolic click and murmur were "due to pericardial roughening" since many of their patients had a "history of acute pericarditis"[7], and the LSM was, as Lewis, MacKenzie and Evans had believed, non-regurgitant and, therefore, innocent. Even though these authors observed the group of characteristics now associated with MVP, chest pain, palpitations, electrocardiographic T wave abnormalities, click, murmur, they did not favour mitral valve disease as an explanation.

Over the years, physicians have described and given names to what they regarded as the "innocent murmur". A long list of well over 100 synonymous names has accumulated. Most innocent murmurs, according to physicians, are heard in systole and are not associated with any disease or abnormality of the heart and its parts. Many of these names for so-called innocent murmurs have, no doubt, been and continue to be unwittingly applied to the murmur of MVP, such names as benign murmur, benign systolic ejection murmur, functional systolic ejection murmur, insignificant murmur, musical murmur, physiologic murmur, twanging string murmur[8] (which resembled Da Costa's "curiously broken, cartilaginous sound"). At least one of these common, so-called "innocent" murmurs, Lewis' "cardiorespiratory murmur", Barlow equated, in his 1963 paper, with the MSC and LSM of MVP. Yet, many doctors remained confused about what they were hearing with their stethoscopes. At the time of Barlow's initial studies, McKusick and Humphries were still calling the MVP murmur the "cardiorespiratory murmur" and claiming it was extracardiac and caused by a "lappet of lung" which in some state of inflation is impinged upon the heart."[9] In 1963, Segal and Likoff[10] from Philadelphia carried out the same cineangiographic studies as Barlow and Criley had done and concluded that LSMs without the clicks were due to mitral incompetence but LSMs with clicks were not due to regurgitation but were innocent, "cardiorespiratory murmurs". In a description almost identical to that of Humphries and McKusick, they said such murmurs were caused by "compression of a lung segment by the left ventricle" or ..."from vibrations of pericardial thickening, pleural or pericardial adhesions".[11] Gallavardin's shaky hypothesis still dominated in certain quarters long after it had outlived all logic.

We might be able to excuse doctors of the thirties for referring to the well known entity of the LSM and click in quaint, unscientific language as "something queer"[12] in the heart but not doctors of the sixties and seventies or even the eighties. Yet, researchers, Hancock and Cohn from Stanford, wrote that, in 1966, even "well-trained" residents, likely in internal medicine or cardiology, reported to them the finding of a "weird sounding heart" which they, obviously, did not equate with the "midsystolic click syndrome".[13] Other doctors were confusing the sounds of MVP with congenital conditions such as patent ductus arteriosus, which is an opening between the aorta and pulmonary artery that should close naturally shortly after birth, pericardial friction rub or just "bizarre unexplained findings".[14]

Understanding of a disease spreads very slowly within the ranks of the medical profession. This explains why it is years before the public actually benefits from research, though the medical profession still makes extravagant claims in the media about the speed with which medical science progresses. Countless individuals are still being told they have completely innocent murmurs most of which are identical. (See Appendix I at the end of the book) Such persons should be examined in the different postures and have an echocardiogram, or even a second opinion, to rule out MVP. My murmur had been given many of these innocent titles, beginning with the internist's vague comments in 1976 on the "noise" and the "queer sound" in my heart. Another cardiologist I saw in 1986 called my PSM a "pericardial friction rub". The echo he ordered showed no prolapse. Was this a technician's error and is this a significant factor in negative diagnoses? My present internist believes that this doctor was mistaking my long, loud PSM for the murmur of pericarditis manifested by a pericardial rub because PSMs are rare in young people with MVP. Obviously this cardiologist was still influenced by the ideas of Gallavardin and others of the past. Another cardiologist, the one quoted at the beginning of this chapter, called my MVP murmur a non-regurgitant, functional outflow murmur. This is equivalent to Dr. Peter Austin's description of a benign systolic ejection murmur or an "innocent" murmur without regurgitation. But, as discussed earlier, the SEM is radically different from either the typical LSM of MVP or the PSM which I had at the time of his examination. The SEM begins, according to many textbooks, after S_1 and increases and decreases with the outward flow or ejection of blood from the ventricles. SEM murmurs have a number of causes, chief among them are aortic or pulmonic stenosis, neither of which has ever been documented in me. Doubts are raised in my mind that doctors are no more skillful at identifying sounds in the heart than were their predecessors during the great debate over mitral incompetence in the *British Medical Journal*.

Barlow's proof that the LSM was a regurgitant murmur was the turning point in the history of MVP. As far as researchers, as opposed to clinicians, were concerned, the confusion surrounding the origin of the clicks and murmurs in systole soon dissolved. Reviews summarizing the history and development of the condition, its symptomatology, complications, prognosis and cause of its underlying pathology followed. The medical journals were deluged with articles on a condition that had been dismissed for over one hundred years as "innocent" or "benign", extracardiac and without evidence of disease of the heart and its valves.

The Naming of MVP

Researchers could not decide on a name for this entity, but, clearly, a single name was necessary to correlate the flood of information that would emerge on MVP. Barlow and co-workers had assembled a set of consistently appearing features into a syndrome: click, mid to late systolic murmur, electrocardiographic and cineangiographic signs.[15] Early in the attempts to describe the abnormalities found in the valves at autopsy, pathologists hit upon names like "parachute deformity of the mitral valve", a term which became so popular that a 1936 specimen of the mitral valve was preserved in the Pathological Museum of St. George's Hospital in London, England.[16] This is proof that the condition was regarded as an aberration, a disease, as early as 1936, and is not such a recent discovery. At autopsy, when the excised heart is artificially filled with a liquid to simulate the maximum pressure in the ventricles just before blood is ejected during systole, the prolapsed valve resembles an inflated parachute and, when collapsed, the elongated chords, looking like parachute strings, fold over upon one another. It is easy to imagine how some excessively long chords could function in this way during the relaxation phase of diastole and gradually with time become fused so as to appear thickened. Another popular name at that time was "blue valve syndrome", so-called since certain staining techniques turned prolapsed valves blue because of accumulated acid muco-polysaccharides in the tissues. This early designation, like the parachute deformity, again suggests that the underlying histological abnormalities were known long before the pathological studies of the sixties and after. "Blue valve syndrome" was abandoned because it was easily confused with another congenital abnormality, that of "chordal insertion into the papillary muscle".[17]

A naming contest ensued. People wishing to learn the important facts about MVP should be familiar with the names by which this disease went for a number of years. MVP has been called Billowing Sail Deformity (Oka and Angrist, 1961)[18], Mid-late Systolic Click and LSM (Barlow et al., 1968)[19], Billowing Mitral Valve Leaflet (Bittar and Sosa, 1968)[20], Ballooning Deformity of Atrioventricular Valves (Pomerance, 1969)[21], Floppy Valve Syndrome (Read et al., 1965)[22], Redundant Cusp Leaflet Syndrome (Hill et al., 1974)[23], Prolapsing Mitral Leaflet Syndrome (Natarajan et al., 1975)[24] and, of course Barlow's Syndrome (Cobbs, 1974)[25]. Although in 1979, Barlow was using the term Billowing Mitral Leaflet Syndrome, the most popular designation and the one seemingly decided upon by all is Mitral Valve Prolapse, a term first used by Criley and co-workers in 1966[26]. Their cineangiographic studies, like Barlow's, showed prolapse of the leaflets coinciding with mitral regurgitation. MVP is a name that allows for degrees of prolapse, since there may only be a click present, while MSC and LSM Syndrome does not.

The Importance of Diagnosing MVP

But, like Shakespeare, one might ask, "What's in a name?" The most important factor which overturned the 100 year old verdict, that the sounds were extracardiac and, thus, innocent, was Barlow's conclusion that there was valvular disease. The moment this was accepted, what had been called a benign condition for over a hundred years or more became a risky one, susceptible to the bacterial infection called IE. However, many of Barlow's contemporaries, such as Humphries, McKusick[27], Segal and Likoff[28], who did not recognize the condition as a disease, did not comment upon this risk in their reports or, therefore, on the need for antibiotic protection. The French, Facquet, Alhomme and Raharison of the Hôpital Tenon in Paris[29], were the first to report cases of IE in the MVP syndrome. They continued, however, to call MVP the Click and LSM syndrome. Old ideas die slow deaths, and the influence of Gallavardin still reigned. Despite the evidence of IE in association with clicks and murmurs, these observers claimed there was no underlying disease of the mitral valve. Though they heard the murmur and the classic click of MVP, they concluded that, because of the variability of this click, the sounds were coming from outside the heart, "d'une origine extracardiaque". These writers do not mention the studies of Barlow, and one wonders if the French had done no further investigation of extra systolic sounds since Gallavardin's influential conclusions. Does this mean that people have an unhealthy reverence for their national heroes or simply that medical knowledge remains tragically isolated within a particular group of doctors, medical centre or country?

Despite the diehards who refused to accept that the entity they had been discussing for a 100 years was, indeed, a disease, a flux of articles in the medical journals repeated Barlow's warning, predicated upon this fact of disease, that the MSC and LSM syndrome posed the risk of IE and, therefore, the necessity of protecting such patients with antibiotics during any procedure that might draw blood and introduce bacteria into the circulation. To list only a few of these important researchers who advocated such protection: LeBauer et al, 1966[30], Linhart and Taylor, 1966[31], Shell et al., 1969[32], Pomerance, 1969[33], Jeresaty, 1971[34], Littler et al., 1973[35], Perloff and Roberts, 1972[36], Pomerance, 1972[37], Kern et al., 1972[38], Hill et al., 1974[39], Kincaid and Botti, 1974[40], Lachman et al., 1975[41], Malcolm et al., 1976[42], Mills et al., 1977 [43], Hammond et al., 1978[44], Weinstein et al., 1979[45], Ringer et al., 1980[46], Shah and Winer, 1981[47], Rajan et al., 1982[48], MacMahon et al., 1987[49]. The list is monumental and shows clearly that the warning was in effect long before my MVP was first diagnosed in 1976 and my illness of 1979-80. In fact, as early as 1949, Harvey had made known, in his important textbook on auscultation of the heart, that the LSM presented the risk of IE, and the patient should be protected with antibiotics.[50]

Progression of Mitral Valve Prolapse

In the absence of IE, MVP is believed to deteriorate slowly. This is why protection from this disease becomes so crucial. Prolapse has been observed to progress from mild to severe during IE as indicated by an increase in the severity of the murmur. Prophylactic antibiotics can prevent this infection and, thus, further valvular deterioration which, either immediately or at some future date, results in cardiac enlargement and failure.

To understand what is meant by deterioration in the MVP syndrome, we might look at the scale described by Robert Jeresaty.[51] There are, according to this writer, four degrees of prolapse. Grade one, with virtually normal leaflets at autopsy but with some histological alterations in the increase in mucopolysaccharides in the valvular tissues, would appear to correlate with "silent" MVP or a click made audible only with pharmacological manoeuvers. No murmur is present. Grade two prolapse is characterized by a click but no mitral regurgitation, grade three by click and mild, mitral regurgitation indicated by a late systolic murmur and grade four by severe prolapse with "ballooned, hooded, floppy" valves at pathology and, in life, moderate to severe regurgitation indicated by a PSM. All categories, Jeresaty points out, share the same pathology, the mucopolysaccharide accumulation or myxomatous degeneration in varying degrees.

Some researchers have studied MVP over long periods of time. One study by Allen, Harris and Aubrey Leatham, published in 1974 [52], involved 62 patients who were followed for a period of 9 to 22 years. The conclusions of the study pointed to MVP as a stable condition. All patients in the study had minimal mitral regurgitation indicated by a LSM, as I had before my root canal work and dental abscess. In 41 of the patients, or about two-thirds, there was no deterioration over an average of 13.8 years, and one patient had retained a LSM for a total of 51 years. The deterioration, documented over a period of 3-18 years in 10 patients, consisted of no more than slight cardiac enlargement on x-ray and the change to "a more even PSM". The description of "a more even PSM" suggests that, in these patients, the PSM was probably heard in only certain examining positions or on certain occasions over many years, but then became constant. Without doubt, there are many people who have had medical histories identical to mine, and it is important to point out here that my murmur changed during my illness and was clearly heard as a PSM by a number of observers during and shortly after discharge from my first hospitalization.

Natural deterioration is believed to occur generally late in life. One patient in this same study was an elderly man whose regurgitation increased at the age of 74 after 11 years of observation. More rapid natural deterioration, where IE has not intervened, is found chiefly in patients with the more pronounced form of the connective tissue disorder that is called Marfan's disease. In the above study, two patients, with obvious skeletal evidence of Marfan's disease, deteriorated in a brief period of time, 3-5 years.

Marfan's Disease and MVP

It was the French physician, Marfan, who, in 1886, gave his name to a set of characteristics not unlike those of MVP. Specific physical features identify the patient with this more severe form of prolapse of the mitral valve, long, spidery fingers, pectus carinatum (a pigeon or shield breast bone that is high and rounded) or pectus excavatum (the indented or depressed sternum, recognized for years in association with the late systolic murmur of mitral incompetence) and a high arched palate which is found in both Marfan's and MVP. Marfan's individuals have an unmistakable tall, thin body with little muscular development, heads much longer than broad, armspans greater than their height, eye problems such as dislocated lens (ectopia lentis) and lateral curvature of the spine with vertebral rotation (kyphoscoliosis).[53]

In Marfan's individuals, the aorta and the aortic valve are afflicted more often than the mitral valve though both can be involved. While the same underlying tissue derangement exists in both MVP and Marfan's disease, the mucoid or myxomatous changes in the latter are more widespread and invasive and frequently result in dilatation of the aorta or an aneurysm in its walls, dissection of the layers of the aorta or pulmonary artery and aortic valve insufficiency. In such cases, the build up of excessive acid mucopolysaccharides so weakens the healthy elastic connective tissues of the medial layer of the aorta or pulmonary artery that they deteriorate and die or necrose, thus the name "cystic medial necrosis of the aorta"[54]. The resultant dilatation and weakening of the aorta and parts of the aortic valve resemble the ballooning or bulging of the mitral valve leaflets in MVP.

Some researchers believe that the presence of mucopolysaccharides in prolapsed valves signifies that MVP is just an undeveloped or latent form, what doctors call a "forme fruste", of Marfan's disease with few, if any, of the major symptoms or features.[55] Others, like Jeresaty, feel there is insufficient evidence to relate MVP and Marfan's disease;[56] though prolapse occurs in Marfan's, the other physical features do not occur in MVP. An individual with Marfan's disease could be recognized on the strength of the physical aberrations alone while a MVP patient could not, since the occulo-skeletal features are far less pronounced. It is appropriate therefore, to stress, once again, that my deterioration took place within one year, in the presence of an obvious oral infection and symptoms of IE and without any evidence of the physical derangements of Marfan's disease. Nor did I have any of the other conditions which share the same connective tissue abnormality that Marfan's and MVP share, such as osteo genesis imperfecta, a congenital disorder characterized by obvious physical derangements such as blue sclerae, deafness, acquired later in life, porotic bones on x-ray, bony protruberances of the skull and a triangular face with more severe cardiac involvement.[57] These diseases underline the stability of the simple form of the MSC and LSM syndrome. Thus it is extremely difficult to accept that my echocardiographic changes, as Dr. Adami stressed, were simply the result of sudden natural deterioration from increased myxomatous tissue in the valve.

It appears that many doctors are unaware that there are degrees of prolapse. Every symptom may, therefore, not be typical of MVP but vary with the extent of myxomatous degeneration. Austin and others whom I saw after my hospitalization emphasized that my symptom of SOB was "typical" of MVP but I had never experienced this before. My principal clinical findings were an increase in mitral regurgitation with corresponding lengthening of my murmur and cardiac enlargement, all of which could have explained my SOB at that time. There are reports of patients with PSMs who are in Class II of the New York Heart Association's classification of heart failure, that is comfortable at rest but symptomatic (manifesting breathlessness) with ordinary activity, which would include climbing of stairs and hills, and who require valvular repair or replacement.[58] "Significant" cardiac enlargement has traditionally been regarded as a sign of deterioration. However, cardiac enlargement in the MVP patients described by Allen et al in 1974, was slight and less than what it might be in association with other causes of regurgitation.[59] Doctors may be looking for significant cardiac enlargement, and, if it is not present, symptoms such as edema and SOB, ordinarily associated with heart failure, will be overlooked in the MVP syndrome as unimportant as they once were to Da Costa.

The Risk of IE in the MVP Syndrome

How great is the risk of IE to the MVP patient? The majority of researchers maintain that the risk is significant. Only a small number of cases have actually been reported in the medical literature. Over a period of twenty years from the publication of the first case by the French writers, Facquet et al, in 1964, to the early eighties only 267 cases of IE and MVP have been documented in the English medical literature according to Baddour and Bisno.[60] IE, however, is not a reportable disease, and, thus, an accurate estimation of its prevalence is unobtainable.[61] Certainly, every diagnosed case of IE with MVP, even where MVP has been documented previously, will not be described in the medical literature. The number of deaths from IE with underlying MVP and the number of undiagnosed mild cases such as mine are not known. Asymptomatic MVP patients with silent prolapse or an isolated click will not likely come to a physician's attention until acute IE is present. But by then the murmur would probably be pansystolic and, thus, attributed to the IE, itself, while no effort would be made to determine the underlying disease of prolapse. Frequently, MVP is first diagnosed at the time of an IE.[62] According to researchers from Stanford, only a small number of MVP patients ever come to medical attention and, therefore, a large population exists with unidentified, subclinical prolapse.[63] The value of identifying these patients is obvious considering the gravity of the risk of IE.

The Systolic Click and IE

The question of whether or not all degrees of prolapse pose the same risk has been discussed in the literature. In his book on MVP, Jeresaty does not recommend antibiotic prophylaxis in patients with "silent" prolapse, that is, no detectable click or murmur, nor in patients with only a click unless dental manipulations or surgery involve an infected site.[64] He bases his opinion on the infrequency of cases of IE in patients with only a click reported in the literature. At the time of his writing, there were only seven cases.[65] However, the cases he describes provoke some questions. One of the patients, a female, presented with IE and a PSM. But five years before this episode, no cardiac abnormality had been noted at her physical examinations. The doctors involved felt that this patient may have had "silent prolapse".[66] Did the IE cause the PSM, and how many people with PSMs or LSMs and IE had undocumented "silent prolapse"?

The latest American Heart Association recommendations for the use of antibiotics in MVP patients, printed in 1984,[67] which Canadian doctors and dentists are required to follow in the absence of any other similar Canadian authority, do not include prolapse with only a click. However, there are American physicians who are emphatic in their recommendation of antibiotic prophylaxis for patients with an isolated click. At Georgetown University, where a case of IE and MVP with click was observed, a female doctor reported that, although she was not taught this ruling in medical school, she was aware that the majority of cardiologists in the Washington, D.C. area advocate prophylaxis with only a click.[68] Again, this suggests that one's fate is bound up inextricably with one's locale.

IE as a Cause of Prolapse

The question of whether IE itself causes prolapse of the valves, or increases the bulging and ballooning, has not been adequately investigated. Researchers only mention the causal relationship in passing, but, in my view, this is an area that requires urgent study. If it could be shown that IE increases or causes the prolapse, more effort would go into identifying and protecting patients with only a click. Some of the documented cases of IE and only a click raise this interesting question of the causal relationship between IE and MVP. In 1968, LeBauer et al[69] described a patient with a click, recorded over a period of six years, in whom a murmur appeared for the first time during the infection on the tenth day of therapy but persisted for the rest of the patient's hospitalization. A month after discharge on a recall visit, this murmur was undetectable. Another case published in 1974 by Kincaid and Botti[70] described a young female patient, eighteen years old, who had no recorded cardiac abnormality, not even a click. During her IE, a LSM was heard for the first time but only with certain pharmacological tests which increased the heart rate. Her murmur did not disappear with treatment but became a PSM. After discharge from hospital, a LSM could be heard but only with isometric hand grip exercises which increase cardiac output by elevating blood pressure and increasing heart rate or increasing the work of the heart. Did the IE make a minor prolapse severe enough to cause leaking and the sound of a murmur in these cases? And would this patient's PSM reappear later on?

In 1975, Lachman and others, including John Barlow, from the Cardiovascular Research unit at Witwatersrand University and the Cardiac Clinic of the Johannesburg General Hospital[71] reported on ten patients of whom seven, without history of any cardiac abnormality, had prolapse detected only at the time of their IE. Eight patients had both a LSM and a click and two had only a click at the time of diagnosis of IE. Only one of the patients developed severe regurgitation during the infection. In support of the fact that IE could have caused an increase in the prolapse, and therefore, a murmur, it might be pointed out that, had the patients' IE been superimposed on a prolapse severe enough to create a LSM, the likelihood is that the LSM would have become a PSM. Did early treatment in these cases prevent progression to the more severe prolapse manifested by a PSM?

In most cases of IE, the crucial concern seems to be to detect the IE early enough to prevent progression of the prolapse and the resultant mitral regurgitation. Dr. Barlow has stated in a recent article that "Excepting patients with Marfan's syndrome, progression to severe mitral regurgitation is uncommon and the majority of patients have little or no increase in the degree of incompetence . . . In the absence of infective endocarditis, we have seldom observed such progression."[72]

IE and the LSM

There are many more reports that document IE in patients with both click and LSM than with just the click. This may suggest that the more severe the prolapse, the greater the risk of IE. Researchers, like Linhart and Taylor, 1966[73] from the University of Florida, as well as Jeresaty[74], believe that such patients likely had a milder prolapse earlier in their history and suffered further damage to their mitral valves during the infection. Linhart et al concluded that, with correct treatment, the murmur can remain the same as it was before the infection.

The burning question of whether IE itself increases the prolapse was raised in a study from Stanford University.[75] This impressive report documents the progression, during IE, of LSMs to PSMs which did not disappear after treatment. This study also indicates the prevalency of IE in the MVP syndrome. One third of the patients with IE in this study conducted over a five year period had underlying MVP.

The disastrous clinical courses of many of the patients in this study, in spite of treatment with intravenous bactericidal drugs, emphasizes the importance of preventing IE in MVP patients. 22 of 25 patients presented with a PSM at the time of detection of IE and, of these, six, all males, were known to have only a LSM before the infection, thus confirming the belief that patients begin with milder forms of prolapse. It also raises the question of whether the MVP syndrome itself is caused by repeated mild episodes of IE that remain undetected as Libman had described throughout his career.

Nine of the patients in the study required mitral valve replacement because of CHF that developed at intervals of from two to twenty years. Recurrences of IE were not uncommon; there were three cases in this Stanford study. This fact suggests that one episode increases the risk of another since further damage of the valve will make the deposition of bacteria and thus the creation of vegetations on the valve that much easier.

The question of whether IE causes the prolapse occurred to these Stanford researchers but they rejected a causal relationship. Only seven of their 25 patients had evidence of prolapse prior to their IE. Six of these patients had a click and a LSM. The other eighteen patients only came to medical attention at the time of their IE when MVP was confirmed by echo. One of the arguments they advanced for rejection of the causal relationship was the old one of histological evidence of myxomatous degeneration but this evidence is inconclusive since there is no way of proving the extent of the tissue disturbance prior to infection or that the accumulation of polysaccharides was not caused by the IE. Because there was an equal number of patients with prolapse and without, who had IE, the Stanford group felt this was "reasonable" evidence that the prolapse was not caused by the IE.

Rather than consider that the patients with PSMs might have had a click and LSM prior to the infection or even "silent prolapse", the authors conclude that the PSM of MVP is more susceptible to IE and that the prolapse in these cases did not become more severe. However, it seems more logical that, if a patient already had severe regurgitation from a severely prolapsed valve, as indicated by a PSM, the vegetations on the valve would then cause heart failure at the time of the illness and not two to twenty years later.

How IE Seeds Itself on the Valve

The Stanford researchers doubt their own conclusion and refer to the seminal works of Simon Rodbard at the University of New York at Buffalo to explain their reasoning.[76] One can see a debate about whether or not IE causes MVP shaping up of the dimensions of that between Evans and his colleagues over the significance of mitral regurgitation. Rodbard's studies show just why the LSM of MVP, as opposed to other cardiac problems, in particular RHD, is so susceptible to bacterial infection. In 1963, Rodbard published a paper with his observations on the relationship between blood velocity and the seeding of bacteria in the heart. He experimented using a permeable tube through which fluid from a high pressure source was driven through a constriction in the tube into a low pressure area. An aerosol containing bacteria injected into the tube allowed him to observe its deposition beyond the constriction. In applying these observations to the heart, Rodbard concluded that the jet stream effect created by blood being forced retrograde at a critical velocity from a high pressure source (i.e.the left ventricle during systole) through a narrow orifice (a small opening in a nearly closed valve) into a low pressure area (atrium) enchanced the seeding process of IE on the atrial surface of the valve. The jet stream effect is analogous to the effect created when one holds a finger over a water faucet turned on full. The jet stream becomes very forceful.

Rodbard's principles can be applied to MVP. Cineangiography demonstrates that the flow of blood backwards into the atrium through the mildly prolapsed valve, as in the case of the LSM, takes the form of a jet stream. In 1966, a group of researchers at the University of Pittsburgh School of Medicine observed "the mitral regurgitant jet being played across the atrium in much the same fashion as one applies paint with a paint spray."[77] And, in 1969, Ariela Pomerance [78] reported on the marked pathological evidence of these "jet lesions" on the atrial walls and anterior mitral cusps of the prolapsed valves from where the blood struck forcefully. It seems that very conscientious medical researchers such as Graham Hayward,[79] only ten years after Barlow's studies which drew attention to the risk of IE, were noting the prevalence of the anatomical sign of the jet lesion from "the posterior cusp defect" of MVP in the presence of vegetations from IE. And, even then, Hayward concluded that such mild lesions as that from the LSM of these prolapsed valves enhanced the vulnerability to the seeding process of IE while severe mitral regurgitation with a large atrium was not found in conjunction with IE. Though Rodbard and Barlow published their observations in the same year, 1963, neither refers to the other, yet Rodbard's conclusions support the theory that MVP with a LSM puts the patient at great risk of IE.

MVP vs Mitral Stenosis as a Risk Factor

Rodbard's studies also overturned the centry old theory that the stenosed valves caused from repeated episodes of rheumatic fever are the most susceptible to IE. Rodbard proved that it is the incompetent, leaky mitral valve from a condition such as MVP that is found more frequently in the presence of vegetations. As evidence, he cited thirty cases in one hospital series of pure mitral incompetence, ten of which developed IE. As well, Cutler's studies in 1958, Rodbard said, showed that bacterial vegetations are found "on incompetent mitral and aortic valves whereas pure acquired stenotic lesions are rarely sites of bacterial invasion."[80]

Another important study in 1977 showed that, in 59 patients[81] who died after anti-microbial treatment for IE, "unequivocal residua of valve infection" was more common in incompetent, regurgitant valves than in narrow, stenosed valves of RHD and, furthermore, was found frequently in prolapsed valves. The authors attribute the deformities of the valve to the IE itself. We are reminded that earlier comparisons of extra systolic sounds, the mid-late systolic murmur of mitral regurgitation, with what was believed to be the graver condition of RHD and valvular stenosis paved the way for years of repudiation of the importance of systolic clicks and murmurs and retarded appreciably the understanding of their true nature.

Paradoxically, Rodbard pointed out that further deformation of the mitral valve by IE actually heals the infection because, once the orifice is widened, the pressure gradient between left ventricle and left atrium diminishes or disappears and, with it, the jet stream mechanism that favours the seeding of bacteria. This could explain the frequency of healing, without treatment, which Libman had described. Several important writers on IE have noted that severe regurgitation and CHF does not appear to predispose the patient to IE. Like these later researchers, Hayward and Rodbard, Libman had observed that patients with mild valvular defects and few or no symptoms were the most susceptible to IE.[82] We can see, then why the Stanford researchers doubted their own hypothesis that the PSM creates greater susceptibility to IE.

It is surprising that this group from Stanford also claimed, without giving supporting data, that 30 to 40 percent of prolapse patients have, on echo, holosystolic murmurs without any sign of bacterial infection.[83] This startling statement contradicts other studies which claim that the PSM with more severe regurgitation is found only in about ten percent of the MVP population and usually in the elderly for reasons already discussed. Can all these pansystolic murmurs with supposedly no history of infection be accounted for? Are they the culmination of a number of episodes of mild, undiagnosed IE treated with oral antibiotics, as I was, or spontaneously healed, as Libman observed? Contrary to what the many doctors said to me, the patient, as Libman's studies showed, does not invariably die immediately from IE. Rodbard's studies support Libman's conviction that mild cases exist which leave the patient with further valvular damage that prepares the way for CHF. Since the PSM can "cure" the infection, as Rodbard hypothesized, perhaps antibiotics cannot take all the credit in every case, and the whole notion of IE as an immediately lethal, very rare disease should be re-examined in an effort to understand MVP. In Libman's experience, IE was a common not a rare disease.[84]

Curiously, the percentage figure that the Stanford group tossed out corresponded with a report from Guy and co-workers[85] in Nova Scotia in 1980 which showed that prolapse was the single most common cause of moderate or severe regurgitation with the clinical sign of a PSM necessitating mitral valve replacement or repair and that 50 percent of these patients had underlying MVP. And, in 1982, a study was published which showed that 62 percent of the patients with severe regurgitation requiring valvular replacement had MVP.[86] The authors of these studies, like Rodbard, regard MVP as superseding RHD as the most common cause for replacement or repair of heart valves because of moderate or severe regurgitation.

It should be overwhelmingly evident from the previous discussion that MVP can no longer be regarded as a benign cardiac condition and the LSM no longer innocent. Many researchers, appreciating just how serious a risk IE is in this syndrome, regard it as a major and frequent complication. A Yale University of Medicine study dramatically concluded that, when IE involves the mitral valve, MVP is *almost always* associated with it and they warned that further studies are needed on the cause and effect relationship between MVP and IE.[87]

In his book, *Infective Endocarditis and Other Intravascular Infections*, published in 1983, Lawrence Freedman stated that the MVP patient's chance of acquiring IE is eight times that of a person with normal valves.[88] Freedman ranked MVP in the high risk category, next to patients with a previous episode of IE, a heart valve prosthesis or coarctation of the aorta.[89] Another recent study done in 1987 warned that the risk of IE for patients with MVP and a murmur is thirteen times greater than that for MVP patients without murmurs.[90]

It, therefore, boggles the mind that, with all the evidence in the medical literature, modern doctors, like their predecessors of over 100 years ago, still declare this syndrome to be insignificant and are still not assessing their patients for MVP and providing them with antibiotic prophylaxis against IE.

14

The War with the Microbes

Below the age of 35 years, 59 percent of patients in the Medical Research Council series were female: over that age 61 percent were male. It will be seen later that part of the reason for this difference is that infection of the mitral valve is far more common in young women.

> J.E. Cates and R.V. Christie. "Subacute Bacterial Endocarditis: Penicillin Trials Committee of The Medical Research Council." (April, 1951) *Quarterly Journal of Medicine* 20 (78): 93-130.

To show how completely *silent* the disease of subacute bacterial endocarditis may be we can quote two cases from the records of the medical examiner. These were young men, apparently in perfect health, who died by violence. The classical pathological picture of subacute bacterial endocarditis was found in the hearts . . . From the foregoing discussion it may be concluded that subacute bacterial endocarditis is probably more common than it has been considered to be in the past . . . it is probable that the well recognized form of the disease with toxic and embolic manifestations represents only one group of patients . . . subacute bacterial endocarditis may be of a *chronic nature* with a continuous and variable attempt at healing by the body. These observations indicate that chronic valvular disease may result from healing or healed bacterial endocarditis.

> Soma Weiss and Cornelius P. Rhoads: "Healing and Healed Vegetative (Subacute Bacterial) Endocarditis, Boston City Hospital." (July 12, 1928) *The New England Journal of Medicine*: 70-74.

There are many distinguished names associated with the study of acute and subacute bacterial endocarditis in the pre-antibiotic era, Glynn, Horder, Hamman, Weiss, Baehr, Craven and Libman, whose work bridged the pre and post-antibiotic eras. Not least among these investigators was the Canadian born Sir William Osler, who once taught medicine at McGill University in Montreal and to whom belongs the following description of the vegetations of bacterial endocarditis:

> The vegetations vary a good deal in appearance and consistence. Soft, greyish-white masses, with roughened friable surfaces, to which thin, blood-clot

adheres, are numerous; or there may be large cauliflower-excrescences, with deep jagged fissures; or, again, long pendulous stalactitic masses . . . and such a long vegetation from an aortic cusp may produce, by contact, a whole series of smaller outgrowths along the ventricular wall. The pressure of the valves against each other, and the action of the blood, tend to loosen and break the vegetations and one can sometimes see where masses have torn off, either entire or by a gradual process of disintegration . . . some vegetations present a remarkable greenish-grey or greenish-yellow colour . . . fibroid induration may take place in the deeper parts, while the superficial portions remain unchanged and necrotic, perhaps also becoming a little harder and shrinking.[1]

This horrifying picture of bacterial vegetations, published in 1885, was found in the heart of an ox. However, IE attacks the human valve in the same way, even today, and the progress of this strange and terrifying disease is identical in human and animal and the outcome can be equally calamitous. Much is known about bacterial endocarditis. In fact, research into this disease has been going on as long as that for extra systolic sounds and in much greater depth largely because, as Libman's studies showed, the disease is very common.

Embolic Nature of IE

The earliest recorded clinical and pathological observations of bacterial endocarditis appeared in a book called, *De Subitaneis Mortibus* or *On Cases of Sudden Death*, written by a Dr. Lancisi and printed in Italy in 1707.[2] The fact that this disease appears in such a book about sudden death reminds us, once again, as does the story of the tennis player in my introduction, that this disease may be absolutely silent with sudden embolic events. IE, however, was not clearly defined until around 1880, at which time the stenotic valves of rheumatic heart disease were regarded as the predisposing factor in about 80 percent of all cases.[3] This was not surprising in view of the fact that narrowing or stenosis of the mitral valve was always thought to be more serious than any lesion which renders the mitral valve incompetent and, therefore, regurgitant. Understanding of the disease developed, according to Osler, because of the work of William S. Kirkes in the middle of the 19thC.[4] Kirkes wrote a treatise on the behaviour of particles of the vegetative, sandwich-like lesions that become detached from their valvular stronghold and circulate in the blood. The idea of endocarditis as an embolic disease thus emerged, and, like Kirkes, Osler and others observed the dangerous effects of the unstable or "friable" vegetations. Pieces, referred to as emboli, break off and travel through the blood stream to lodge in the arteries of the heart or other organs, brain, kidneys or spleen. They may cause death or only localized damage when the blood supply is blocked off and surrounding tissues, starved of oxygen, die, the whole process being called an infarction.

The Vegetations of IE

Emanuel Libman, likely the most important figure in the study of bacterial endocarditis, was indebted to Osler and dedicated his 1941 textbook on SBE to him "whose stimulation led to the studies upon which this volume is based". Libman described vegetations in the human that were identical to those Osler had described in the ox. They were green, pink, red or greyish-white, and the valves often appeared "worm-eaten" or like "sharkskin".[5] Though modern descriptions are not as colourful, "cauliflowers" and "stalactites" are still among the pathological findings and, whether in human or animal, Osler's and Libman's observations on the colour, size and consistency of the vegetations have remained the same throughout the century. Favoured adjectives are bulky, friable, calcified, granular, tiny, pinpointed, rough, smooth and greyish-white. The last, greyish-white, was the colour which Libman attributed to healed vegetations, and is evidence that modern researchers are seeing healed vegetations, likely without knowing that they are.

As I pointed out in my introduction, young, healthy persons, such as the tennis player, can die of something that very closely resembles a heart attack or a stroke but is, in fact, endocarditis. If a patient with MVP dies suddenly, and the attending physician says the cause of death is a heart attack or some other common catch-all diagnosis, relatives should request to see the pathological report. Being able to recognize a description of this disease then becomes absolutely essential.

Pre-Antibiotic Treatments of IE

Modern researchers consider the term "infective endocarditis", first used by Glynn in 1903[6] and then revived by Thayer in 1931[7], is more accurate for this disease because an agent, other than bacteria, for example, fungi of the candida or aspergillus species, may be the etiologic factor[8]. But, no matter what the definition, the disease is not transmissible and thus "infective" does not mean contagious.

Other modern researchers object to the division of IE into acute and subacute forms because the mistaken notion is created that the latter cannot be explosive or lethal. But it is the subacute forms that linger for long periods of time and are likely those cases that heal naturally without antibiotic treatment, leaving the patient with CHF. Even though there has been much opposition to the idea of spontaneous cure, Libman's studies in the pre-antibiotic era offer convincing evidence that spontaneous recovery did occur in 20-25 percent of mild, subacute cases.[9] As in the case of MVP, Libman's contemporaries cried nonsense, that survival was rare and occurred in only 1 percent of cases.[10] We know for a fact that the "cures" in the range of 4 to 6.5 percent of cases which were attributed to sulpha drugs and heparin, a mucopolysaccharide that acts as an anti-coagulant, existing naturally in the lungs and the liver[11], must have been examples of spontaneous or natural healing since these drugs are now known to be totally ineffective against IE. The physicians, with whom I discussed my case, denied that I could have survived without immediate and prolonged treatment with massive doses of antimicrobials administered intravenously, but the literature of the past emphatically refutes this belief.

Understanding of disease proceeds slowly and not altogether logically as is demonstrated in the case of MVP. No medical efforts to triumph over death could be more outrageously inhumane than those early pre-antibiotic attempts to halt microbial ravage. And, as in the case of modern medicine, these early efforts were directed not at prevention but at salvation, no matter what the cost in terms of human suffering. Heavy metals, prominent in these treatment regimes, were injected into the dying in combination with nitrates or sulphur. A favorite instrument of torture was arsenic,[12] a poison which has always enjoyed a long and historic association with acts of depravity, being the favoured murder weapon of church, government or commerce, and the method our male dominated societies used in the past to force the "milk and roses" complexion upon women to recreate them in their own idealistic conception of beauty.[13]

Though such intramuscular injections of carbolic acid, arsenic, mercury and even sterile turpentine and milk failed miserably and caused much additional suffering, the ingenuity of the medical profession was without limit. With the logic of a Lewis, MacKenzie or Evans attacking mitral regurgitation, a "dehydration" treatment with mercurial diuretics, such as "salyrgan", was administered to the moribund in an effort to render the host environment "less favorable to the organisms", and, in the astonishing words of Paul White, he who had demonstrated such reasonableness in the matter of systolic clicks and murmurs, was "the most imaginative".[14]

These salvationist treatments paled in comparison with the cruel, primitive immunization tactics. Inconceivable as it may seem, doctors even injected patients with anti-streptococcal horse and goat serum or guinea pig blood infected with "spirochaeta morsus-muris". This seemingly harmless, rather musical sounding medical term, which probably impressed the uninformed patient with its Latin ring, translates into ratbite fever. The result was, of course, an acute case of that disease while the IE remained uncured.[15] Somewhat contrasting fare was the patently ludicrous injections of large doses of vitamin C[16], an innocuous treatment which likely would appeal to modern lovers of natural healing. It is not surprising that, according to one review, 246 of 250 patients, four being lost to follow-up, subjected to these "curative" toxins expired, their sufferings multiplied by increased "chills, heightened fever, nausea, vomiting, burns, abscesses, deafness and prostration."[17]

The microbial war reached an absurd peak of immorality with "frantic and pathetic appeals", often just naked monetary bribes, through the media, radio and newspaper, for blood transfusions from donors who had survived streptococcus viridans endocarditis.[18] But it was not until the availability of penicillin to the public in 1945 and the subsequent development of other chemotherapeutic agents that the course of the war with the microbes changed.

Host-Invader Relationship

To understand IE, one must understand the delicate truce between the host, human, and the invader, bacteria. The word, "host", used by infectious disease specialists, is particularly appropriate. The human body provides an hospitable habitat for the continued existence of its guests, the parasitic bacteria, aerobes, that live on the skin, or anerobes that live within the oxygenless environment of the mucous membrane-lined body cavities such as the mouth and intestinal tract. The host and the bacteria have formed a symbiotic relationship in which they share the same nutrition and waste disposal system. Most importantly, the human host provides the bacteria with the opportunity for reproduction and protection from enemies, and certain microorganisms assist the host in the decomposition of food and the production of waste materials. It is a relationship that exists for the life of the host, unless the microbes transgress the barriers of their respective territories, within or on the body. When they invade the bloodstream as in IE, these symbionts then become pathogens that can destroy their beneficial habitat and bring death to their host and themselves.[19]

Identification of Microscopic Bacteria

The microscope has permitted the identification of the bacteria that causes IE. According to shape and behaviour, there are four major groups of bacteria: the oval or sperical-shaped cocci, the rod-like bacilli, the spiral or spirilla and the comma-shaped vibrios. Cocci and bacilli can occur singly or in pairs (diplococci), chains (streptococci) and clusters (staphylococci). The streptococci and staphylococci are the most important types of microorganisms. Together, they are responsible for 80-85 percent of all cases of IE[20], and, in the case of MVP, the bacteria in 46 percent of cases is streptococcus viridans. [21] To assure that the most effective bactericidal weapons are used in the fight against IE, researchers had to further distinguish these microorganisms into two groups of bacteria called gram-positive and gram-negative. Bacteria cells, heat-fixed on a microscope slide, are stained with methyl violet which causes them to turn blue. If, after other steps of treatment and a final wash with alcohol, they are decolorized, they are then said to be gram-negative and, if they retain the dye colour, possibly because of their thick cell walls impervious to solvents, they are gram-positive. This technique is named after its inventor, the Danish bacteriologist, Christian Gram. Antimicrobials which attack gram positive bacteria may be less effective or totally ineffective in the fight against gram negative microorganisms, hence the necessity of knowing this essential fact.

Breaching the Barrier

There are specific, well-known procedures that can cause IE. Individuals who have no obvious or microscopic abnormality of the heart or valves are not at risk, but, even in susceptible persons, IE cannot occur unless the barrier of bacteria-resistant epithelial tissues of the body's outer skin or the special endothelium lining the mouth, hollow organs such as the bladder, the respiratory, gastrointestinal or genitourinary tracts is broken, permitting bacteria access to the bloodstream. Such breaches in these barriers are thus potentially hazardous to patients with MVP or others with cardiac abnormalities such as mitral stenosis from RHD or certain congenital cardiac defects. If appropriate protection with antibiotics is instituted prior to the invasive event, the bacteria will be killed before they can gain a foothold on damaged valves. The bacteria which causes a systemic infection such as IE are associated with their source, with what is called in the medical literature, the "portal of entry" to the bloodstream and are named accordingly. For example, a staphylococcus epidermis indicates that the origin of the bacteria is the skin (epidermis) and a streptococcus faecalis (from faeces or feces) endocarditis indicates that the origin of the bacteria is the gastrointestinal tract, specifically, the colon, the sigmoid colon or the rectum.

Procedures that Cause IE

The ways in which IE can be contracted are numerous and, unfortunately, modern technology has greatly multiplied them. They include any investigative or surgical procedures involving the naso or oropharynx (mouth, teeth, upper respiratory tract), gastrointestinal (stomach and intestines), genitourinary or urogenital tracts and the cardio-renal system.[22]

Gastrointestinal Procedures

Rectosigmoidoscopy or **sigmoidoscopy** can cause a bacteremia according to Lawrence Freedman who has stated that "Virtually any procedure which traumatizes the normal (not to speak of diseased) epithelium in man is capable of inducing discharge of bacteria into the bloodstream."[23] Sigmoidoscopy is a procedure allowing the visual examination of the lower 10-12 inches of the large intestine and rectum which includes the sigmoid flexure, the S-shaped terminal portion of the colon that links with the rectum. A proctoscope is used if only the rectum is examined. Either a flexible fiberoptic or rigid tube with illuminating and magnifying devices may be used. Mechanical trauma to the epithelial tissues during investigative procedures can happen and, thus, as Freedman said, may also be more risky when tissues are diseased by an ulcerative colitis or hemorrhoids. Just as with the bronchoscopy examination, there may be additional risk in these procedures if the instrument for examination is made of a rigid rather than a flexible fiberoptic material because tearing of the tissues is more likely to occur.[24] A case of IE developing after rectal biopsy, rigid sigmoidoscopy and barium enema has been reported in the medical literature.[25]

Colonoscopy, an examination of the entire some fifty inches of the large intestine, and the barium enema x-ray, which is usually done prior to this test, can also cause a bloodstream bacteremia.[26] While the incidence of bacteremia is said to be low with the colonoscopy, the barium enema has been shown to cause a greater bacteremia than the sigmoidoscopy.[27] Barium, which is injected into the large intestine via the rectum, is used as a contrast material for the purpose of taking x-rays. The pressure of the fluid itself and abrasions from the tip of the enema tube could force bacteria into the bloodstream.[28] Barium enema and proctoscopy were two procedures which I underwent without antibiotic protection at the Mayo Clinic. Ideally, if there is no tearing of the tissues and no bleeding, IE will not occur. This cannot, however, be guaranteeed and that is why antibiotic protection is important.

Other procedures known to facilitate the entrance of bacteria into the bloodstream are as follows:[29]

1) tissue biopsies of the liver, in particular, and of the uterus or kidneys
2) urologic procedures such as surgery or investigative instrumentation of the urethra (dilatation), the small canal that conveys the urine from the bladder to the exterior opening, of the ureter or of the bladder, that is cystoscopy which is a visual examination of the bladder
3) prostatectomy (removal of a part or all of the prostate gland)
4) peritoneal dialysis or lavage of abdominal cavity and viscera
5) hemodialysis (mechanical filtering of impurities from the blood when the kidneys do not function)
6) surgical insertion of a pacemaker to regulate the heartbeat
7) replacement of natural heart valves with prosthetic devices
8) indwelling IV catheters (e.g. nutritional or antimicrobial purposes)
9) cardiac catheterization of the left ventricle
10) blood and platelet transfusion.

By virtue of their sex, women with MVP have extended risks which the quotation from the British Medical Research Council Series on IE at the beginning of the chapter appears to verify. The following are known to cause a bacteremia:

1) intrauterine contraceptive devices[30], [31](cases of IE have been reported in the medical literature)
2) cesarian section
3) induced or spontaneous abortion
4) dilatation and curettage (D&C)
5) pelvic infection
6) menstruation [32]
7) punch biopsy of the cervix
8) normal vaginal delivery[33]

A group, including Dr. John Barlow, from the University of the Witwatersrand and Johannesburg Hospitals have reported IE in the MVP syndrome after curettage following a spontaneous abortion and after a normal pregnancy and delivery.[34] Osler noted in 1885 that endocarditis may "attack" pregnant women and run a rapid course leading to abortion." Childbirth fever, the cause of death in many women, was, of course, IE as Osler had correctly observed.[35]

It is not automatic for a MVP patient to be protected in the above situations. In 1986, a gynecologist and a cardiologist, when asked, said I did not require ABP for an intrauterine biopsy, even though both were fully aware of my medical history. While the uterus itself may be free of bacteria, it is possible that microorganisms from the skin or genitalia could be introduced into this sterile area during the procedure.

The Oral Route

A great many of the microorganisms responsible for IE live in the mouth and upper respiratory tract. Almost any oral procedure or septic condition of the mouth can cause a bacteremia and, thus, the risk of IE. Investigations of the mouth, nose or throat such as **nasotracheal intubation or nasotracheal suctions** which involve the insertion of tubes via the mouth and nose or **bronchoscopy**[36], especially if the bronchoscope is rigid, are dangerous. In one study, the use of a rigid bronchoscope caused a fever in 24 of 52 patients and 15.4 percent of patients had positive blood cultures. No bacteria was produced when a flexible instrument was used.[37]

Tonsillitis

Spontaneous infection of the upper respiratory tract occurs far more commonly than with the above manipulations. Medical researchers have observed the strong association between tonsillitis and IE for well over 80 years. I, myself, and many of the people with MVP who have written to me in response to my article on MVP in *Healthsharing* magazine, had a history of two and three episodes of tonsillitis a year into adulthood when the tonsils were removed. In 1903, Glynn, in the Lumleian lectures delivered at The Royal College of Physicians and Surgeons in London, England, stated that "pathogenic organisms found in the mouth and adjoining cavities are recognized agents of infection and cases of infective endocarditis are reported to have followed abrasions of the lips, inflammation of the tonsils and diseased conditions of the mucous membranes of the nasal sinuses and the middle ear."[38]

Glynn's colleagues, Horder, Libman and Osler, frequently reported cases of IE in association with tonsillitis. Among his observations on spontaneous cures, Libman described a case of a patient in whom classic symptoms of IE, fever, splenomegaly, anemia and Osler's nodes, began and disappeared simultaneously within a month with recovery from tonsillitis. A recurrence of the tonsillitis brought the same symptoms of IE, but, after the removal of the tonsils, the patient remained well.[39] In 1937, Hamman observed that, in fatal cases of IE, the tonsils were enlarged and scarred and the superificial cervical nodes, the glands at the angles of the jaws, were also enlarged.[40] It was significant that, during my illness, one observer noted enlargement of the superficial cervical nodes and recorded this in my medical records.

Even after the widespread use of penicillin, tonsillitis, with or without a history of rheumatic fever, has remained prevalent in the histories of patients with IE.[41] Specific microorganisms known to cause IE, such as haemophilus aphrophilus have been isolated from tonsils, gums and between the teeth.[42] Because this particular haemophilus species requires a high concentration of CO_2 for growth in the customary media, it is called aphrophilus from the Greek word, aphros, for froth or bubbling, as is found in the fermentation of wine. The haemophilus microorganisms have been found in as much as one third of all oral clinical specimens.[43] In 1981, a case was reported in *The Canadian Medical Association Journal* describing IE in a patient with one swollen tonsil covered with white exudate.[44] And researchers from the University of Gottingen in Germany have reported a tonsillitis-endocarditis syndrome in the dog. Beta haemolytic streptococci were isolated from the tonsils and heart valves of 4.4 percent or 54 of 1225 dogs which died from acute cardiac failure resulting from IE initiated by tonsillitis. The report also stated that acute cases often become chronic, responding to antibiotic treatment and, in one case, after tonsillectomy, the animal became a high achievement dog.[45]

Tonsillectomy

It was Libman who pointed out that tonsillectomy is a prophylactic measure to prevent IE in patients with chronic severe tonsillitis. However, tonsillectomy, itself, is extremely dangerous without antibiotic coverage. The rate at which microorganisms shower the blood stream during tonsillectomy is almost equal to that in tooth extraction.[46] There are many reports, past and current, of IE following tonsillectomy. Bacteremia following tonsillectomy has been noted in as many as 38 percent of cases, but there are many researchers, for example, Everett and Hirschman (1977), who feel this figure is on the low side since many of the reports appeared before anaerobic techniques for culturing bacteria were available.[47]

Septic Conditions of the Mouth and IE

Dental manipulations figure prominently in anyone's life. But, when they involve infected teeth or tissues, the procedures are particularly risky. In 1935 and 1939, Okell and Elliott conducted experiments that demonstrated, for the first time, that the mere rocking of a tooth with forceps could send a shower of bacteria into the blood stream in 86 percent of 21 cases when severe gum disease was present compared with only 25 percent of cases in which there was no gum disease. They also showed that, even in the absence of any trauma, there was leakage of bacteria into the blood stream in patients with severe oral infection.[48]

Dental Hygiene and IE

Modern dental hygiene products that are designed to keep teeth clean and gums healthy such as oral irrigation devices, wooden or rubber stimulators and dental floss can be dangerous if blood is drawn and, especially, if the gums are in a diseased state. I personally have heard of a case of an individual who contracted IE from an oral irrigation device. In studies comparing the incidence of bacteremia after a variety of dental manipulations, it was found that 50 percent of 30 patients with severe gingivitis had a bacteremia after the use of an oral irrigation device compared to only 7 percent of 30 patients with mild gingivitis in another group.[49] My dentist, knowing I had MVP and a history highly suspicious for IE, still recommended the purchase of such a device. Light or deep cleaning and scaling of dental plaque, another preventative measure, can also cause a bacteremia.[50]

Even such ordinary, innocent actions as chewing and brushing can be hazardous to the health of the MVP patient if a septic condition exists in the mouth. After Okell and Elliott's studies, Murray and Moosneck, a year later in 1940, showed that chewing sticky substances such as a one inch cube of paraffin for one half hour produced a bacteremia in 55 percent of 336 patients with different degrees of dental caries and gum disease[51]. Other researchers have reported that chewing hard candy such as "mint lump" for ten minutes caused bloodstream bacteremia. Blood cultures taken prior to and after the chewing were positive in 2 of 5 patients with pyorrhea or purulent infection of the gums. There was *no bacteria* in the blood of patients without gum disease.[52] Chewing hard, sticky and, one might add, sugary substances, when there is infection in the oral cavity, whether gum disease or a root abscess, can be risky for persons with MVP.

Dental Caries

Numerous cases of IE have been reported in the pre and post antibiotic literature in patients with tooth decay. Early researchers regularly described the condition of their patients' teeth whether or not a connection was made with IE. While the most common microorganism in the pre-antibiotic era was strep. viridans, modern research has pinpointed other microorganisms in dental plaque that cause both decay and IE, such as strep. mutans and the haemophilus species. The name, haemophilus, comes from the Greek word, "haemo", for blood and "philos" for loving, signifying, literally, that this microorganism forms a special bond with the blood to facilitate its growth. These types of bacteria are both normal inhabitants of the oral cavity. Strep. mutans which has a peculiar, indisputable affinity for smooth surfaces like dental enamel, causes tooth decay. In the presence of sucrose, this microorganism forms other sugars, glucan or fructose, which promote the quality of adherence.[53] Thus, the dangers of eating sugary substances are obvious.

The haemophilus species, frequently associated with IE and tonsillitis in the earlier literature, also show a distinct attraction for the smooth surfaces of teeth, but, curiously, few reports of haemophili causing IE have appeared in the post antibiotic era until just recently[54] when cases of hemophilus endocarditis were reported in MVP patients, one in association with an infected wisdom tooth. [55] A 1974 report[56] from the Pathology Department of the Royal Dental Hospital in London, England showed that the average concentration of the haemophilus species in saliva is very high. Haemophilus parainfluenzae, one of the varieties of the Haemophili, is, in fact, the principal species found in saliva, dental plaque and the gingival crevice and, when pus is present, haemophilus parahaemolyticus is found. Once again, an unhealthy mouth is a health hazard to the MVP patient.

Extraction, Endodontal Work and Dental Cleaning

If the gentle actions for which our teeth were designed can cause a bacteremia, it is not difficult to imagine the danger of violent trauma, such as extraction or endodontal interventions. Most researchers agree that exodontic and endodontic procedures are the most likely to cause a significant bacteremia. IE caused by extraction of teeth was noted very early in the medical literature, and, once again, in the presence of infection of the teeth or gum tissues, the danger is multiplied. Okell's 1930 studies compared the incidence of bacteremia in clean and septic mouths in 138 patients after extraction and found positive cultures in 75 percent of those patients with marked gum disease but in only 34 percent without detectable gum disease.[57] A 1978 study indicated that the incidence of bacteremia after extraction in patients with periodontal disease can be as high as 80 percent.[58]

However, many modern researchers believe there is a bacteremia every time a tooth is extracted, whether oral infection exists or not. For instance, Bender and colleagues at the Albert Einstein Medical Centre in Philadelphia showed that the incidence of bacteremia increases with the size of the blood sample taken and with the severity of the extraction. They found positive cultures, in the case of multiple extractions, in 93.4 percent of patients, but, with milder, single extractions, only 68.7 percent of the patients had bacteria in their blood. The bacteria in the blood increased with the size of the blood sample, and these authors suggested that, if blood samples of 25 to 50 ml be taken, positive cultures would exist in 100 percent of extractions.[59] During my first hospitalization, only three samples of blood were taken for culturing, and one of these was partially spilled on the bedclothes.

Numerous cases of IE in association with tooth extraction have been reported in the literature. In 1956, Hobson and Juel from the Radcliff Infirmary at Oxford reviewed the literature on IE for a period of twenty years from 1930 to 1951 and concluded that "in varying proportions of cases in all published series a dental extraction has been specifically identified as the causa causans."[60] Contemporary studies confirm that, of all the dental manipulations that have caused IE, 12[61] to 25[62] percent have been related to tooth extraction where antibiotic coverage was not provided during the procedure. Even when I was finally hospitalized for the extraction of my tooth, coverage was not started until after the extraction.

Periodontal Surgery

Periodontal procedures, involving surgery on bone or gums, such as gingivectomy (surgical excision of the gums), which I underwent when the endodontist and periodontist were searching for the cracked root, carry as great a risk of IE as extraction. One study at The National Heart Institute at Bethesda, Maryland showed that both extractions and periodontal procedures produced strep. viridans and other bacteria, including strains resistant to penicillin, in 80 percent of patients.[63]

Endodontic Procedures

There is a strong association between endodontic procedures and IE, and the skill of the endodontist is a more significant factor in this than in any other type of dental procedure. Studies have confirmed that, whether the pulp is vital or necrotic, positive blood cultures will occur when root canal manipulations extend beyond the opening of the root canal[64] as discussed earlier in this book. The periapical abscesses that can result from the root canal work itself or from cracked roots are resistant to oral antibiotics since pus and necrotic tissue simply absorb these drugs without healing while favouring the growth of resistant organisms which then leak out [65] into the bloodstream. Prevention of pulpitis is essential in susceptible patients, and, if inflammation occurs, immediate elimination of necrotic tissue by root canal treatment or extraction is imperative. Retention of a seriously infected tooth, as in my case, for prolonged periods of time exposes the patient to a major risk.

It is well documented in the medical literature that any kind of manipulation of an infected area, whether tonsils, gums, joints, prostate gland or boils for example, can produce a bacteremia. In 1977, Everett and co-workers compared the incidence of bacteremia in these different infected sites and found it was greater following surgery on the bones and soft tissues of the face, hence teeth, gums or tonsils.[66] Purulent lesions in the periodontal tissues, of the kind I suffered, as pathologist, W. Sims, from the Royal Dental Hospital in London, England pointed out in his 1974 study, are a constant source of bacteremia and indicate deeper infection from necrotic tissues, whether "dead teeth, dead bone or other tissue or simply dead space around teeth."[67] Surgery on infected lesions of any kind in the mouth is extremely risky for the MVP patient when appropriate antibiotic coverage is not provided.

Numerous reports indicate that strep. viridans, a common inhabitant of the indigenous flora of the oral cavity, still accounts for 35-50 percent of cases of IE [68] and, more specifically, a dental focus of infection, including that from extraction, is responsible in about 45 percent of all cases of IE[69]. Though strep.

viridans accounted for about 90 percent of all cases in the pre-antibiotic era, other organisms of the oral cavity, especially those associated with teeth, such as the haemophili and strep. mutans have emerged, in the modern era, as significant pathogens and, if included, might suggest a higher incidence of teeth involvement in IE than 10-50 percent. As already pointed out, streptococci and staphylococci together account for about 80-85 percent of all cases of IE and, in the case of a recurrent IE, 94 percent of cases are caused by bacteria in the oral cavity according to Welton's studies in 1979.[70]

Pathogenesis of IE

The inception and development of the disease of IE is a fascinating subject. Its course supports the hypothesis that prolapsed valves themselves may be caused by bacteria. Long before the introduction of antibiotics, it was observed that abnormal or damaged endothelium, no matter how minimal, exposes the underlying collagen, the connective tissue that gives form and structure to the valves, and encourages the adherence to and colonization of microorganisms on the valves. Endothelium, a special kind of tissue composed of a thin, smooth layer of cells, lines the heart, lymph vessels, blood vessels and arteries and covers the valves. Early pathological studies demonstrated that there was often nothing more than a mere microscopic "roughening" of the endothelial surface of the valves in the presence of the vegetations of IE.[71]

In 1927, Grant and colleagues described the two kinds of abnormalities of the valvular surface in cases of IE, recessions, in the form of crevices and pockets, or projections, which were named "endocardial tags" in 1856 by a Dr. Lambl. These doctors imagined that the recessions or pits offered a shelter or nest for the bacteria to gain a foothold and multiply.[72] These descriptions may seem somewhat clumsy and "mechanical"; however, the belief that endothelium must be damaged before vegetations can adhere to the valves still exists today.

Rheumatic Heart Disease (RHD) and MVP

The prevailing view over the last century has been that the fibrosed valves of rheumatic heart disease were considered the most vulnerable to IE, just as the murmur of mitral stenosis was considered the most serious. In his Gulstonian Lectures on Malignant Endocarditis, Osler pointed out that Sir James Paget, the British surgeon and pathologist (1814-1899), first drew attention to the frequency with which the sclerotic or scarred and malformed valves of RHD were attacked by IE.[73] Sclerosis means literally hardening, as in the disease multiple sclerosis which gets its name from the sclerosed or scarred areas of nerve fibers found throughout the central nervous system. Sclerosis or scarring is the end-product of the proliferation of fibrous connective tissue that takes place during the healing of inflamed tissues.

However, a closer look at early pathological descriptions of valves attacked by IE shows that, in many cases, the underlying valvular abnormalities were similar to those now known to exist in prolapsed valves rather than valves damaged by RHD. Osler[74] and Glynn [75] observed that sclerotic valves affected by IE showed thickening in the majority of cases. Modern studies describe thickening as a classic pathological feature of prolapsed valves. Some of the words chosen by the early pathologists to describe the underlying valvular pathology in the presence of IE, are virtually identical to modern terminology for prolapsed valves. In 1885, Glynn, for example, reported on the common finding of swelling of the valvular tissues, of "benign excrescences" in "lax and flaccid" valves which crowded together and weighed down the whole valvular apparatus.[76] Modern pathological reports stress the bulging, stretching and heaviness of "floppy" valves. And Grant's "raised and undercut folds of endocardium on the surface of thickened cusps" [77] could be the "folding and convolution" and "upward doming of the cusp" in the modern pathological descriptions of prolapsed valves.[78] The word, "ridges" which Grant and colleagues used in 1927,[79] is almost synonymous with the word, "pleating",[80] used in the 1982 Merck Manual description of prolapsed valves. In modern studies, prolapsed valves are frequently described as "translucent and gelatinous" as well as "white and opaque" from fibrosis.[81], [82] One is tempted to ask if the "milk spots"[83] of fibrosis Glynn remarked upon and the "translucency" Osler referred to [84] in their discussions of IE were, in reality, evidence of prolapse in connection with IE rather than rheumatic heart disease as was thought. And, most fascinating, Grant's "endocardial tags" on the surface of the valves were "gelatinous" and "translucent" or "dense and white".[85] These are the precise words used to describe the malformations of prolapsed valves.

Evidence of IE in Early Studies of Irritable Heart and Effort Syndrome

One could go back even further and ask whether Da Costa was, in fact, describing mild cases of IE in soldiers with a symptom complex now indisputably believed to be that of MVP. As is widely known, MVP often comes to light for the first time only during an episode of IE. Information on an insignificant murmur or no murmur at all may have been documented prior to the infection. Many of the soldiers Da Costa described complained of the onset of symptoms of palpitation, chest pain and shortness of breath with a bout of fever and diarrhea. These could very well have been signs of IE. Da Costa noted simultaneously the unusual midsystolic auscultatory signs. When the illness abated, the patient's symptoms and clinical findings did not disappear. Were these fevers, gastrointestinal disturbances and diarrhea plus the clinical findings, especially of murmurs, indicative of mild IE of the sort Libman described fifty years later? Surface wounds or even severe disease of the teeth and periodontal tissues which were spongy and bleeding from scurvy could have been the precipitating factor. Da Costa was not likely familiar with IE in 1861 since it had not yet been described in the literature.

Interestingly, Da Costa described the case of a young man with many symptoms and clinical findings identical to those of MVP, including small chest dimensions, who died from a combination of fever, cardiac hypertrophy and strangulated hernia which could imply an embolic episode. At autopsy, there was a suspicious piece of evidence pointing to IE, that of "a clot entwined in the mitral valve."[86] One is reminded of the way in which the tennis player, whom I described in my introduction, died. Was this a vegetation or was it simply a thrombus associated with MVP? More will be said later of the risk of embolism in the MVP syndrome.

Da Costa frequently reported finding considerable quantities of oxalate of lime in the urine of men in whom the onset of cardiac symptoms coincided with that of fever and diarrhea.[87] Oxalate of lime is a salt sediment from Oxallic acid which is excreted from the kidneys of patients with nephritis or gastroenteritis and nephritis. Nephritis particularly affects the glomeruli, and glomerulonephritis is virtually a universal finding in IE.[88] Oxalic acid is found in fungi of the genus aspergillus. Is it too tenuous to suggest that these were mild cases of IE, spontaneously healed, of the fungal type, the aspergillus species, from acute or chronic inflammation of the sinuses, bronchi, lungs or contaminated skin wounds that would leave the soldiers with a chronic nephritis? Aspergillus fumigatus is known to produce a nephrotoxic reaction in kidney cells.

Lewis had observed that, by far, bacterial infection of some kind brought on the "effort syndrome". 181 of 558 or 33 percent of soldiers had symptoms dating from an infectious disease characterized by fever of unknown origin, influenza, dysentery or tonsillitis.[89] Lewis compared the incidence of infectious disease or serious illness in the heart with gun shot wounds and found that almost 80 percent of those with effort syndrome had suffered some kind of serious illness while only 18 percent of the gun shot wound cases had a previous significant illness. [90] He also observed that men went about with chronic SBE, lasting many months, while they fought in the frontline trenches.[91] These past reports go a long way towards dispelling the popular view among doctors I spoke to that IE ends immediately and invariably in death.

The cardiac symptom complex Da Costa, Lewis and others frequently described began then, in the majority of cases, with a febrile illness very much resembling Libman's mild cases of IE. Given that they were talking about MVP, it is conceivable that many early pathological descriptions of valvular deformities in the presence of vegetations were, in fact, evidence of the acid mucopolysaccharides of prolapsed valves and not signs of rheumatic heart disease as was originally thought. Lewis had reported on the widened, relaxed mitral rings at autopsy in patients with Soldiers' Heart,[92] a common feature in the autopsied specimens from patients who have died suddenly of MVP.[93] And, though Gross and Fried, in 1937, believed that the fibrosed valves of rheumatic fever were the sites of the vegetations of IE, many of their necropsy specimens manifested "a widening of the vascularized spongiosa layer." [94] This pathological feature of extensive spongiosa is what characterizes MVP and indicates excessive mucopolysaccharides in the valvular tissue which causes it to stretch, balloon and fold.

The Pathology of MVP and RHD

The question of the true relationship between RHD and MVP, which these older studies raise, remains as yet unravelled. A full understanding of the cause of prolapsed valves is not likely to be reached unless the intricate triad of RHD, IE and MVP is studied in depth. Pathological studies have traditionally associated fibrous tissue in the valves with RHD, yet John Barlow has observed a case of a woman who, in life, had only a mid-systolic click, and, at autopsy, had a single fibrosed chordae.[95] However, confusion arises because mid-systolic clicks have also been found in RHD. In 1976, Barlow and others from the University of Witwatersrand studied 12,050 black children, between the ages of 2 and 18, from the economically deprived township of Soweto and found the click and/or LSM in 168 for an incidence of 13.99 per 1000 rising to 29.41 per 1000 children at the age of 17. 123 or 73 percent had the click and 8 or 5 percent the LSM while 37 or 22 percent had both click and murmur. In the same study RHD was found in 6.9 of 1000 children aged 2 to 18 and 19.2 of 1000 children in the seventh grade. RHD is traditionally associated with poverty and overcrowding. Barlow concluded that "against the background of low socio-economic status in Soweto and the high prevalence of rheumatic heart disease, it is possible that an unknown and probably large number of chidren with LSMs or non-ejection systolic clicks have mild rheumatic heart disease."[96] The studies of Barlow and others at the University of Witwatersrand suggest that there is a definite connection between RHD and MVP and also that the prevalence of MVP may be a factor of the socio-economic condition, specifically poverty.

Recently, pathologists from St. George's Hospital in London, England, brought forward evidence that there is a connection, though that remains as yet not fully understood, between RHD and MVP. Their pathological investigations show that the fibrosis, normally an indicator of RHD, is also present in the majority of prolapsed valves, and that this "very considerable secondary fibrosis" has often caused confusion and "an erroneous diagnosis of rheumatic disease."[97] In 1975, Luxton et al also stated that the calcification and fibrosis, formerly regarded as unique to RHD, are also found in prolapsed valves.[98] Modern research thus supports what I have theorized from a reading of the early pathological studies of Osler, Glynn, Grant and others, specifically that the underlying condition, in many cases of IE, was, in all probability that of MVP rather than RHD or of MVP in conjunction with RHD.

According to Barlow, the rheumatic process could produce a click and LSM just as the myxomatous process of MVP can. He has found that 20-25 percent of MVP adults have a documented history of acute rheumatic fever.[99] The latest research strengthens the idea of a relationship between RHD and MVP and even raises the question of whether or not the two conditions co-exist and are initiated by the same sequence of events. In 1980 a group of children with MVP were tested for antibody to a specific streptococcus Group A that remains elevated in the blood for many years after acute rheumatic fever. 34.9 percent had evidence consistent with prior acute rheumatic fever and 61.9 percent had experienced important streptococcal infection, suggesting a "rheumatic etiology exists in a large proportion of children with MVP." [100] I, myself, and many of the men and women who wrote to me, have had a prolonged history of streptococcal infection, tonsillitis, all during childhood and adolescence.

Experimental Studies on Healing in IE

There are many experimental studies currently being undertaken of the pathogenesis of IE using the rabbit model. Such efforts are not new. They are a revival of past attempts, like Barlow's experiments to prove the LSM regurgitant, and they emphasize the circular and repetitive nature of medical research. In 1906 and 1907, Horder described how IE could be initiated in the rabbit by the intravenous injection of saprophytic streptococcus from human saliva or faeces,[101] and, in 1927, Grant et al stated that "the surest method of producing a bacterial endocarditis in animals is by injuring the valves and subsequently introducing organisms into the blood stream."[102]

Grant's inspiration did not find fruit until the late sixties. Lawrence Freedman and a team from Yale University observed that catheters inserted into the body could cause systemic infection and hence IE in man. Subsequently, this Yale team described a technique for inserting catheters into the right and left ventricles of the rabbit, moving them back and forth to injure the valvular endothelium, thus simulating the damage of a disease like MVP, and then injecting bacteria via the catheter into the heart.[103] The progress of the disease and the effects of various pharmacological manoeuvers, such as anti-microbials, could be studied.

In Lawrence Freedman's view, valvular abnormalities, even mildly damaged endothelium as was found in the older studies of IE, disturb the flow of blood in the heart and, whenever blood flow is interrupted or slowed down, the clotting potential or the coagulability factor of the blood, is increased. Whether or not a valvular injury has been made, as in the case of the experimental rabbit studies, the introduction of a polyethyline catheter, or any foreign body into the heart, such as pacemakers or prosthetic valves, stimulates local coagulation of blood. The consequence is the formation of thrombi or clots which Freedman calls non-bacterial thrombotic vegetations (NBTVs), and which he regards as an absolute prerequisite for the establishment of IE. These thrombi contain the same cellular substances, platelets and fibrin that result from the interaction between fibrinogen and thrombin in the blood, as the bacterial thrombotic vegetations contain. The rabbit studies showed that when bacteria is introduced, via the catheter, these non-bacterial thrombi attract bacteria or become infected and thus IE is established.[104]

These animal studies revealed several startling facts. As confirmation of

Libman's ideas, healing, without antibiotics, does take place and, Freedman explains, "consists of progressive endothelialization of the surface of the vegetation, phagocytosis of bacterial debris and calcification and fibroblastic organization." [105] This suggests that the establishment of fibrosed material in the valve, which, in the past was said to characterize the effects of rheumatic fever, is part of the healing process of IE. The bacterial vegetations are coated with endothelial tissue, which, in turn, seal off the bacteria. The whole process might be compared to the grain of irritating sand that is coated with protective secretions from inside the oyster shell, thus forming a pearl. In fact, even the catheter inserted in the heart of the rabbit is endothelialized. The fibrosis and calcification, characteristic of the healing process, could thus be common to both RHD and prolapsed valves and could explain the progression of the prolapse to the "floppy" valve stage as a result of repeated IE episodes involving the valve.

The British researchers, Durack, Beeson and Petersdorf[106], who have carried out the same experiments in the rabbit as the Yale group, have observed the healing process more closely and have found that it takes place in the oldest and deepest parts of the vegetative layer which grows by accretions of platelets and fibrin and is continuously endothelialized or covered with new endothelial tissue. There is a startling absence of leukocytes and phagocytes in these vegetations, indicating that the body's natural defences are unable to penetrate the fibrin-platelet vegetation. Likewise, antibiotics can only affect the younger microorganisms in the vegetations on the outer surfaces of the valves. The older bacteria, deep within the vegetation, enter a resting phase which begins as early as two days after innoculation with bacteria. Evidence of healing, that is death or sterilization of the bacteria, is provided by staining methods and by observation of the calcification of necrotic tissue and bacteria. In part, the healing is natural, due to aging and crowding and thus limited nutrition. A population explosion so to speak, leads to the death of the bacteria by starvation since deep-seated bacteria would not be bathed by the nutritious blood. It is a process akin to Darwinian natural selection, the death of the less fit or less adaptable bacteria. Unfortunately, however, as Durak points out, the older colonies deep within the vegetations contain foci of live bacteria and there is continuous regrowth since the bacteria is only in a resting stage. Thus the mechanism for relapse or reawakening of dormant bacteria is created.

In these animal studies, spontaneous healing took place largely in the tricuspid valve of the right side of the heart. However, there was evidence of healing in the left side as well. In the right side of the heart about 25 percent of the infected vegetations became sterilized in the rabbit models.[107] If the animal survived long enough, there was some healing in the left heart according to the British team. For instance in their studies, one of the 57 test animals with left sided IE had no signs of infection at necropsy.[108] A single vegetation on the aortic valve was sterile. This suggests that, in humans, in longstanding cases of mild subacute infection, the chance of survival would be greater as Libman and other older researchers have reported in cases that lasted anywhere up to three years. Nevertheless, the greater danger of left sided infection underlines the serious nature of the risk of IE in the MVP syndrome. It was also observed from these experimental animal studies that the size of the vegetative lesions diminished with the administration of antibiotics [109] and thus healing would be more likely.

Platelets and the Infectious Process

The pathogenesis of IE cannot be understood without a knowledge of how blood platelets behave in the formation of thrombi. Platelets, as is commonly known, play a crucial role in arresting bleeding. The platelets release a factor, a lipoprotein, which reacts with plasma factors to stimulate prothrombin production and thus clotting activity. They clump together or aggregate at the site of the injury to create a hemostatic plug and prevent further bleeding. We, therefore, think of platelets as lifesaving, one of the body's primary defence mechanisms against severe blood loss and death.

However, scientists have discovered that platelets have an alternative fascinating role: they can be injurious and even destructive to the human host. The formation of NBTVs, of course, would be impossible without platelets which along with fibrin form a stable clot. It is the inherent property of stickiness of the platelets, their ability to aggregate, that contributes ultimately to our destruction when we acquire a bacterial infection of the heart. The presence of microorganisms, bacterial pathogens, especially staphylococci and streptococci, actually stimulate the platelets to clump together to form a vegetation which becomes the necessary shelter for the protection of the bacteria.

The extent of the platelet aggregation depends on the ratio of the number of bacteria to the number of platelets. As the platelets come together to form a thrombus, the bacteria are incorporated in large numbers inside this growing vegetation. Our own natural defences then turn against us and act in defence of the bacteria that can destroy us by offering a "protected sanctuary", impenetrable to the body's natural weapons, the phagocytes and leukocytes, neither of which are found in necropsied specimens of vegetations, and to bactericidal drugs. C. C. Clawson describes his observations on the assistance of the platelets in the endocarditic process:

> True phagocytosis or ingestion was extremely rare; rather the microbes came to lie between the aggregated platelets, yet in a position segregated from the surrounding media. The bacteria retained normal fine structure, appearing viable for a period in excess of an hour. This indicated that there was no detrimental influence from this duration of residence within the platelet aggregates. Quantative culturing confirmed this by yielding nearly 100 percent of the initial counts of Staph. aureus, Strep. pyogenes or E coli. The latter findings are in agreement with those of experimental endocarditis which suggest that the bacteria find a protected sanctuary within the platelet-fibrin vegetations.[110]

Bacteria and Endotoxins

The end-products of bacterial decomposition during an IE provoke some intriguing reflections on the pathogenesis of prolapsed valves. When bacteria die or decompose deep within the vegetation, they release endotoxins or poisons. Curiously, certain by-products of bacterial decomposition, specifically the polysaccharides, are found normally in the intercellular ground substance of human tissues, in particular in valvular tissue. Polysaccharides are the threatening substances mysteriously increased to the point of overwhelming the sturdier fibrosa or collagen tissue in prolapsed valves and they are what make the valve stretch and balloon. "Polysaccharides", according to Wannamaker and Parker, "are the principal substances mediating the attachment of bacteria to surfaces and to each other in both gram negative and gram positive species."[111]

Present on the surfaces of certain streptococci and forming the capsule of the bacteria is a substance called hyaluronic acid which is composed of viscous mucopolysaccharide, the substance accused of disrupting valvular architecture. Hyaluronic acid has antiphagocytic properties and thus works against the defence activities of the body. Furthermore, hyaluronidase, an enzyme which exists in some strains of pathogenic bacteria, including Strep. and Staph., facilitates the microorganism's ability to produce disease by breaking down the barriers of the hyaluronic acid capsule or polysaccharide capsule of the bacteria, thus promoting the spread of the bacteria into the cells and valvular tissues.

The question raised in my mind is: do these bi-products of the decomposition of the older bacteria deep within the vegetation then become part of the increased mucopolysaccharide spongiosa layer which causes the valves to prolapse? And is this an ongoing or chronic process of repeated attacks of mild bacterial endocarditis, the sort Libman described, with natural healing and consequent accumulation within the valve of mucopolysaccharide from decomposed bacteria, leading, ultimately, in such individuals, to an increasingly severe form of "floppy" valve? In other words, one could envision polysaccharides begetting polysaccharides via bacterial decomposition and hence the progression of the bulging and ballooning of the prolapsed valves.

In the future, research may show that the increased spongiosa in prolapsed valves is evidence, not of congenital abnormality, but of repeated episodes of IE, spontaneously resolved or contained by the natural defences of the body or contained enough to postpone death by the use of oral antibiotics for some other assumed illness. Even more fascinating proof that MVP could be caused by IE might exist in the latest observations provided by electron microscopy of floppy mitral valve leaflets removed at surgery. Deposits of platelets, and sometimes fibrin as well, have been observed on the damaged endothelial surfaces of the valves.[112] Platelets and fibrin are the materials that compose the vegetations, and it is the platelets, like the polysaccharides that assist the bacteria in adhering to the valvular surfaces.

The whole question of IE raises another issue. A topic of great interest recently in the medical literature is the finding that MVP patients have a greater susceptibility to thrombus formation, Freedman's NBTVs. The incidence of stroke or cerebral embolism is four times greater in MVP patients than in the normal population.[113] Thus the same mechanism that is believed to create a susceptibility to IE also creates susceptibility to non-bacterial thrombotic events such as cerebral embolism. It is believed that the more dense the spongiosa layer in the prolapsed valves or the greater the acid mucopolysaccharide content, the greater the stretching of valvular tissue and hence the greater the prolapse and leaking of blood. In line with my suggestion regarding bacterial endotoxins, is it possible that MVP individuals develop a greater propensity for stroke as the murmur and prolapse become more severe as a result of episodes of unrecognized IE which could increase the acid mucopolysaccharides and hence the prolapse and with it the potential for the blood to coagulate in the left side of the heart? Further studies are necessary to answer some of these questions and to explain the cause of prolapsed valves.

15

Signs of Infective Endocarditis

Delay in diagnosis will, of course, vary from patient to patient depending on his concern about symptoms which might seem no more serious than those of "flu".

> Lawrence Freedman: *Infective Endocarditis and Other Intravascular Infections* (New York: Plenum Medical Book Company, 1982), p. 79.

Generally, mild mitral regurgitation causes no physiological difficulty and no symptoms . . . the chief danger is bacterial endocarditis, the incidence of which, however, is impossible to obtain from present data.

> B.W. Cobbs: "Clinical Recognition and Medical Management of Rheumatic Heart Disease and Other Acquired Valvular Disease" in Hurst, J.W. et al. *The Heart* (New York: McGraw-Hill Book Co., 1974), p. 866.

In cases of valvular damage or death from IE, the doctor's usual defense is to say that bacterial endocarditis could not be identified and that it is an extremely difficult disease to detect. However, this is simply not true, and, in the first fifty years of this century, IE was not a difficult disease to detect. There are a whole host of physical and laboratory signs of IE. In fact, there are likely more ways of identifying this disease than there are for detecting many other diseases.

IE is commonly overlooked or mistaken for other diseases of a far less damaging nature. I had contemplated confining the clinical and laboratory signs of IE to an appendix at the end of my book. However, I chose not to because I believe this information is, in no way, supplementary to the main issues here. To put this information at the end would suggest that it is not absolutely necessary for the patient to know. But, if the doctor cannot identify IE, the patient had better be able to do so, and, if the doctor is not familiar with all the tests to uncover the disease, the patient should have the knowledge to be able to suggest them.

This chapter is a summary of the symptoms which the patient might report to his doctor who should then, if he is astute, look for the clinical and laboratory abnormalities, the non-specific, those that can be found in other illnesses, and the specific, those found only in IE. These signs are not arranged in order of importance or prevalence, and the whole picture must be taken into account, especially the source of the infection. I cannot emphasize strongly enough how important it is for individuals with MVP, for individuals with any susceptible cardiac disorder, to be familiar with these signs. Such knowledge can mean the difference between a normal life and one greatly compromised by valvular damage and/or renal dysfunction, between the freedom and security of having one's own valve instead of an artificial or animal tissue valve and, ultimately, between life and death.

The primary signs of IE are the same as they were in the first half of the century although, in the modern era, a greater number of laboratory diagnostic tests are available. It is hoped that the patient, especially one with a known MVP, who thoroughly familiarizes him or herself with these signs, will be able to protest vigorously and effectively, by demanding a thorough investigation as outlined in this chapter, when a diagnosis of "flu"[1], viral infection, even the common cold, sore throat or tonsillitis, in the presence of high fever, or a diagnosis of psychiatric illness is made.

Positive Blood Culture

It goes without saying that the positive blood culture is definitive for IE but, in 10-20 percent of cases, and perhaps more, the cultures are negative;[2] that is, in the presence of accepted nutritional requirements, microorganisms cannot be grown from the patient's blood in the laboratory. The positive blood culture should be the first thing the doctor looks for, though this is frequently not the case as will be discussed in the chapter on problems in diagnosing IE. The blood is cultured to confirm a **suspected** IE in the presence of any of the other signs. Bacteria is not routinely sought in blood samples. The physician must first suspect that there is an IE before he will think to request the lab to do specific tests to verify the presence or absence of bacteria or fungi in the blood. His suspicions can only be based on his clinical observations made during the physical examination and on the patient's report of symptoms, not on laboratory signs. As has been said, "The single most important factor in the diagnosis of IE is a high index of suspicion."[3] Without that suspicion, no blood cultures, nor any other test, will be done. But it must be stressed that a negative blood culture does not rule out IE. Dr. Austin did not suspect IE in my case and, thus, he did not order any blood tests, in spite of my complaints of fever, tachycardia, chest pain and a source of infection clearly related to ongoing dental manipulations. His lack of suspicion is all the more incomprehensible in view of the fact that he heard, on that visit, a change in my murmur and had ordered an x-ray which showed a definite increase in the size of my heart over the previous year.

Non-specific Compaints

The following symptoms[4] can be found in many illnesses and are not specific for IE though they constitute very significant clues: 1) fever 2) pallor 3)chills 4) sweats, especially night sweats 5) unusual fatigue 6) exhaustion 7) diarrhea 8) vomiting 9) persistent headache, especially if the patient does not have a history of headache 10) loss of appetite 11) anemia 12) general malaise 13) weight loss 14) cough 15) chest pain 16) abdominal pain 17) musculoskeletal arthralgias 18) peculiar visual disturbances.

Fever of Unknown Origin (FUO)

The normal body temperature is 37°C or 98.6°F. The individual with habitual fever unrelated to illness is very rare. Though fever is a non-specific sign, a doctor should suspect IE in all cases of "fever of undetermined origin"[5], particularly in the presence of a murmur or in the presence of MVP. There is disagreement in the literature as to what temperature constitutes a fever. *The Merck Manual of Diagnosis and Therapy* states fever as 37.8°C (100°F) orally or 38.2°C (100.8°F) rectally.[6] There are reports of IE in the medical literature in patients with temperatures as low as 37.2°C and even 36.4°C[7]. Temperatures may vary in the same individual with spikes in the afternoon.[8] Some writers, like Barlow, Lakier and Mazansky of the Johannesburg Hospital, suggest that any temperature above 37°C is cause for investigation for IE in the right setting[9] and that would mean in the presence of valvular abnormalities such as MVP. Fever was detected only rectally in one of their patients with IE, even though he was dyspneic or breathless at rest. One of the dentists I saw while I had a periodontal abscess, insisted a temperature of 38.5°C did not indicate fever.

Again we should look at the literature of the past. It has something to teach us. Osler pointed out long ago in 1885 that fever in the course of an IE is **variable, intermittent, high, low or absent**.[10] And, according to many modern writers, fever is absent especially in the elderly, in patients with uremia, CHF or in those who have taken oral antibiotics, corticosteroids[11] or anti-inflammatory drugs such as Tylenol. Some writers say the fever should be more than one week in duration, while others believe more than three.[12] The point I am making here is that the patient should not accept a doctor's opinion that IE is not present on the basis of an absence of fever.

Heart Signs

Murmurs

The existence of a FUO of a week's duration in a patient with a known click and/or murmur is highly suspicious of IE while fever and the sudden appearance of a click and/or murmur, never documented previously in a patient who has regular check-ups, in my view, should be "virtually diagnostic" of IE, as is fever in the presence of a new murmur, for example, an aortic murmur in a patient with a known mitral murmur.[13] However, murmurs may be absent in right-sided, tricuspid valve endocarditis[14] such as may develop in a drug abuser.

Changing Murmurs

Changes in the character of heart sounds and murmurs is common in IE.[15] Of most importance to the MVP patient is the "changing" murmur. Both the old and the modern literature document such changes, especially that from a LSM to a PSM in the presence of fever and other symptoms of IE. In a MVP patient, such a change in the mitral murmur points strongly to IE. During infection, murmurs may change in intensity or loudness and quality.[16] According to researchers, intensity or loudness is graded on a scale of 1 to 6. 1)faint, heard only with special effort 2)faint but readily recognized. 3) prominent but not loud 4)loud 5)very loud and 6) exceptionally loud, can be heard with the stethoscope just removed from the chest wall.[17] During IE, changes may occur in frequency (pitch) or configuration (shape). If one is a musician, there will be no difficulty understanding the term "shape". The shape of a murmur may be crescendo, decrescendo, crescendo-decrescendo or (diamond-shaped), plateau or plateau with crescendo in LS.[18] There are many words to describe the auditory character of murmurs, for example, rough, blowing, honking, rumbling, grunting, musical, harsh, whooping, squeaky, buzzing or scratchy.[19] All of these descriptions, especially honking, blowing, whooping and musical, have been used to describe the MVP murmur[20] and, in Cates' and Christie's 1951 Pencillin Trials, known mitral murmurs were observed, during IE, to change, becoming "louder, high-pitched and musical."[21] The direction of radiation of the murmur may alter. For example, a strictly apical systolic murmur of MVP may become louder during infection and radiate to the patient's back, the armpit or neck. In 15 percent of patients with IE, no murmur may exist on the first examination for illness and, in particular, the murmur may not be heard in the early stages of the disease,[22] even though there is fever and a positive culture. Any of these changes in a MVP murmur, especially a change in duration from a LSM to a PSM, should alert the physician to the possibility of IE. In my case, as in others, the classic changing murmur, in a setting typical for IE, was simply disregarded as unimportant because it was the murmur of MVP.

Rhythm Disturbances

Tachycardia is very common with IE especially in the presence of high fever and, in one hospital series, fever and tachycardia were found in 92.6 percent of patients.[23] This could be a strong clue that the patient has IE, if other signs are present. Unfortunately, my cardiologist had considered the excessive tachycardia I suffered during my illness to be nothing more than a few, benign palpitations, what medical textbooks describe as "a common, disagreeable, subjective phenomenon . . . an awareness of the beating of the heart".[24] This description, indeed, suits the rapid heart beat caused by strong exercise, sexual intercourse or fear, for example, but not the kind suffered during a potentially crippling disease. As an undergraduate at University, when I had to deliver a paper before my fellow students, I experienced such benign "palpitations" which I dismissed, without further thought, as evidence of fear, and, indeed, a "nuisance", the word favoured by Austin. This is the only situation in which this term, "nuisance", might be justifiably applied. When I described the two episodes of rapid heart beat that I experienced in 1979 to doctors, I used the word, "flutter", prior to ever having read anything in the medical literature. "Flutter" is the actual word cardiologists have chosen to refer to either atrial or ventricular tachycardia in the range of 250-350 beats/min or 200/300 beats/min respectively. [25] It was this type of rapid heart beat I experienced during my illness. However, the episodes recurred frequently, preventing me from lying down to sleep.

Cardiac Enlargement

Any change in the size or shape of the heart may be a clue to IE. An increase of more than **two cm**. in the transverse diameter of the heart is classified as significant and under **two cm**. a minor enlargement. Increases under **one** cm. are rejected as unimportant.[26] In my case, Dr. Austin, who had noted a tiny, undersized heart in 1976 and 1978, considered a 2.5 cm. increase in the transverse diameter of my heart in 1979 as "minor" and, since he did no blood tests, he obviously did not think of this increase in heart size as a clue to IE, even though other symptoms and a known source of infection were part of the picture.

Sudden cardiac enlargement can be caused by acute regurgitation due to vegetations on the valves, a pericarditis, myocarditis or mural endocarditis in association with bacterial infection. Any word ending in "itis" means inflammation and that of the myocardium or heart muscle, myocarditis, while that of the outer fibrous sac or pericardium, pericarditis. Acute pericarditis is accompanied by a pericardial effusion, an increase in the fluid surrounding the heart, thus causing enlargement in the cardiac silhouette. Enlargement of the entire heart or of one chamber will show up on x-ray but is less likely to show up on the electrocardiogram. However, my electrocardiogram showed ST segment depression at rest during my infection. The ST segment is that portion of the heart's electrical activity which occurs between depolarization, that causes ventricular contraction, and repolarization, an electrical phenomenon represented by the T wave on the electrocardiogram, that prepares the ventricles for the next contraction. ST segment depression can mean hypertrophy, left ventricular strain[27] and ischemia from an inadequate blood supply to the heart muscle.

In 1980, a study done in Massachusetts described cardiomegaly in a MVP patient who had vegetations only on the walls of the heart or a mural endocarditis (from the Latin murus=wall). No vegetations were found on the valves or chordae.[28] Cardiac enlargement has been found in certain studies in 75 percent of patients during IE and is generally present in mural endocarditis.[29] If doctors look for valvular vegetations on echo in a case of mural endocarditis they could misdiagnose the patient's illness.

A study at the University of Minnesota Hospital showed that 22.9 and 27.1 percent of IE patients at autopsy had evidence of septic myocarditis and pericarditis respectively. Usually an abscess within the heart is the cause, but this may go undetected. Such abscesses have been found in over 60 percent of patients with IE.[30] The incidence of pericarditis in IE varies from 4 to 27 percent.[31] Pericarditis can develop if a myocardial infarction involves the pericardial walls, and myocardial infarction has been found in 40-60 percent of autopsied patients with IE.[32] One should recall the tennis player described in my introduction. The fact that pericarditis is so prevalent in IE recalls the older idea that the MSC and LSM were caused when the pericardium adhered to the lungs during an infectious episode. It then becomes a question once again of whether MVP is caused by chronic or repeated attacks of mild IE that are accompanied by a pericarditis. The earlier researchers may have been confronted with pericarditis in association with an IE, which went undetected as Libman had suggested was frequently the case.

In 1950, Sheldon and Golden described twelve autopsy cases of IE where abscesses of the valve rings had been healed inadvertently by antibiotics. 86 percent of all fatal cases of IE from 1947 to 1951 in their study revealed "ill-defined swellings" in the mitral and aortic valve rings which were proven to be healed abscesses.[33] The thickening or nodules on my tricuspid valve, which were seen on echo during my third hospitalization, were, in all likelihood, the "ill-defined swellings" of healed tricuspid valve ring abscesses and not myxomatous tissue deterioration as was suggested to me. My tricuspid murmur and a recent echocardiogram, which showed healed vegetations on the mitral valve and tricuspid valve ring, would appear to verify this. As I have already pointed out, in 25 percent of laboratory rabbits in experimental studies, tricuspid valve vegetations heal spontaneously.

All the above findings in IE, myocarditis, pericarditis, cardiac enlargement and abscesses on the valve rings or in the heart, may be the primary evidence of IE or they may be in association with typical valvular vegetations. Other signs may be less prominent or even absent altogether.

Peripheral Signs

There may be pallor of the skin, mucous membranes of the mouth and the conjunctiva of the eye in addition to the following five classic external signs of the skin and nails: petechiae, Osler's Nodes, Janeway's lesions, clubbing and splinter hemorrhages. Modern researchers believe that these external signs have decreased in the antibiotic era. However, doctors may simply be overlooking them, especially if IE never occurs to them or if they attempt to confirm it solely by echocardiogram which does not always show vegetations or, if oral antibiotics have been administered early in the disease, before diagnosis, these highly specific clinical findings, diagnostic of IE, may not be evident.

Petechiae

Petechiae are minute, rounded, red spots with pale, whitish or yellowish centres. They are often found in the conjunctiva of the eyes, the lids, the fundus, (the posterior portion of the interior of the eye which can only be seen on opthalmoscopic examination), the oral mucosa of the mouth, both the hard and soft palate, and on the hands or feet. These hemorrhages when found in the eyes are called Roth spots.[34] They are small, sometimes flame-shaped with pale centres. Red, non-blanching petechiae may become brown and barely visible within several days. They are the most common skin lesion, and it was Libman who first drew attention to the fact that they could represent either embolization or the leakage of blood from capillaries injured by inflammation.[35] Though reportedly less frequent in the antibiotic era, a 70.4 percent incidence of this kind of skin manifestation has been reported in a study done at the University of Minnesota in 1961.[36]

Osler's Nodes

These tender, painful skin lesions were named after Sir William Osler who emphasized that they were highly specific for IE and rarely found in any other disease. These lesions are nodular, small, firm, raised, reddish-purple spots sometimes with a whitish centre. They occur on the fingertips, the pads of the toes, soles of the feet, the skin of the lower arm and, occasionally, on the sides of the fingers. Because they can disappear within hours or several days, the French called them "nodosités cutanées éphémères."[37] They are more frequent in longstanding, subacute rather than acute cases. Recent attempts to culture these nodes confirm the truth of Osler's observation that they are minute emboli which contain bacteria rather than a "perivasculitis resulting from an immunologic reaction to the pathogenic organism" in association with non-bacterial emboli.[38] Once again, the past reasserts itself, suggesting strongly that doctors avail themselves of the knowledge about IE that has accumulated for almost a century.

Janeway's Lesions

These spots on the skin were named after Dr. George Janeway, Emanuel Libman's teacher. In 1897, Janeway described them as abundant, small hemorrhages, slightly nodular, in the palms of the hands and the soles of the feet but rarely on the arms, legs or trunk. Libman added that they are red, 1-4 mm. in diameter, either macular (flat) or papular (circumscribed, solid, raised) and blanch on pressure or when the extremities are raised. An isolated few can be easily overlooked since the margins of these nodes are not distinguishable from the surrounding skin. Unlike Osler's lesions, they are not painful or tender.[39] Doctors today often consider these skin lesions to be confined to the pre-antibiotic era but, according to a 1982 paper from the Mayo Clinic, most patients with IE have either arthralgias or peripheral signs such as Janeway's lesions.[40]

Clubbing of the Fingers

Clubbing is considered the most useful of these external signs because, according to relatively recent research at St. Bartholomew's Hospital in London, England, it is "so rarely found in diseases with which IE can be confused."[41] Clubbing may be described as a broadening and thickening of the soft tissues of the ends of the fingers and toes with loss of the angle of the nailbed. Clubbing also occurs in a congenital lung disease called bronchiecstasis in which the bronchi become dilated and distorted. Fibrosis eventually destroys the lung tissue and leads to pulmonary hypertension. However, Libman noted that the clubbing of IE is much milder than that of bronchiectasis.[42] According to both pre and post antibiotic writers, the true clubbing of IE is distinguished by the margin of red skin around the nails, what researchers at The Royal College of Physicians and Surgeons of London, England, described as a "boggy, edematous nail-bed" indicative of active infection.[43] Though clubbing is said to be found in only 10-20 percent of cases of IE in the antibiotic era and is largely found in longstanding, chronic cases[44], there is a great deal of confusion over its identification. Again, because clubbing is not thought to be a prominent sign in the modern era, it is frequently overlooked, though in a 1978 textbook on IE, clubbing was said to occur in as much as 52 percent of subacute cases of the disease.[45]

Splinter Hemorrhages

Like the hemorrhagic spots in the eyes, these are tiny blood clots or emboli which may have broken off from the valve and travelled through the bloodstream to lodge in the fingernails or they may be explained as immunologic phenomena. They are distinguishable from the trauma of injury because they are located at a distance from the ends of the fingernails and are longitudinal, reddish-black and splinter-shaped.

Splenomegaly

The enlargement of the spleen occurs most frequently in chronic cases and has been reported in approximately 60 percent of patients according to a study by Barlow and co-workers.[46] The incidence of spleen enlargement may be considerably underrated. Libman found splenomegaly in 80-90 percent of cases of IE and pointed out that, though the spleen may not be felt, it may still be enlarged.[47] There is every reason to believe the accuracy of Libman's facts since doctors in his time were much more skilful at palpating organs than doctors today who rely heavily on technology as a diagnostic tool especially in the case of IE. The confusion over whether or not my spleen was enlarged is a fact in support of this opinion. But despite our sophisticated scanning technology used to calculate spleen size, if a doctor does not order a spleen scan, in a questionable case where a spleen cannot be felt, technology is of no use. A moderate increase in size may not make the spleen palpable or the spleen may not descend because of adhesions to the diaphragm as a result of the infection, just as the pericardium may adhere to the lungs during inflammation.

Infected emboli may lodge in the spleen, as in the heart, other organs or fingernails, cutting off the blood supply in the area and destroying surrounding tissue. These emboli to the spleen cause local tenderness or pain in the left upper quadrant of the abdomen with radiation to the shoulder. I had a type of pain fitting this description, but Dr. Austin told me it was an atypical chest pain associated with MVP. This emphasizes that there are possibly many symptoms attributed wrongly to MVP that perhaps ought to become clues to other diseases. Small infarcts in any organ can be asymptomatic. The greatest danger is that the spleen may rupture causing hemorrhage and death. Even while IE may seem to be under control, an abscess may develop in the area of an infarction, causing a peritonitis or inflammation of the serous membrane lining the abdominal cavity. In one series of IE cases, splenic infarction was found in 41 of 78 patients, or over fifty percent, who had died, suggesting that splenic emboli are infrequently detected during life.[48]

Extra Cardiac Manifestations

Many modern researchers believe that extra-cardiac signs of the musculoskeletal, renal and neurological kind have only recently emerged as indicators of IE and that they now overshadow the more classic skin signs so emphasized in the pre-antibiotic era. Those who hold this opinion are eager to point out that IE is a changing disease but this is an attitude that engenders confusion in diagnosis and a tendency to overlook the obvious signs. As well, a thorough search of the medical literature reveals that these signs are not new and do not represent a changed picture of IE, that, in fact, the writers of the pre-antibiotic era, Libman, Horder, Osler and Glynn have all reported at great length on the rheumatic, renal and neurological phenomena of IE.

Musculoskeletal Manifestations

"Rheumatic endocarditis", a term frequently used in the earlier writings, suggests the thin line between acute, inflammatory rheumatic disorders of a streptococcal origin, such as rheumatic fever (RF), and IE. In the pre-antibiotic era, Horder published an important paper on 150 patients who died from IE, 66 of whom had joint pains and 22 of whom had swollen joints.[49] In one modern review of 1977, Churchill, Geraci and Hunder from the Mayo Clinic reported that 44 percent or 84 of 192 patients with IE had either arthralgias (joint pains without inflammation), myalgias (muscle pains) arthritis (inflammation with swollen joints) and low back pain.[50]

Arthralgias

This is the most common musculo-skeletal sign of IE. It occured in about 32 of the 84 patients or 38 percent in the Mayo study. In some of these patients, the pain migrated from one joint to another.

Arthritis

Arthritis with inflamed, swollen and painful joints occured in 31 percent of the patients in the Mayo study. If a swollen, painful joint is the only symptom a patient has, IE may only be detected by **arthrocentesis** which involves puncturing the joint and aspirating the synovial fluid for analysis of bacterial content. The synovial fluid is the clear, thick, lubricating secretion from the membrane that lines joints, bursa (the sac that contains fluid located over bony parts of the body especially knees and elbows) and tendons. In 1978, Good and co-workers of the Ann Arbor Veterans Administration Hospital in Michigan, described migratory arthritis in a MVP patient with IE. Positive synovial cultures were followed by negative ones 36 hours later that complicated the diagnostic process. These authors advised early arthrocentesis before defense mechanisms or immunologic reactions intervene and render the cultures negative, thus causing further delay in the diagnosis.[51] For the same reason, Osler's nodes should be cultured early. But, of course, once again, the doctor must suspect IE before he will be prompted to order an arthrocentesis. It is not likely that the timid patient with only fever and an isolated swollen joint will demand arthrocentesis as a test for IE.

The authors of the Mayo study maintain that the development of acute synovitis in specific joints which are not frequently involved alone in more common forms of arthritis such as "rheumatoid arthritis" should arouse suspicion of IE. These commonly affected joints are a single metacarpophalangeal joint of the fingers, the sternoclavicular joint and the acromioclavicular joint that unites two bones of the shoulder, the acromion and clavicle.[52] It was Libman who drew attention to tenderness or soreness of the sternum.[53] A case I have already discussed reported by Kincaid and Botti[54] described a

MVP patient with a swollen, inflamed ankle, fever and chills as her only symptoms of IE. This patient did not even have a murmur.

Low Back Pain

Churchill and colleagues reported this symptom in 23 percent of their patients.[55] There may be spinal tenderness and decreased motion, pain in the paraspinal muscles, or simply muscle spasms in the lumbar area. This last type of pain was the **only** sign in one patient for three months prior to the diagnosis of IE. Other causes of low back pain can be ruled out if the patient has not suffered either previous back strain, degenerative joint or disc disease or previous episodes of back pain from an old injury and if x-rays are normal or exhibit minimal degenerative arthritis.

Vertebral Osteomyelitis

This is another type of back pain indicative of IE. It is caused by microorganisms that invade the bone marrow and create inflammation within the spinal column. Commonly, the microorganisms are candida or staphylococcus aureus but may also be strep. viridans. In his book, *Infective Endocarditis and Other Intravascular Infections*, Lawrence Freedman pointed out that it is likely that "osteomyelitis due to viridans streptococci is always an indication of the presence of IE."[56] In 1980 a case was described in the medical literature with symptoms of tenderness over the spine, spasm of the paravertebral musculature, erosive changes in the vertebral discs on x-ray, elevated gamma serum globulin and small pericardial effusion with minimal cardiomegaly. While the authors of this study rated vertebral osteomyelitis as extremely rare, they were of the opinion that low back pain accounts for 25-33 percent of all complaints of a musculoskeletal nature in IE.[57] Fungal infection with the candida species, for example, can be caused by indwelling catheters or from surgery to replace natural valves with prosthetic ones. A 1976 report [58] described the case of a woman who had developed thrombophlebitis in her arm from an intravenous catheter, just as I had on my first hospitalization. However, there was no IE in the case of this woman, only a pyogenic vertebral osteomyelitis, since she had no pre-existant valvular lesion.

In cases of fungal endocarditis, no matter what the cause, blood cultures are often negative and, thus, many cultures may be required to detect bacteria and, even then, the blood may remain sterile. Frequently, a cure is thought to have been obtained with antimicrobial treatment, but, quite often, there is relapse after substantial periods of time have passed indicating the fungal endocarditis was not really cured, but had remained dormant so that symptoms were suppressed. Patients with fungal endocarditis, therefore, require long follow-up. Freedman reported that he had seen "staphylococcal osteomyelitis with recurrences after an interval of twenty years with the same phage-type bacterium"[59] in patients supposedly cured of candida infection. Phage bacteria are bacteria infested with ultramicroscopic tad-pole microorganisms. Some staphylococci bacteria, so infested, become antibiotic resistant. Freedman's observations show that the agents of vertebral osteomyelitis can remain quiescent for long periods of time, only to reactivate at a later date. Since I developed thrombophlebitis from an IV catheter in my arm and had an elevated serum gamma globulin and recurrent, severe low back pain for which there was no history of injury but which resembled the painful symptoms described in these reports, while I had signs of chronic IE, I naturally wondered if there was a vertebral osteomyelitis or if the healed tricuspid vegetations had been caused by infection from the IV catheter. At the time of the episode of severe, disabling low back pain, my x-ray findings were interpreted as "degenerative osteoarthritis" the result, it was stressed, of normal wear and tear on the spine, but it is known in the medical literature that signs on x-ray of vertebral osteomyelitis can be mistaken for "degenerative osteoarthritis"[60]

Myalgias or Muscle Pains

Myalgias or muscle pains have been found in 19 percent of IE patients according to Churchill and co-workers from the Mayo Clinic.[61] Their patients reported pain localized to thighs and calves, and one patient had right thigh pain for three months before a diagnosis of IE was made. This was the only symptom this patient had of IE. This suggests, once again, the importance of looking for IE when an at risk patient, such as a MVP patient, reports pain of this nature. It is believed that this type of myalgia may be caused by an embolus in a small muscular artery or arteriole with resultant muscle cell destruction. What must be stressed is that myalgias of this kind may be mistaken for other diseases such as "collagen vascular disease", an inherited disorder of the connective tissue, as this report indicated.

Hypertrophic Osteoarthropathy

Hypertrophic osteoarthropathy is another type of musculoskeletal pain associated with IE that can be mistaken for rheumatoid arthritis. The periosteum, the fibrous membrane covering the surfaces of bones, becomes inflamed. There is new bone formation, arthritis and clubbing of the fingers. A patient with IE manifesting as Hypertrophic Osteoarthropathy was reported in the *Annals of Internal Medicine*.[62] He complained of constant aching pain that prevented walking and sleeping but was unrelated to motion and was made more severe by local pressure. The pain began in his finger tips and toes, increased in severity and extended up to the elbows and knees, and his finger tips were described as bulbously enlarged, extremely tender and soft at the nail beds. X-rays showed periosteal thickening along the shafts of the metacarpals, the radius, ulna, tibia and fibula. The writers, McCord and Moberly, in their conclusion, remarked that symptoms of hypertrophic osteoarthropathy of a chronic nature can be mistaken for rheumatoid arthritis. A 1974 study from The Massachusetts General Hospital described the death of a MVP patient whose IE was misdiagnosed as rheumatoid arthritis which was treated accordingly.[63]

Neurologic Manifestations of IE

Like most other signs of IE, cerebral vascular involvement was discussed at great length in the earlier, pre-antibiotic literature and its frequency emphasized. The incidence today remains the same as it was when Osler first stressed cerebral events in 1885.[64] Early appearing complications of a neuropsychiatric nature are of less severity, and, therefore, prompt diagnosis and treatment can prevent major brain damage or death. Classic reviews, such as that of Irwin Ziment of the UCLA School of Medicine in 1969, which showed cerebral involvement to vary dramatically from as low as 9 to as high as 80 percent of patients with IE, are still regarded by researchers of the eighties as valid.[65] Where the mitral valve is involved, the frequency of cerebral complications is greatly increased, 52 percent compared to 28 percent with aortic valve infection.[66] This means MVP patients have a greater risk of brain damage. Confirmation of cerebral involvement can be made by cerebral spinal fluid analysis, but the danger is that the results, as in the case of blood cultures, may be negative for bacteria or for other abnormalities. The use of the modern CAT scan (computerized axial tomography) is also a means of early diagnosis, and some researchers consider it superior to cerebral spinal fluid analysis.[67] The CAT scan is a type of moving x-ray which, like ventricular cineangiography, also requires the injection of contrast dyes to view certain body organs such as liver and kidneys. It allows the inner geography of the body to be photographed, and pictures can be taken of a specific area of the body while others are blurred. The computer is then used to reconstruct the body section from scanned radiographs and convert it to video images.

Warning Signs of Central Nervous System Involvement (CNS)

Some reports on IE indicate there may be only "severe, unremitting, localized headache"[68]. Other signs of brain involvement appear to be of a purely psychological or neurotic nature and, therein, lies the danger. These signs are decreased concentration, lethargy, insomnia, vertigo, irritability, confusion, disorientation, psychosis, neurosis, auditory and visual hallucinations, emotional lability, personality or behavioural changes, euphoria, delirium and depression. All these signs may predict a cerebral vascular catastrophe,[69] but they have, unfortunately, been mistaken for psychiatric or neurotic illness.[70] It must be stressed that symptoms of cerebral dysfunction, especially if they are minor, are often completely overlooked and, if they are the only sign or one of a few signs not readily recognized as a manifestation of IE, the diagnosis will likely be missed. Patients have been mistakenly admitted for psychiatric and neurologic investigation, thus delaying treatment and, in the words of one important researcher from UCLA medical school, Irwin Ziment, "It is not known what proportion of patients with such toxic symptoms actually do have organic brain lesions secondary to bacterial endocarditis."[71] He warns doctors to pay more attention to these seemingly psychological abnormalities. It may be recalled here that, when I reported chest pain for the first time, which was in addition to the other symptoms that rounded out a picture of IE, my cardiologist interpreted my complaints as evidence of "pathological anxiety" and a "labile mentality".

Principal Ways in Which The Brain is Affected

Cerebral Embolism

Cerebral Embolism is the most common neurologic complication.[72] A clot of blood or embolus (pl.emboli) can block an artery in the brain just as it can the heart and, when it does, it is called an embolism. Major emboli occur in about 6-31 percent of cases [73]. One of the most important causes of cerebral emboli, when the mitral valve is involved, is atrial fibrillation. This is a chaotic, irregular heart rhythm which has been described as "analogous to numerous pebbles being thrown into different areas of the same pool at once."[74] In IE, the emboli are pieces of the bacterial vegetations which break off from the valve and travel through the circulation to lodge in the arteries of the brain just as they can in any other organ, such as the spleen, kidneys, heart. Occlusion of an artery in the brain is commonly referred to as a "stroke". Damage, logically, depends on the size of the embolus. Some emboli are so small that the damage is "silent" and the patient is unaware. There may be only minor symptoms such as stiff neck or headache. Multiple cerebral emboli may cause symptoms of toxemia: headache, impaired concentration, lethargy, drowsiness, insomnia, dizziness, vertigo or irritability, as already mentioned, but a large embolus may cause a major cerebral vascular disaster with varying degrees of paralysis, speech loss and coma or death just as in the case of non-bacterial emboli which cause strokes. If the cranial nerves are involved or the retinal arteries of the eye, there may be visual disturbances such as blurring and dimming, double vision, dark spots in the visual field (scotoma), blindness in one or both eyes, unequal pupils or paralysis of the face, palate, tongue, larynx or eyes. Cerebral emboli may also impair motor control with symptoms of tremor, muscular incoordination, Parkinsonism, convulsions, chorea (irregular, involuntary actions of the muscles of the extremities and face), hiccuping from brain stem emboli, vomiting, chewing, excessive scratching, rhythmic tongue protrusion and spasms of the muscles.[75]

Mycotic Aneurysms

Mycotic aneurysms are associated almost exclusively with IE but are said to be less common than emboli, occurring in 2-10 percent of cases of IE.[76] The word, aneurysm, applies to a ballooning or dilatation of an artery which can ultimately burst. Some reviewers of the cerebral complications in IE consider this incidence to be falsely low because aneurysms, unlike emboli, are not as easy to detect. Doctors miss them both in life and at autopsy when rupture and hemorrhage have obscured the true cause of the patient's death. As well, minor aneurysms can heal with antimicrobial treatment and, so, at autopsy, no longer contain bacteria that would identify IE, if the aneurysm had been the only sign of this disease.[77] Aneurysms may be multiple or single and generally result from an infected embolus lodging in the walls of an artery or its vasa vasorum, that is one of the many small blood vessels in arteries and their corresponding veins. The word, mycotic, implies infection with a variety of microorganisms, including the streptococcus, the staphylococcus and fungi. Aneurysms may occur in the arteries of other organs as well. The formation of an aneurysm is similar to the creation of a vegetation in that it grows through the adherence of platelets and fibrin. The walls of the artery become weakened from distension and balloon outward until they leak or rupture, causing bleeding or hemorrhage, usually massive, into the subarachnoid space (that is the area between two of the membranes, the arachnoid and pia mater, which cover the brain and spinal column), the cerebral tissues or ventricles.[78] A minor leak may not be fatal, but massive rupture means death. Cerebral aneurysms are generally asymptomatic or without major symptoms until rupture occurs.[79] Thus mortality is extremely high, occurring in about 60 percent of cases.[80] But symptoms of "severe, unremitting localized headache" have been reported just as they have for emboli and, with early antimicrobial treatment, cerebral damage or death can be avoided.

Brain abscesses

These abscesses are caused by septic emboli discharged from the heart valves or other sites of vegetations such as walls of the ventricles of the heart. Multiple micro-abscesses are usually symptomless, but large ones can cause seizures and convulsions, and larger emboli result in serious brain damage. The symptoms are basically the same as for other cerebral complications. Unlike mycotic aneurysms, the abscesses occur outside the arteries, in the surrounding perivascular tissues or structures. The larger abscesses with serious clinical symptoms are more common in acute than subacute IE. The abscess initially causes inflammation with gradual necrosis of the tissue, similar to an infarction in any other organ of the body. At pathology, bacteria is found in these brain abscesses.[81]

Meningoencephalitis

According to many researchers, this is the most common CNS complication in IE. This is a general inflammation of the brain and its membranous coverings called the meninges, that is the dura and pia mater and the arachnoid. The inflammation itself is usually the response of the surrounding tissues of the brain to a mycotic aneurysm or an embolus[82]. The symptoms are the same as for any toxic complication in the brain, and, generally, the neck becomes rigid. There may be cerebral edema, congestion and frequent hemorrhages of different sizes. Inflammation of the meninges alone, **meningitis**, rarely occurs in IE and, if it does, it usually occurs with SBE. If meningitis is the only symptom, IE may go unrecognized with fatal consequences. I know personally of a case, which will be discussed in the next chapter, of an individual whose IE was mistaken for an uncomplicated meningitis. One of the problems in detecting the **meningitis** associated with IE is sterile cerebral spinal fluid. The meningitis may subside without antibiotic treatment[83], but this does not mean that the patient will survive since, if there is an endocarditis of the valve that goes unrecognized, treatment is withheld and graver complications will develop affecting other body organs.

Long-term Results of Cerebral Complications in IE

One of the strongest reasons for avoiding IE is that, even with antimicrobial treatment and the eradication of bacteria from the blood, the after-effects, of an immunological nature, of the disease remain. Studies have shown that as many as 51 percent of individuals who suffered from IE, with or without detectable cerebral emboli, may still die up to five years after treatment from recurring cerebral emboli that have their origin in an uneradicated mycotic aneurysm just as they may die from congestive heart failure.[84] Individuals who recovered from a mild case of IE, or have been inadvertently treated with oral antibiotics without a diagnosis, would suffer the same fate as those whose IE was recognized and treated. However, their late complications would not be attributed to a healed IE but simply to stroke or some other cerebral vascular complication. Pathological examination of the brains of a group of patients, who died some years later of neurologic complications after presumed treatment of their IE, revealed a slowly developing "proliferative endarteritis" or an inflammation of the inner lining of the cerebral arteries which caused narrowing of those arteries and lead to thrombotic occlusion of the vessels.[85] Ziment et al, who have done much research on IE and the cerebral complications, explained that this late developing endarteritis may be the reaction of host-defense mechanisms responding not to emboli or actual bacteria but to the products of bacterial decomposition, the toxins which must then still be in the blood.[86] It is interesting, too, that Libman had also explained such late cerebral events in terms of an immunological vasculitis. This explains why IE is classified as one of the immune diseases. The explanation of researchers such as Ziment et al would seem to support my theory of how the continued presence of endotoxin of the polysaccharide kind, in some way altered to become acid mucopolysaccharide, could cause proliferation of this substance in prolapsed valves during and after an IE.

Renal Complications — Glomerulonephritis

Each of the two bean shaped kidneys are made up of two million functional units called nephrons. Each nephron contains a glomerular capillary network enclosed in a capsule (Bowman's capsule) and is attached to two uriniferous tubules. The function of the glomeruli (sg. glomerulus) is the ultrafiltration of impurities from the blood while that of the tubules is reabsorption of water and solutes back into the system and selection of certain solutes for secretion along with the urine.[87] In IE, it is the glomeruli that become diseased with eventual destruction over short or long periods of time of the glomerular capsule. The medical profession has long known that inflammatory disease involving the glomeruli or glomerulonephritis, acute, subacute or chronic, is most commonly caused by the streptococcus or other bacteria.[88] Glomerular involvement in IE was described very early in the medical literature, in 1910 by Lohlein and in 1912 by Baehr, and Bell's long comprehensive discussion in 1932 hinted at the immunological nature of the glomerular lesions, thus pointing to the direction modern research would take.[89] It is now well established that the glomerular damage occurring in IE is of an immunological nature precipitated by the presence of bacteria in the blood. The bacteria stimulates the body's immunological defenses, and repetitive stimulation, even in the absence of the antigen, perpetuates and maintains the nephritis found in IE.

Immunoelectrophoresis

In the experimental laboratory, glomerulonephritis is now one of the most completely understood of the auto-immune diseases. In auto-immune diseases, tissue damage is the result of the body's inability to distinguish "self" from antigen. The term "auto-immune" is misleading because it suggests "self-protection" when, in fact, the process is one of self-destruction. The body endeavors initially to defend itself from the invader-antigen by producing antibodies in the cells of the reticuloendothelial system, specifically the thymus, bone marrow, lymph nodes and spleen. An antibody or immunoglobulin is a "glycoprotein", composed of a carbohydrate and a protein, that reacts specifically with antigens in the blood.[90] Immunoglobulins differ in molecular size and weight. The bigger and heavier, the less mobility and, therefore, they can be detected in the blood by the speed at which they move through an electrical field when stimulated by an electrical charge. This process of detecting immunoglobulins is called **electrophoresis**. The three main globulin groups are the alpha, beta and gamma, so named from the first three letters of the

Greek alphabet. The alpha and beta globulins can be fractioned into fast and slow alphas called alpha one and two and beta one and two. The three main immunoglobulins, which contain all the known antibody molecules, according to the Swedish researcher, Jan Waldenstrom, and which are adopted by the World Health Organization (WHO) are IgG, IgA and IgM.[91] It was the IgG that was found in my blood on electrophoresis at the Mayo clinic, though subsequently since my first experience with IE, all the immunoglobulins have shown increases at one time or another. In any case, a standard urinalysis is an insensitive test for glomerulonephritis that may only show up much later after the episode of IE.

During IE, the kidneys, like any other organ are targets for emboli containing bacteria. The damage to renal tissue has lead Libman and others to describe the "flea bitten kidney".[92] However, the most frequent kind of damage is immunological rather than embolic and is in the form of a more diffuse nephritis caused by the deposition of immunoglobulins in the glomerular basement membrane of the nephrons in the kidney. These immunoglobulins are detectable on immunoelectrophoresis of biopsied kidney tissues. The glomerular membrane is the middle of three layers of the glomerular capillary and it functions as a barrier in the filtration process.[93] The immunoglobulins are established in the glomeruli by means of circulating immune complexes (CICs). Simply put, the circulating immune complex is the union resulting from the binding of the host's antibody (Ab) with the antigen (Ag) or the causative microorganism. The protective resources of the body join with the invading enemy. This Ag-Ab union or CIC circulates in the blood serum of patients with IE in 90 percent of cases,[94] and CIC mediated disease is known to continue "even after sterilization of infected cardiac vegetations," a fact which only confirms Libman's studies.[95] This is why renal disease, after cure of IE, continues to progress.

Researchers believe that, in the early stages of infection, during the time between the introduction of the antigen into the blood stream and the detection of the responding antibodies in the serum, the gamma M immunoglobulin is predominant but, as the immune response progresses, gamma G immunoglobulins supplant the gamma M.[96] This may explain why IgG is the most frequently isolated immunoglobulin, found on electrophoresis of glomerular basement tissue in 70 percent of patients with IE and glomerulonephritis.[97] It is the immunoglobulin, rather than the antigen, of the immune complex that is generally recovered from kidney tissue although, in 1971, Kaufman et al were able to find streptococcal antigen as well as immunoglobulin in the renal lesions.[98] This would go a long way towards proving that chronic glomerulonephritis is caused by the original disease of IE. Most researchers believe that immunoglobulin IgG is somehow altered by the original infecting microorganism to become the antigen[99] that is deposited in the kidneys because the body loses its capacity to distinguish its own defense mechanisms from the antigen, hence the understanding of glomerulonephritis as an auto-immune disease.

Generally in IE there is a polyclonal hypergammaglobulinemia, that is all the immunoglobulins are increased, but there are cases of patients whose blood shows on electrophoresis only a monoclonal immunoglobulin spike. A study done in Paris, France reported that three of five patients with IE had only monoclonal immunoglobulin IgG or a monoclonal gammopathy on electrophoresis.[100] It was exactly this IgG that was discovered in my blood at the Mayo Clinic.

Monoclonal Gammopathy

IgG is associated in most medical people's minds with myeloma or cancer of the bone marrow. When this immunoglobulin showed up in my blood, repeat tests were done for myeloma. Myeloma comes from the Greek word, **myelos**, meaning bone marrow, but the term no longer means only bone marrow cancer but refers to the proliferation of abnormal plasma cells. Evidently, a past IE was not thought of in association with the increase in immunoglobulin IgG in my blood. Both the cardiologist and the internist admitted that an IgG immunoglobulin could be a leftover from a previous IE, but they denied that IE was a likely cause of my problems. However, there may be yet another explanation for the increase in immunoglobulin IgG. Subsequent urinalyses during and after my "infection" have shown increasing urinary protein that is now over the supposedly normal limit. My internist believes that a certain amount of protein in the urine is normal, and that everybody leaks some protein. However, the opinions expressed in the medical literature do not on the whole support his opinion, and a popular book written for the lay public, *Medical Access* by Richard Saul Wurman, states categorically that there should be no protein in the urine.[101]

It is also well known that the monoclonal immunoglobulin, IgG, which doctors believe to be most characteristic of multiple myeloma, is also found in the serum of patients with proteinuria and glomerulonephritis.[102] Most frequently, this is misinterpreted by doctors as a "benign monoclonal antibody".[103] It seems more logical, given my suspicious history, that the IgG points, not to multiple myeloma nor benign monoclonal antibody, but to a chronic glomerulonephritis. Symptoms of renal disease do not manifest until about 50 percent of the kidney has become non-functional[104] and this takes place only over a long period of time.

Signs of Renal Involvement in IE

There are many people with chronic kidney disease today who suffer greatly. What is the cause? Did they have an IE that was not diagnosed as in my case? In 1932, E.T. Bell, one of the most distinguished early writers on the subject of the glomerulonephritis of IE, emphasized that this complication was more common than embolism.[105] Modern writers, such as Lawrence Freedman, confirm that the renal disease associated with the deposition of CICs is "a universal histological finding in patients with IE" whether or not the renal disease produces symptoms.[106]

Although the glomerulonephritis of IE may be completely undetectable except by electrophoresis of biopsied kidney tissue,[107] in acute cases, there are more obvious signs in the urine such as an abnormal sediment, protein, blood, red and white blood cells and casts[108]. Casts are actually tissue molds, produced by the "solidification of protein" in the nephron, which take on the shape of their origins. Red Blood cell casts indicate the glomerular origin of the bleeding, and leukocytes and white blood cell casts indicate the inflammatory nature of the glomerular infection.[109] There may also be evidence of greatly diminished urinary output, and blood tests may show the retention of waste materials, nitrogenous compounds.[110] These nitrogenus substances are urea nitrogen, an end product of protein metabolism, and creatinine, which is a normal constitutent of blood and urine and a waste product of creatine. Urea nitrogen and creatinine are filtered from the blood by the kidneys and excreted in the urine in constant amounts. Tests for creatinine in urine are done over a 24 hr. period along with a blood test to measure blood urea nitrogen or BUN. Normal serum creatinine is 0.7-1.5 mg/100 ml.[111] In renal disease, potassium, sodium, calcium, glucose and fatty acids may be increased in the blood, and, in acute glomerulonephritis, there is increased cryofibrinogen in the plasma, decreased complement and increased cryoglobulins, particularly in SBE.[112]

Other Laboratory Abnormalities in IE

The white blood cells or leukocytes which fight infection may be elevated. The normal count is 5000-10000/cu. mm. However, WBCs are known to be normal in 50 percent of patients with IE.[113]

Circulating Immune Complexes (CICs)

CICs are a positive sign of glomerulonephritis and, along with clinical findings, CICS are an indication of acute IE.[114] In the first report on CICs in 1976 by Bayer and colleagues at the Wadsworth Veterans Administration Hospital in Los Angeles, 28 of 29 patients or 97 percent with active IE had high levels of CICs in their serum. The longer the illness, the greater the number.[115]

Erythrocyte Sedimentation Rate (ESR)

ESR is defined as the rate at which the red corpuscles in fluid blood, to which anticoagulant has been added, separate from the plasma and settle at the bottom of a glass test tube to form a packed column. [116] This rate may be increased in IE as well as other diseases. The distance the RBCs fall is measured over a period of one hour, and the final calculation is called the

ESR. An elevated sed rate or ESR indicates an increase in fibrinogen, a blood clotting factor, and gamma globulins or immunoglobulins and points to the need for more specific tests for CICs.[117] However, an increased sed rate is not specific for IE.

Rheumatoid Factor (RF)

RF, long thought to be present only in rheumatoid arthritis, is now known to be elevated in many diseases including IE.[118] RF is a protein substance that acts as an anti-gamma globulin and is specifically produced in the body to react against human immunoglobulin. It was first observed in 1940 that the serum of patients with rheumatoid arthritis (RA) would cause sheep red blood cells to agglutinate or stick together.[119] It was also noted that the serum of patients with RA caused streptococcal bacteria to agglutinate by binding with a specific antibody in the serum,[120] and, logically, this would assist in the formation of vegetations. RF is sometimes called an "autoantibody" because it interferes with certain gamma globulins in their role of phagocytosing or destroying bacteria and thus perpetuates disease. For this reason, they are often referred to as anti-gamma globulins. The constant production of CICs provokes the formation of RF which appears in about 50 percent of patients who have had IE for longer than six weeks compared with only 6 percent of cases of early detection.[121]

Hypocomplementemia

Complement is a substance with enzymatic properties that exists in the blood and serum and is decreased or depleted in IE, especially if there is glomerulonephritis.[122] "Hypo" means under production or a deficiency. Low serum complement is related to the all important CICs. Complement is another weapon in the body's defense artillery, functioning bactericidally as an anti-pathogen in association with antibodies. In the laboratory, complement is fractioned into C1, C2, C3, C4 for analysis and any one of these fractions may be depressed in the serum of IE patients.

Cryoglobulinemia

In IE, cryo (cold) precipitable globulins are present in the blood. These substances are globulins that clump together in colder environments, at temperatures less than 37°C, and, therefore, become crystalline, sticking to the walls of test tubes rather than settling to the bottom of a glass tube as red blood cells do when the sed rate is increased. Cryoglobulins are believed to be circulating immune complexes, either polyclonal (mixed IgG, IgA or IgM immunoglobulins) or monoclonal, usually IgG. Cryoglobulinemia is found in 80-90 percent of IE patients.[123]

Heart Antibody (Hab)

Hab is present in patients with IE and was found in 62 percent of patients in one 1977 study.[124] It is said to disappear from the blood after cure with antimicrobials. Hab is an indication of the degree of myocardial cell damage inflicted by the infective process and is usually found in patients with IE and CHF and could show up if there is myocarditis. No doubt, the persistence of this antiheart antibody after antibacterial treatment indicates the permanent, irremediable damage done by the IE. Hab has been observed to result from auto-immune abnormalities in rheumatic fever and supports, therefore, the notion that damage to organs of the body can continue long after the bacterial antigen has disappeared from the blood since the damage is brought about by continued stimulation of the immune system. One wonders then if the cardiomyopathy that certain researchers believe underlies MVP is not in some way connected immunologically to a previous IE. On two occasions, cardiologists have made the statement that I must have suffered from a previous myocarditis though no explanation was given for their opinion. In similar fashion, multiple myeloma, manifested by an IgG monoclonal antibody, is also believed to be caused by chronic over-stimulation of the lymphoreticuloendothelial system which has produced the immunoglobulins in the first place.[125] It might not then be unreasonable to ask whether cancer can be caused by an infection of the gravity of IE which in turn causes chronic stimulation of the immunoglobulins of the body's defense system. In other words, the body's defenses do not turn off once the danger is passed.

Immunological sequelae persist as a consequence of IE, even after healing. Libman described patients with positive cultures and other classic signs of IE who passed out of the acute stage into what he called the "bacteria free stage" when clinical signs of IE and positive cultures were no longer evident. These patients had a chronic illness that persisted for years, manifested by a variety of symptoms: persistent splenomegaly, clubbing, both of which I continue to have, progressive anemia, embolic accidents, endarteritis, which was discussed under neurologic signs of IE, mycotic aneurysms, hepatic cirrhosis and, in particular, myocardial and/or renal insufficiency, due to subacute or chronic glomerulonephritis, both of which eventually lead to death.[126]

In 1965, Cordeiro and co-workers of Lisbon, Portugal suggested that Libman's bacteria free stage is equivalent to the modern second phase of IE which they call the immunological phase. In this stage, the patient has a mixture of chronic infection and immunologic disease. Most doctors do not believe there is such a phase as Libman described. However, Cordeiro et al [127] described this stage in a 1965 paper as "characterized by nephropathy (which is generally a proliferative glomerular lesion), dysproteinemia (abnormalities in blood proteins such as the benign monoclonal immunoglobulin G and monoclonal M component, both of which have been found on electrophoresis in my blood), anemia and vascular fragility."[128] What this means is that the patient has kidney disease, immunoglobulin abnormalities and a tendency to hemorrhage, for example as manifested by purpura or skin lesions of the lower extremities. In addition, Cordeiro et al warned that "there is little tendency to cure; antibiotics are ineffective and mortality is high. We believe that most of the cases that get to the second phase have a relatively long period of pyrexia in the first phase, due either to late diagnosis or inefficient treatment."

The signs I have described here do not represent all the signs of IE, but they are those to which much attention has been given in the medical literature. I have described these signs of IE in great detail because there is much evidence that IE is a disease that is frequently misdiagnosed or simply overlooked and because there is some indication in the research to suggest that bacterial infection, specifically a mild IE, lays the groundwork for other diseases, particularly glomerulonephritis. The symptoms of IE can range from none, as in the case of the young tennis player whose death without an autopsy would certainly have been classified as a myocardial infarction, to non-specific, to many classic signs such as changing murmurs, new murmurs, splenomegaly, cardiac enlargement, tachycardia and any of the laboratory signs described here. If there is a murmur and fever and blood cultures are negative, an exhaustive search should be made for these other signs to complete the picture, though experts in IE warn treatment should not be delayed until positive identification of a microorganism. However, if the patient has no symptoms or clinical signs the doctor can spot, he is not likely to order any lab tests of blood or urine. Then it is crucial for the patient to know all about IE, what tests should be done in order to uncover this disease and be confident in demanding that these tests be done. Tests of body fluids are non-invasive and can save the life of the patient with IE. To protect oneself from this disease or any other disease, the patient must become an informed, medically literate individual.

16

The Differential Diagnosis

Endocarditis Caused By M[6]

We recently treated a young woman with endocarditis caused by this organism
. . . The patient was a 31 year old female with known mitral valve prolapse
who was admitted to the hospital on 30 April, 1982 because of fever. Five
months before admission she had dental cleaning without anti-microbial
prophylaxis . . . her illness was characterized by fever, rigors, headache,
myalgias, and anorexia. One week before admission, outpatient blood cultures
were processed in another laboratory and were reported to be sterile. On
admission to the hospital, she was febrile 39°C, normotensive, and had a
pulse rate of 100 per min. There was a petechial lesion on the right conjunctiva
but no other peripheral stigmata of endocarditis. There was a grade IV/
VI holosystolic murmur at the apex with radiation to the axilla . . . A chest
x-ray showed a normal heart size and contour but with plethoric lung fields,
suggesting early left ventricular failure. The electrocardiogram showed sinus
rhythm and diffuse ST elevation consistent with pericarditis. Two dimen-
sional echo demonstrated . . . a large vegetation on the mitral valve. Therapy
was started with 4×10^6 units of penicillin G intravenously every 4 hr and
100 mg. of gentamycin IV every 8 hr . . . fever promptly remitted. The
following day, six blood cultures . . . indicated microbial growth, and gram
stain showed small gram negative coccobacilli which stained unevenly. Two
days after admission, she became oliguric and creatinine rose to 3.6 mg./
dl. The urine had protein, hemegranular casts, and low sodium concentration
and it was felt she had immune-complex nephritis. The previous antibiotics
were discontinued: ampicillin (2G intravenously every 4 hr) was instituted
. . . over the next few days, she remained afebrile and renal function improved,
but progressive left ventricular failure developed . . . on hospital day 12,
a prosthetic mitral valve was inserted because of the continued cardiac failure.

A.E. Simor and I.E. Salit. "Endocarditis Caused by M[6]." (May,
1983) Journal of Clinical Microbiology 17 (5): 931-933.[1]

From the preceding chapter, it is obvious that a great deal is known about
IE, its risk factors and signs and symptoms. It is not a mysterious disease;

it is not, as I will show later, even a rare disease. There are thousands of articles about IE in the medical journals. The few hundred or more which I have read represent only the tip of the iceberg. The opinions of many doctors about this disease are, therefore, astonishing. Doctors have told me that, despite my MVP, my risk of contracting IE from any surgical or dental procedures was "next-to-nothing".

In the spring of 1983, an article of mine on MVP, the first written by a lay person and possibly the first to appear in the lay literature, was printed in the Canadian magazine, *Healthsharing*, which has a wide circulation in Canada and the United States. Accompanying that article was a questionnaire which solicited information from people with MVP. In addition, I broadcasted my project over "Metro Morning", a local radio station. From these two sources, I received only 33 replies. This number is insignificant in terms of the numbers of people with MVP and suggests that there are, as researchers believe, thousands of people who have unidentified MVP or murmurs which they have been told are insignificant.

From my small survey, however, I acquired some very important facts. Of the 33 respondents, sixteen did not have antibiotic prophylaxis against IE. Fifteen had a history of strep throat or tonsillitis and 8 suffered some febrile illness that closely resembled IE but remained unidentified, though typical symptoms of MVP dated from the time of the illness. Most startling of all, there were, among the 33 individuals, ten episodes of IE, two occurring in the same person. In the majority of these people, MVP was diagnosed only after 1979, despite the fact that the signs of this disease and the examining techniques for uncovering it have been known since 1963 and even well before that time.

The following stories, communicated to me, of the experiences of individuals with MVP offer some very disturbing facts. These patients had not, of course, been protected with antibiotics during risky situations such as dental interventions, and their IE went undiagnosed for long periods of time resulting in severe damage to heart valves or valve replacement.

Jeff

In January of 1979, the year I became ill, Jeff was first told he had MVP. He was 47 years old at the time but had been aware of a "click" since he was 19 when he submitted to a medical examination for the airforce. At some point between the ages of 19 and 47, he must have acquired a murmur. Not long after he learned of his MVP, in September of 1979, he contracted acute IE and was admitted to hospital. He had not been provided with antibiotic prophylaxis for any dental or medical interventions, and his fever was said to be of unknown origin. From his communication, it appears he was treated for an appropriate length of time, six weeks, though he was unaware of the kind of antimicrobial used in his treatment. Upon his release from hospital, in November, he succumbed to a mycotic aneurysm of the brain, a complication of IE which I discussed in the previous chapter. He remained unconscious for one week during which time he suffered from emboli to his legs. A clamp, he was told, was placed on the cerebral artery to stop the bleeding into his brain, and his life was "saved" a second time. His doctors told him an embolus from the infected valve had lodged in the walls of a cerebral artery during the acute infection. Mycotic aneurysms are, as I pointed out, usually associated with longstanding IE. Had Jeff, in fact, had his IE long before his admission to hospital? Was it the result of a dental intervention so far removed from the acute episode of IE as to appear unrelated? There is no indication that Jeff had antibiotic protection prior to his IE even though such protection had been advocated by hundreds of researchers, including Barlow, long before 1979. Why was Jeff's murmur not diagnosed until 1979? Was Jeff's IE actually the cause of his MVP murmur and the reason for its appearance in January of 1979? Had he had several mild episodes of IE in the years between 19 and 47 which finally culminated in an acute episode that created a murmur in addition to the click? Though he says he suffers from no after effects, he is taking 125 mg of Hydrochlorothiazide (HydroDIURIL) daily. This is a very high dosage of diuretic, but Jeff appears to be unaware that this drug is prescribed for congestive heart failure or renal failure, both of which are the sequelae of an IE. In other words, he has fluid overload, but his doctor has only told him that he has elevated blood pressure. Jeff does not appear to be aware that his current health is in any way the result of damage done by the IE.

Gail

Gail's story is similar to mine in that she suffered from a long, complicated illness which began in 1975 with a fever which may have been related to dental work. Her history, like mine, includes repeated episodes of sore throat and tonsillitis. Her initial fever was accompanied by an episode of extreme SOB and severe neck pain, a triad of signs which could mean IE, but this disease was apparently never suggested. At some point in her lengthy illness, she was found to have a change in her murmur, an enlargement of her heart and spleen and clubbing of her fingernails. These same signs, which I had, are, of course, classic signs of IE. Differential diagnoses were hypothesized, and she was told she had a respiratory infection (which may have been pneumococcal endocarditis) and, two years after the precipitating febrile event, chronic obstructive lung disease. Her SOB continued and she collapsed one evening from excessively rapid heart beat. It may be remembered that tachycardia is a symptom of IE in ninety percent of cases. When Gail recovered, she suffered daily from chest pain and SOB, as well as episodes of visual disturbances and elevated blood pressure. She was admitted to the Coronary Care unit and woke up three times with SOB and eventual loss of consciousness. It was shortly after this experience that she was sent to a cardiologist who gave her an echocardiogram and a stress test and told her she had MVP but was too young for angina. This was three years after the initial febrile event. Subsequently, a great deal of confusion arose over the nature of her symptoms which were primarily SOB and episodes of near fainting. Cardiac catheterization was done, and she was told she did not have MVP. Other cardiologists apparently disagreed with this. At some point, a psychiatrist was brought into the picture, and Gail was described as "a difficult, manipulative person," who was "emotionally labile", a description which matched Dr. Austin's portrait of me at the time of my fever, abscessed tooth, tachycardia, enlarged heart and change in murmur. Gail was eventually sent to a neurologist who told her she was "just getting old". In May of 1983, since her MVP was by now officially recognized, Gail was finally given antibiotic protection for dental work, but, unfortunately, only for fillings and extractions, not for cleanings. Gail, however, now has heart failure at the young age of forty-nine and has had to cease working as a nurse. Her case demonstrates the confusion surrounding MVP and underlines once again the curious causal relationship between IE, MVP and CHF.

Jack

Jack, a man in his fifties, had a history of rheumatic fever and a murmur which was called a "noise" in his heart. In 1963, the year Barlow warned that MVP created a risk of IE, Jack developed a fever of undetermined origin with chest pain, cold sweats and emboli in his legs, but his blood tests were negative. When a causative microorganism, strep viridans, was finally grown from his blood, he was treated in hospital for one month, not with IV anti-microbials, but four intramuscular shots of Pen G. He recovered and was given daily penicillin prophylaxis of one-half million units because of his history of rheumatic fever. However, it is known that low levels of ABP for the prevention of RHD are ineffective against IE[1] and may only encourage resistant strains of more common bacteria. In 1981, Jack again developed a fever, in association with periodontal surgery, which was diagnosed as "flu". Weeks went by with spiking afternoon temperatures. He was taken off his daily prophylaxis which had been masking the bacteria, and blood cultures became positive at which point he was admitted to hospital for IV antibiotic treatment. His **MVP** was then identified for the first time. Jack now has SOB and is on diuretics for fluid retention both of which mean his heart is failing, although his doctor has never told him he has congestive heart failure (CHF) or even glomerulonephritis (GN) which he could also have. Jack is reluctant to admit that he has breathlessness and a lack of strength and does not appear to know that the deterioration in his health is related to his bouts of IE. Another bout of IE and he will require valve replacement according to his doctor. Jack's case is an example of IE being mistaken for "flu" and an example of the dangers of daily penicillin prophylaxis in the encouragement of resistant strains of bacteria or unusual microorganisms.

Doug

Doug, a man in his early thirties, had always been very active in sports. He was tall and well built with no obvious physical signs of MVP. He had never been told he had a heart murmur and claimed he was without symptoms. When I questioned him closely, however, he did reveal that he had experienced dizziness, almost complete black-outs, when he stood up. He didn't think this was worth mentioning because he believed everyone had this. The medical name for this classic sign of MVP is orthostatic hypotension which refers to a fall in blood pressure when body position is changed from the sitting to the standing. In September of 1988, while at work, he noticed unusual fatigue which increased over the months and was accompanied by very heavy night sweats. He, however, continued to engage in sports. Local doctors were unable to tell him what was wrong, and he was sent for tests to a neighbouring city. At no time were any blood tests done. He became increasingly unwell, lost 40 pounds and developed massive left sided headache which was, in all likelihood, an embolic episode or some other cerebral complication of IE. The doctors' differential diagnosis was, at one point, meningitis. Though, as I have pointed out, meningitis can be a sign of IE, if other signs are present, the medical examiners did not think of this disease. In January of 1989, five months later, he saw a specialist in his area once again. This doctor listened to Doug's heart and told him he had a murmur which was then identified as MVP, presumably by echocardiogram. He was, at last, told he had IE and was admitted to his local hospital. However, like the tennis player described in my introduction, Doug was active, playing hockey the day before his admission to hospital. Unfortunately, he was treated for only two weeks with IV anti-microbial drugs and, with the appearance of cure, was released prematurely from hospital. Shortly after, he developed severe, unrelievable pain in his left forearm. Again, no local doctors could identify the problem and he was sent to Toronto where he was found to have an embolus in association with his uncured IE. His valve was then replaced with a porcine tissue valve, and the embolus was removed from his arm. There is a very disturbing aspect to Doug's case. Doug claimed that he experienced no shortness of breath. One is likely to believe this since Doug said he played hockey right up until his admission,and left ventricular failure (LVF) never appeared to be a part of his medical picture. Nevertheless, he was told that a large vegetation had ripped away his valve, which was said to be hanging by a thread, and that he would not survive without valve replacement. This exact same echocardiographic picture was given to Margo whose story I relate next. Margo, however, was dying of left ventricular failure, was too weak to get out of bed and required oxygen. My question relates to whether or not valve replacement is becoming the standard treatment for IE no matter what the medical picture? More will be said of this later. Doug's endocarditis took place in 1988, twenty-five years after MVP was unequivocally shown to pose the risk of IE, a fact which should be astonishing to anyone who has read this book. Several questions remain unanswered. When did Doug acquire his murmur? At the time of his IE when he may have had only a click? MVP frequently comes to the attention of medical examiners, as I've shown from a study of the medical research, only at the time of an IE. Or had Doug's general physician, like Austin, simply ignored Doug's MVP murmur, not believing it required protection from IE? Why were blood tests not done? Was Doug's IE undiagnosed because it was in the setting of MVP which is believed, even today, to be an innocent clinical finding? After his release from hospital, several doctors invited Doug to a discussion of his illness. At no time was MVP mentioned as the precipitating factor. When he asked, he was only told that he had a stretched valve. Stretching, as I have discussed, is a characteristic of the increased mucopolysaccharides of prolapsed valves. Why was his MVP ignored or downplayed in importance at this discussion? This issue will be addressed later in this book.

Margo

Margo is the young woman in the case quoted at the beginning of the chapter. The day that article was printed in *The Journal of Clinical Microbiology*, Margo became a statistic. At the time she was stricken with IE in April of 1982, she was just beginning a successful legal career. In 1979, the year I contracted IE, Margo's GP told her that she had a "harmless" murmur which he only later identified by echocardiogram as MVP, even though he had recorded the gold standard, the auscultatory sign of a mid-systolic click, in his notes.

Like all the specialists I had seen, Margo's GP gave her a two or three line description of a completely harmless, congenital condition found mainly in woman of a certain body type, specifically women on the tall, thin side, though there are many women with MVP who are short, of normal weight or overweight. He told her this condition would not affect her life whatsoever and she should not give it a second thought. Margo recalls that he placed great emphasis on the insignificance of MVP. What was most disturbing was his declaration that MVP had only suddenly, in the eighties, become very common in young women. Either her GP was unaware of the hundred years of research that preceded the identification of the MVP syndrome or he chose to ignore it in order to impress upon Margo the absolute unimportance of MVP. While he gave advice regarding antibiotic protection, it was inadequate advice. Certain uncommon events, root canal work and abortion, required the use of antibiotics he said, though he at no time explained the reason for this and never mentioned IE. He requested Margo to convey this information to her dentist. Thus Margo received only slightly more information than I had received from Austin and Rhodes. And, as Doug's case demonstrates, the current treatment of MVP, in the late eighties, is the same as that which Margo and I received in the late seventies and early eighties.

The information which Margo received was of little use to her. She was a modern, sophisticated woman who used contraceptive devices. Abortion was highly unlikely. She was also very much opposed to it. Generally, root canal work is only necessary for people whose teeth have not been properly cared for, as in my case, in childhood and adolescence and is frequently the result of heavy fillings. Margo came from an upper middle class family of medical people. Her father was a retired internist, her brother a general physician, her sister a nurse and her brother-in-law a dentist. All her life, she had had excellent dental care. In fact, her GP had so convinced Margo of the insignificance of MVP that she told no one in her family.

Margo informed her dentist of her GP's specific recommendations. Like Slapek and Cohen, her dentist recorded Margo's prolapse in his records but did not discuss coverage with her for any other dental interventions, such as fillings, scaling, cleaning or periodontal surgery. In fact, the matter was ignored as in my case, even though her dentist would, like mine, have recently received his College's Dispatch, dated August 1979, reminding him that he should follow the American Heart Association (AHA) recommendations regarding the use of antibiotic prophylaxis with MVP and a murmur.

Medical researchers have never explained why IE can develop in one person and not another with the same valvular disease and no protection or why one occasion and not another would cause an IE. It was not until the second visit for a routine cleaning in November of 1981 that Margo became ill. The first sign, as in Doug's case, was fatigue. Margo attributed this to a fast-paced career and social life. Margo's fatigue increased and towards the end of March, 1982, signs of a persistent illness, not unlike the flu, became apparent, exhaustion, anorexia, headaches, chills and fever. Margo began to stay away from work, a few days in bed, a few days in the office. Her alarm increased when she experienced visual disturbances that left her partially blind in both eyes for a period of twenty minutes. Her opthamologist refused to see her on an emergency basis, because blindness appeared in both eyes, and directed her to see her GP. The opinion of the opthamologist reflects a major deficiency in the modern health care system, the lack of co-operation and communication between the physicians who look after different parts of the body. Teeth, eyes, heart, brain are all treated separately as though they belonged to different people. Margo was an uninformed patient like myself, and, therefore, a relationship between teeth, eyes and heart was unthinkable just as it was for me.

A routine five to ten minute visit with her GP in which she related her symptoms produced no diagnosis. Blood tests showed nothing. He said that she had flu, and bed rest would cure her instantaneously. Much later, during the course of a malpractice suit, Margo would at last have access to her hospital and doctors' medical records which clearly showed that her test results of April 12 were far from normal. They showed protein and blood in the urine, elevated ESR, lowered platelets and an increase in the white blood cells or leukocytes, especially the neutrophils. An increase in the neutrophilic bands is highly indicative of an acute bacterial infection because it means that the neutrophils do not have a chance to mature. The bone marrow sends out incompletely developed neutrophils in response to the urgent demands imposed by infection.

The grave danger is that the body will be depleted of mature neutrophils. Such a situation is called neutropenia which is frequently associated with IE. Death from overwhelming infection thus ensues.

Margo's condition deteriorated inexorably. Chills and fever increased with afternoon temperatures spiking to 102° F which Margo began recording. Severe tremors kept her awake at night and she was unable to go to work. Because her GP impressed upon her that she had flu, she did not tell any members of her family who were scattered about Canada and the United States. Margo's weight dropped noticeably. She became completely bedridden, and friends brought her food. Headaches, chest pain and tachycardia developed along with severe chills which doctors call "rigors", so-named because the muscle stiffening and rigidity resembles the rigormortis that sets in after death. These were signs of impending doom.

Margo saw her GP again on April 23 and related her symptoms in great detail, as I had done to Austin. However, he still insisted she had nothing more than flu and added that her hectic lifestyle was prolonging her illness. Margo got the impression that her doctor felt her symptoms were psychosomatic. Once again, in Margo's case, as in Gail's and mine, the doctor created a portrait of the neurotic female, "mentally labile" and "pathologically anxious". Later, she would find that she had been called "hysterical" in her medical records. Her GP's medicine was "reassurance", the same which Gail and I and many other women with MVP receive. Later that day, the GP called Margo to tell her that a second set of blood tests, done at a different lab, showed nothing. Margo's medical records indicate that her GP, at this point, had actually thought of IE though he never mentioned this disease to her. His differential diagnosis remained that of flu with a preference for mononucleosis or a stubborn virus. Nothing short of a positive blood test would convince him of IE.

Margo's friends urged her to ignore her GP's advice and go to a hospital emergency. She, at first, refused, because she said she would appear even "more neurotic". She also refused to allow her friends to contact either her father in Florida or her brother in California. Instead, Margo called her GP again. He was away and sent his replacement out to her apartment. This doctor spent five to ten minutes examining her and declared there was nothing seriously wrong. She was reacting "hysterically" to a harmless, common garden-variety type of flu he told her. This left Margo without any hope whatsoever of getting help.

Margo's brother stopped unexpectedly in Toronto on his way home to Montreal. His visit with his sister was not intended to be a medical examination and he had not even brought a stethoscope. However, he was alarmed by her appearance and her symptoms even though he knew nothing of her MVP. Margo, of course, like myself, had made no connection between the teeth and the heart and, so, could not tell her brother of the dangers that her pre-existing condition might have posed. Margo's brother discussed her illness with their father who had practiced in the pre-antibiotic era. He knew that an FUO of prolonged duration should be thoroughly investigated for IE. Margo's brother called her GP and asked if he had ruled out SBE. He replied that Margo's cultures were negative and her blood platelets were too low for IE. He, however, agreed to see Margo once more on April 29th. Another blood sample proved to be negative but, because Margo's hemoglobin was very low, he now urged her to go to the emergency ward of Richview Hospital, the hospital where Dr. Cofman had ejected me.

Margo arrived at the hospital in the afternoon of April 29, 1982, two weeks after my discharge from my third hospitalization with splenomegaly and tricuspid abnormalities, all of which simply registered the confusion surrounding MVP at that time. There was no bed available for Margo at Richview. The initial examination in the emergency ward of the hospital would have been conclusive enough to convince an Osler, Glynn, Horder or Libman or even a lay person, after reading this book, of IE. Apart from the FUO and chills, there was a long, loud pansystolic murmur, Grade III/VI with radiation to the axilla, swollen supra clavicular nodes, pallor, fatigue, weakness, weight loss, anemia, anorexia, rigors, SOB, chest pain, diffuse myalgias, diarrhea, non-productive cough, headaches, Roth spots or petechiae in the right conjunctiva of her eye, clubbing of the fingernails and oliguria or fluid retention, indicative of kidney involvement. Her preliminary lab tests also showed distinct abnor-malities, lowered hemoglobin and platelets, neutrophilia or greatly increased white blood cells, elevated ESR and liver function, blood and protein in the urine and electrocardiographic signs of pericarditis.

But Richview refused to admit Margo. A friend called Margo's father who then spoke with his old friend who was Chief of Surgery at that hospital. Margo was finally admitted. One can only shudder at what might happen to the individual who does not have a doctor in the family who could come, not once but twice, to the rescue in such a desperate situation.

However, in spite of violent chills, rigors, temperatures oscillating wildly between 35.8°C and 42°C and blood pressure plunging to 90/52, Margo was shelved, without treatment, into an emergency cubicle in the corridor where she spent the entire night on a stretcher. At 9:15 p.m., she was given only an anti-pyrexial drug, Tylenol, which could be purchased over the counter. The Tylenol increased her rigors unbearably. Two blood samples, instead of the usual eight, were collected, and fluid input and output were monitored.

At 8:00 a.m. Margo was admitted to a room, and, at 9 a.m., doctors appeared to have recognized a kidney problem because the urogenital team was sent to her room. Certain tests were done, routine and microscopic cultures and electrophoresis of urine. At 11:00 a.m., the Infectious Disease (ID) team was consulted, and differential diagnoses were once again postulated: collagen vascular disease, lupus erhythematosus, which was favoured, even though distinctive skin lesions identify this disease and murmurs are not characteristic unless IE is present, lymphoma (cancer) and ordinary sepsis ("flu"). The ID resident and the cardiologist agreed that antibiotics should be withheld until the patient's SBE was confirmed by echo. Once again, the reliance on the technological wonders of the machine. It was of no consequence that the echocardiogram cannot accurately distinguish between the lumps and bumps of MVP and the vegetations of IE, nor record vegetations smaller than 2 mm.

In that 24 hr. delay, Margo's BP plunged to 70/40 and her temperature to 34.9° C. But blankets, not antibiotics, were piled upon the dying woman. In that time, Margo's murmur changed, became louder, going from II to IV/VI. An x-ray revealed fluid in Margo's lungs and early signs of left ventricular failure. At 1:30 p.m., Margo was wheeled back into her room. The echo had revealed a large vegetation on the anterior mitral leaflet. Doctors now took a closer look at the longstanding signs: nailpolish was removed and splinter hemorrhages noted, along with clubbing, a petechial lesion in the right conjunctiva of her eye and the intensification of the MVP murmur.

At 8 p.m. April 30, approximately seven months after her illness began with the cleaning of her teeth, and over 24 hours after admission, treatment was begun, and Margo was given pen G, 3.5 million units IV every 4 hr. and gentamycin, 100 mg IV every 8 hrs. to coincide with every second dose of penicillin. Other laboratory tests were done, rheumatoid factor, CICs.

After the flurry subsided, Margo was left alone to sort out what had happened to her. She was engulfed by an overwhelming feeling of shock and bewilderment. She was also greatly stressed because there was very little she could understand. It was the stress of impotency, of being completely at the mercy of other people's knowledge. Her comprehension of what all this meant was not increased by the succession of neophytes who filed into her room, interns who wanted to get a crack at a living specimen of this rare disease they likely had been taught had been expunged, along with leprosy, the black death or bubonic plague by the miracles of medical science. They rhymed off their list of formula questions including whether she had SOB, a symptom which would have been obvious to anyone in her presence for any length of time.

After 24 hours of treatment, Margo's condition had not improved. Her kidney function continued to deteriorate, and a cardiology resident, for the first time, raised the question of GN in the medical record. He placed a question mark beside her treatment regime of pen G and gentamycin but he did not appear to have conveyed this to others or, if he did, no notice was taken of his opinion.

On day two of antimicrobial treatment, the cultures were reported positive for a gram negative coccobacillus of the Kingella species, the dentrificans. This identification, it turned out, was incorrect. The patient's fever subsided or "defervesced" as the medical report says. There were, as yet, no signs of acute CHF or emboli. However, complications ensued. There was severe oliguria and a sharp rise in serum creatinine from 1.1 mg/dl to 3.6 mg/dl (dl=100 milliters). Normal creatinine is .7 to 1.5 mg/dl. There was other evidence of renal failure: active urinary sediment, 3 plus protein in urine, many red blood cells and granular casts, a few white blood cell casts and a BUN of 40 mg/dl. Normal is 10-20 mg/dl. An elevated BUN or blood urea nitrogen means that the body is retaining the poisonous waste products, the urea of normal protein metabolism, because the kidneys are unable to excrete them. There were also the signs of left ventricular failure.

A renal consultation followed. The decision, however, was not to switch to a different antimicrobial nor to change the present levels of drugs. Instead fluid intake was restricted to 400 cc per day and protein and sodium ingestion were reduced while sodium excretion was to be closely monitored. If a further deterioration in renal function took place over the next 48 hours, tobramycin was to replace the gentamycin. Margo was admitted to Intensive Care on May 3. Kidney dialysis was postponed until after a trial of Lasix which Margo said truly made her feel as if she were dying.

The causes of her renal failure were then discussed, and, once again, the differential diagnosis was noted in her medical records. Her kidney failure was caused possibly by acute tubular necrosis (ATN) which means that the renal tubules are being destroyed. The same kind of ischemic changes that can affect the arteries in the heart can affect the renal tubules. The tissues die from a lack of nutrition because of a severe reduction in blood perfusion or from the presence of toxins. The other possible cause of Margo's kidney failure, according to a member of the renal team, was GN indicated by decreased excretion of sodium. A question was asked in her medical records. Was left ventricular dysfunction, occasioned by valvular vegetations, or underlying GN, secondary to IE, causing the renal failure?

Margo remained in IC while the Renal, Cardiac and Infectious Disease teams pondered the problem. The microorganism was again identified incorrectly as "cardio bacterium hominis", a gram negative microorganism. Such microorganisms, doctors believe, are associated with larger vegetations and renal failure. Inevitably, however, the suspicion that renal failure was precipitated by the drug combination of Pen G and gentamycin arose. It was then that Margo's doctors switched immediately to ampicillin. Correspondingly they recognized that GN was more likely than ATN. Nevertheless, it was underlined in her medical records that pen G and gentamycin had been "almost certainly adequate" and, until the organism was better identified in the laboratory, ampicillin, 2 gm. IV every six hours was to be the method of treatment.

Once ampicillin replaced the pen G and gentamycin, Margo's renal function improved dramatically according to her medical records. Blood pressure increased significantly and peripheral edema resolved. Creatinine dropped from 3.6 to 2.6, and BUN from a high of 56 to 40. But, in spite of renal improvement, Margo was dying from left ventricular failure. Severe shortness of breath forced her to sleep in the sitting position and oxygen was required. A second critical question was asked in her records. What was causing the pulmonary edema? The heart or the kidneys? Was the cause left ventricular dysfunction secondary to valve vegetations or fluid overload with circulatory congestion from the failing kidneys? Ampicillin was increased from 8 gm. per day to 12 gm. with rapid renal recovery.

On May 7, 1982, the entire team held a consultation, and different drugs, digoxin, digitalis, were tried to combat impending death but these weapons were puny against an acute case of IE. LVF continued to progress relentlessly with lethal arrhythmias and a new third heart sound. The miraculous engine of salvation, the deus ex machina, creaked into strategic position ready to snatch the victim from the jaws of death. The natural valve would be excised and replaced with a technological wonder, a spanking new Ionesco-Shiley prosthesis made of calf tissue. Animal tissue valves, her doctors believed, did not, like synthetic substances, require anti-coagulants, important if Margo would wish to have children later. The operation was scheduled for Tuesday, May 11, 1982 at another hospital, the same where my enlarged spleen was identified as a misplaced kidney.

In the twilight of her long struggle, still uninformed and completely bewildered, Margo refused to sign the consent form for the open heart surgery. She had not been told the choice was surgery or death, nor anything of the quality of life after the operation. She had not entered the hospital to have her chest sawed open. She had entered the hospital with flu. She could not imagine open heart surgery with valve replacement anymore than she could imagine that the teeth and the heart were connected. Margo was, like myself, like all the other cases described here, like most people, completely uninformed.

Margo's father was called for his oral consent, but all doctors involved knew that was not, from a legal standpoint, good enough. The patient's written consent was required. Her refusal brought her cardiologist rushing angrily to her bed-side. His message was brutal. It was surgery or death. Family and friends begged the terrified young woman to submit while fiercely determined staff wheeled her to the operating room. Outside the OR doors, Margo's resistance shattered like glass and she feebly scribbled her name as consent to this enormous violation of her body. And, in reality, her scrawled, uninformed signature was nothing more than the primitive "x" of a medieval peasant.

17

Straw Men in the Wind

However, these diagnoses appear to be "straw men in the wind" when one views the subsequent course of events . . .

> B. Castleman and B. McNeely. "Case Records of the Massachusetts General Hospital." (August 1, 1968) *The New England Journal of Medicine* 279 (5): 260-266.

Among the sleuths of the cardiovascular world are the radiologists, whose challenge it is to record visually the inner workings of the complex blood-pumping network. Within the last decade or two, they have been given tools that make the stethoscope and electrocardiogram, valuable though they are, seem like tin lizzies.

> August 1983, *Readers' Digest*, p. 82

I believe without question, that the stethoscope is the best instrument to detect mitral valve prolapse and the good thing, it does not cost the patient one cent.

> W.P. Harvey in M.D. Cheitlin and R.C. Byrd. "Prolapsed Mitral Valve: The Commonest Valve Disease?" (January 8, 1984) *Current Problems in Cardiology* 10: 1-54.

"Every available orifice is used to gather information about a patient's illness and, when nature has failed to supply an opening, enterprising physicians have made their own."[1] These are the words of doctors, Beaty and Petersdorf, of the University of Washington School of Medicine in Seattle in their report on the iatrogenic factor in infectious diseases such as IE. The word, "iatrogenic", is derived from the Greek word, "iatros", which means physician, and refers to injury or disease caused by the interventions of physicians. A report by these authors revealed that 20 percent of 1000 hospital admissions over an eight month period resulted in hospital acquired iatrogenic disease. Drugs were the cause in 51 percent of cases, and incorrect diagnostic or therapeutic procedures in 24 percent.[2]

It would take Margo a long time, as it did me, to realize that her illness was iatrogenic in origin. After her surgery that "saved her life", her only feeling was unquestioning gratitude and admiration for her surgeon. Not until she realized that her life should never have had to be "saved" did she, in fact, become angry and set about challenging the powerful medical establishment. I, too, had gone through the same emotional process of initial gratitude for finally securing the attention of medical people and being admitted at last to hospital for an investigation after a year of an unidentified illness.

But all the suffering was not over for Margo. She would find that replacement of her valve did not end her horrifying ordeal. There followed weeks of pain from infection in the incision, pleurisy, serious arrhythmia, visits to the plastic surgeon and the open heart surgeon and another month in hospital. Margo required two years of psychiatric treatment for depression. Her personal life and her career were dramatically affected. Her animal tissue valve would eventually have to be replaced. She would then be much older so that a second operation would naturally take a heavier toll on her health. Of course, all the risks of open heart surgery remain, the physical and psychological trauma, the risk of brain damage, paralysis or death on the operating table.

Contrary to the information Margo's doctors gave her, replacement of the natural valve with an animal tissue valve does not prevent the formation of emboli. Margo has experienced episodes of retinal emboli with partial blindness in one eye. It is, therefore, necessary after all for her to take anti-coagulants for the rest of her life. In spite of these drugs, she has experienced episodes of retinal emboli. According to recent reports, the Ionesco-Shiley bovine valve in the mitral position, which Margo has, carries a higher risk of thromboembolism than other valves in other positions. Only 71 percent of patients with these valves are free of embolism at the end of three to four years.[3] Anti-coagulants have serious side effects such as cerebral hemorrhage, and thus sports that could cause injury are particularly dangerous as is any kind of accident, domestic or otherwise. Visits to the dentist are affairs fraught with danger and anxiety for Margo. She must have IV antibiotics followed by oral penicillin. Intramuscular injections cannot be used because of the possibility, once again, of anti-coagulant related hemorrhage. Pregnancy is thus out of the question unless Margo wishes to take the risk of going off the anti-coagulants. And contraceptive methods, such as the IUD, as I've already pointed out, can cause IE, and, when there is a prosthetic valve, the risk is even greater. As well, oral contraceptives enhance the risk of thromboembolism.

Though her surgeon might have joked insensitively when she awoke from surgery, "I bet you wish you had hair on your chest now," Margo has suffered from extreme psychological distress over the scar on her chest. She feels that she is less attractive, not only because of the appearance of this considerable scar, but also from knowing that her possible early death makes her a bad investment, from an emotional standpoint, as either a mother or a lifetime partner.

When Margo began investigating her illness she met the same conspiracy of silence as I had. Doctors invariably interpret a patient's independent efforts to gather personal health information as the prelude to a malpractice suit which, in fact, Margo had undertaken against her dentist and general physicians. Of course, she, like I, met with little success. Malpractice litigation, as already discussed, is a despairing, unsuccessful battle for most people because doctors will do everything possible to prevent access to the truth, to the information in the medical record and will protect their colleagues. In both our cases, doctors even went to the extreme of expressing opinions that were completely contrary to the findings of medical research. Such a search for personal health information often becomes a marathon of fabrication. Judges, it will be remembered, almost always favour doctors and, in any issue of credibility, the doctor's testimony and that of his expert witnesses is frequently accepted over that of the patient.

For example, in his official Statement of Defence, her GP claimed that he had fully instructed Margo with respect to *all* dental procedures, not just root canal treatments. Her dentist, likewise, testified, in his Statement of Defence, that Margo had not informed him of her heart murmur or of her GP's advice regarding prophylaxis. Her GP further claimed that Margo's murmur had not changed to a PSM from the LSM which he had heard on other occasions and which corresponded to the late systolic prolapse of the 1979 echo he had ordered. On her April 29th visit, a day before admission to hospital, he claimed he heard a 2/6 systolic ejection murmur (SEM) which is often regarded as an "innocent" murmur. Some doctors in emergency also described such a murmur along with a PSM. A second murmur, which observers called a SEM, was also heard on my admission to the TMSC, in addition to the LSM, though only months later a PSM was heard. Doctors say that the SEM can indicate turbulence in association with enlargement of the aortic root. This was the description given to my MVP murmur many years ago, in 1974, when it was first heard but this diagnosis has subsequently been ruled out countless times. Were the observers, in my case, hearing a tricuspid murmur caused by an IE? The important question is whether doctors can, even currently, distinguish between the SEM and the LSM of MVP, or between an innocent murmur, if such exists, and a MVP murmur. Such confusion over what a doctor hears with his stethoscope must mean that many MVP patients remain unidentified and, therefore, unprotected during risky surgical or dental procedures. And the public must ask whether modern doctors are, in fact, losing their skill with the stethoscope because of the reliance on the echocardiogram and other diagnostic technologies?

Her GP had not, of course, told Margo that her murmur was a LSM. Doctors do not give specific details like this or use medical terms with patients. He told her only that it was an "innocent" murmur. Everyone who has read this book now knows that a LSM is a regurgitant murmur and is, therefore, not an innocent murmur. When Margo had gained some knowledge after her surgery, she asked her cardiologist if she had had a regurgitant murmur prior to her IE. He told her that the echocardiogram her GP had done had not shown regurgitation. However, there was the sign of late systolic dipping or late systolic prolapse which means regurgitation, and the LSM, which her GP heard with his stethoscope, by definition, is a regurgitant murmur. This was, of course, exactly the question for which I struggled to find the answer over several years. Did I have a regurgitant murmur prior to my febrile illness in association with an abscessed tooth? However, the uninformed patient could only draw one conclusion from the information provided by this cardiologist: she did not have a regurgitant murmur prior to her infection. She had nothing to go on except what this doctor had told her, and, since medical opinion does not appear to be uniform about the use of ABP when only a click of MVP is present, she could only imagine, from his assessment, that she had been in no need of ABP when her teeth were cleaned.

Furthermore, like Rhodes, her cardiologist claimed that the use of ABP with MVP was his own **personal** opinion and that of Richview; it was not, he stressed, the "norm" in Toronto. Only five years earlier in 1978, he claimed, doctors did not recommend ABP with MVP. But, as I've pointed out, warnings were very clearly made in 1963 by Barlow and appeared consistently in the medical literature from many medical centres all over the world. The GP and the dentist would then be exonerated because they were abiding by the standards of their locale. The cardiologist claimed that Margo's GP was correct in prescribing this protection only for root canal treatments because other "minor" events such as cleaning were no more risky than brushing, flossing or chewing. Margo was, therefore, to understand that she had got her IE from one of these routine practices. She did not, of course, know that there had never been any actual reports of patients with healthy mouths contracting IE from chewing, flossing or brushing, despite evidence that these events can release bacteria into the blood stream. This was the opinion, the cardiologist testified, of many respected "medical men" who would never adopt such rigid precautionary measures regarding an innocent condition like MVP. He strenuously denied that any of his colleagues had done anything wrong. Margo had just been "unlucky", he said, and, furthermore, he warned her, unequivocally, "I'm not going to ruin any man's career over you."

The relationship between the doctor and the patient is one of master and servant. It is a relationship between the privileged and the underprivileged. The inequality is most evident in the matter of access to personal medical information. In many places in Canada and the US, the patient does not have a legally protected right to this information though he or she may not realize this. Doctors, other than the treating doctor, however, believe they have an inalienable right to everything in the medical record and all they require is the patient's signature which few refuse. The inequality became frankly evident to Margo when her cardiologist asked her if he could use her case in a presentation to a group of doctors which included a very well known cardiologist from the United States who had written textbooks. The cardiologist promised Margo she could stay for the discussion which would follow her examination before the other doctors. The discussion he said would include information about MVP and ABP. Against the advice of her psychiatrist, and only because she wanted to be present for the lecture afterwards, Margo gave her consent.

Prior to the lecture, Margo innocently asked one of the doctors, who would have the honour of presenting her to the group, if he would meet with her. They agreed to meet fifteen minutes before the presentation, but this doctor reneged, hastily promising a meeting afterwards. To Margo's astonishment, her GP had been invited to the presentation as if to show approval of his treatment methods. But this wasn't the first shock. After the patient had been presented and examined before all the doctors and at the commencement of the discussion, her cardiologist ordered Margo to leave the room. She protested, but he refused to allow her to stay. Her body could be used for a physical examination for study purposes, in the way a dummy might be, but she, herself, was not allowed the right to hear the discussion which was of such crucial interest to her.

After this humiliating and frustrating event, Margo tried once more to arrange a meeting with the doctor who had promised to talk with her, but he failed a second time to show up. The cardiologist finally met with Margo after she had telephoned him, but he told her nothing of any importance had been discussed and the opinion of the group, uniformly, was that no medical proof existed to show the risk of IE was greater with MVP. What is even more astounding is that the American doctor had written a textbook which included a short discussion of MVP and the warning that it required antibiotic protection for dental interventions. And this doctor was present at this seminar!

When Margo finally talked on the telephone to the doctor who had failed to meet her, he defended both her GP's and her dentist's treatment. Her blood results and urinalysis, on her visits with her GP, he said, were all normal though, in fact, her medical records would show this to be untrue. At that time, however, she did not have access to them. The blood cultures her GP had ordered were all negative, the doctor said, and cultures, he insisted, were always positive, no matter what time of the day they were taken. He then warned that Margo could not prove that the cleaning of her teeth five months earlier had actually caused her IE. And such a rare microorganism as the M^6 isolated from Margo's blood, he declared, would stump the best of labs. And, as though he were a judge, he ruled finally that her disease was caused by vigorous flossing and bleeding gums. As proof, he cited her solitary bout of periodontitis in the past. His verdict implied that Margo had this disease at the time of her dental cleaning but was unaware of it. Neither the cardiologist, the surgeon nor this doctor were named as defendants in Margo's malpractice suit, yet, nevertheless, all acted defensively, confusing her with misinformation for the purpose, by the admission of at least one of them, of protecting their brothers.

But the questions concerning Margo's case do not end with the matter of antibiotic coverage for a risky condition. Margo's hospital records, when carefully examined, raise some thorny issues which should be of interest to anyone entering hospital for treatment of IE. Apart from the refusal to accept clinical evidence of IE on admission to emergency, there was the matter of the 24 hour delay until there was echo confirmation of vegetations on the valve. As I have pointed out, the echocardiogram is not reliable in the identification of vegetations, and research strongly advises that treatment be based on the whole picture, whether or not vegetations are present on echo. Any delay in treatment could be crucial in acute cases. Reliance on technology rather than on the doctor's bedside diagnostic skills is not advantageous according to a study from the Harbour University of California and Los Angeles Medical Centre. This study examines the usefulness of the echocardiogram in verifying the presence of vegetations and concludes that echo was unnecessary in the case of 24 patients with IE. All had one or two of twelve obvious clinical signs of IE used as criteria. A positive blood culture was found in 23 of 24 patients and emboli to the lungs found in 17 of 24. Echo was unnecessary in two-thirds of the cases of IE.[4] If waiting for echo confirmation delays treatment, then reliance upon this diagnostic equipment is hazardous.

In the matter of Margo's antimicrobial treatment in hospital, there could well be some other questions. The choice of combination pen G and gentamycin, which was likely used in an effort to cover both gram positive and gram negative bacteria in a case of negative cultures,[5] had some serious drawbacks. Penicillin G or "penicillin notatum", the original penicillin made naturally from mold, at one time effective against both gram positive and gram negative microbes, is now only largely effective against gram positive microorganisms.[6] But even then there are gram positive "resistant" staphylococcal strains as well, and, in hospitalized patients, the incidence of these resistant strains has been shown to be as high as 90-95 percent.[7] Pen G is inactivated by enzymes called penicillinases which are excreted by certain bacteria. This is the same substance used to destroy penicillin in blood cultures rendered sterile by oral administration of antibiotics prior to a diagnosis of IE. Penicillinases are produced by resistant strains of gram positive staphylococci and many of the gram negative microorganisms.[8] Gentamycin, an aminoglycoside, is used to treat serious gram negative infections. Pharmacologists point out that, in cases of IE with unidentifiable microorganisms, physicians will treat with gentamycin and a penicillinase-resistant penicillin which pen G is not [9]. Therefore, it is curious this drug was chosen.

It appears from the medical records that streptococcus viridans was the bacteria first thought of. In the past, strep. viridans was believed to be the most common microorganism, implicated in almost 100 percent of cases of IE of dental origin, but not today. It would appear then that penicillin G was chosen because strep. viridans is a gram positive microorganism which does not produce the penicillinase enzyme that inactivates pen G.[10] Such a choice suggests that, initially, a gram negative microorganism was not considered. Unfortunately, the most overlooked microorganisms in the laboratory are, in fact, the slow growing, fastidious gram negative ones. Margo's consistently negative blood cultures suggested this and, therefore, treatment with one of the semisynthetic, broad spectrum antibiotics, such as ampicillin, which have been specifically developed to destroy both gram negative and gram positive microorganisms in dubious, longstanding cases like Margo's.

The antimicrobials used also suggest that glomerulonephritis in association with IE was not immediately suspected. The medical and pharmacological literature distinctly warns that both pen G[11] and gentamycin [12] are highly toxic and can precipitate renal failure in the presence of serious renal impairment which Margo clearly demonstrated on admission. Penicillin G is rapidly excreted through the kidneys. Thus, much larger amounts of this drug with more frequent administration are also required to maintain the necessary levels in the body to kill the microbes. Researchers suggest that, in cases of SBE and fulminating infections, as much as 24 gm. daily of pen G may have to be given.[13] But Margo was given only 12 gm. the same dosage as she was later to receive of the semisynthetic penicillin, ampicillin, a drug which is not excreted primarily through the kidneys, and is, therefore, safer in cases of kidney impairment.[14]

The renal involvement in the elimination of a particular drug from the body can vary from 0 to 100 percent.[15] In the presence of kidney disease, the maximum elimination capacity is rapidly reached and hence renal shutdown can occur as it did in Margo's case. Gentamycin can be particularly dangerous. Its chief characteristic is its almost total elimination by filtration through the glomeruli, which are, without question, always damaged to some degree in IE. Little, if any, of gentamycin is absorbed by the renal tubules.[16] Although pen G is excreted extremely rapidly through the kidneys, it is believed that only about 10 percent of this drug is eliminated by glomerular filtration and about 90 percent by tubular secretion.[17] Though ATN or acute tubular necrosis is uncommon in IE, Margo's physicians first assumed this was the cause of her renal failure likely because they had used pen G. At one point, during her progression towards renal failure, tobramycin, another aminoglycoside used to combat gram negative bacteria, was proposed as a substitute for gentamycin. That it is eliminated from the body in the same way as gentamycin, by filtration through the glomeruli, suggests that, at this point, glomerulonephritis was still not thought of in conjunction with IE. Impairment of renal function is less, however, with tobramycin than gentamycin.[18] It was thought that this alternate drug would do the same job, specifically, cover a possible gram negative bacteria, while being less toxic to the kidneys. However the switch does not appear to have been made, and, eventually, ampicillin was chosen.

Gentamycin must be administered in very small amounts. According to Goodman and Gilman, "the recommended parenteral dose for administration in patients with normal renal function is 0.8 to 1.2 mg/kg per day, given in two to four equally divided and spaced doses."[19] Thus it is administered according to the body weight. This dosage may be increased, provided renal function is normal, to 5 mg/kg per day when life is threatened. A kilogram is equivalent to 2.2 pounds. Margo's weight was about 120 pounds or about 54.5 kg, possibly less since she had lost a great deal of weight. At the higher limits of the recommended average dose, 1.2 mg/kg, she should have received about 65.4 mg of gentamycin a day, considering that her renal function was seriously impaired. However, Margo received 100 mg every eight hours or 300 mg per day, a dosage that far exceeded the recommended dose of 65.4 mg per day for patients with normal renal function. Her dosage was more in accord with the maximum dosage recommended for life threatening disease, 5 mg/kg, when renal function is normal.

It must be stressed that Margo never, at any time, had normal renal function. On admission she had oliguria, blood and protein in her urine. While kidney involvement was recognized, the opinion seemed to be that the IE involved the tubules rather than the glomeruli. Immune complex glomerulonephritis occurs universally in IE and varies in degree from the merely histological to the severely dysfunctional. An early check for CICs on admission might have pointed to glomerulonephritis, but this was delayed until renal involvement had progressed to failure.

One of the most convincing pieces of evidence that gentamycin could have been the cause of Margo's renal failure was the striking increase in her BUN which rose from 10 on admission to 41 after the administration of pen G and gentamycin. This is double the normal limit. Retention of nitrogenous compounds in the blood, with resultant elevation of the BUN level, is a known adverse effect of gentamycin therapy specifically because this drug affects the rate at which toxic elements are filtered out of the blood by the glomeruli.[20] Further evidence that renal failure could have been precipitated by this drug in combination with pen G was the immediate tripling of the creatinine level from 1.1 on admission to 3.6 mg/dl, almost three times the normal amount. Just before switching to a less toxic drug, ampicillin, creatinine soared to 7.3 and BUN to 55, dangerously high levels indicating complete shutdown of the kidneys and poisoning of the entire circulatory system.

During the pen G and gentamycin therapy, cardiac and pulmonary function deteriorated markedly. While on admission, Margo's chest was said to be clear, according to her medical records, after administration of these drugs, her chest x-ray showed evidence of pulmonary edema, described as a fine reticular pattern (or network of fluid invasion), particularly noticeable in the lower left lobe of the lung. The lungs were also said to show signs of thickening suggestive of left ventricular failure, and there were pleural and pericardial effusions and dilatation of the left atrium and ventricle, though the increase in heart size, as in my case, was said to be within normal limits. Again this raises the question of the smaller than normal heart size in MVP patients and the possibility that heart failure might, simply on the basis of size, be more common in MVP patients than in those without. What is most curious is that, in spite of continued reports of good left ventricular function on echo, Margo's pulmonary edema worsened with severe shortness of breath and rales (rahls), that is abnormal sounds heard, on auscultation, in the lungs and indicating the presence of excess fluid.

It appears from Margo's medical records that the question was, in fact, raised as to whether the pulmonary edema was cardiac in origin, since left ventricular function was good, or was secondary to the circulatory congestion caused from the failing kidneys. One then asks, if the kidney problem had been appropriately addressed at the outset, would valve replacement have been necessary to prevent death? Because Margo's heart would have already been considerably compromised or overworked by the increased regurgitation due to a prolapsing valve made worse by the vegetations from the IE, the added burden of extra fluid in the circulatory system from the failing kidneys would have been the "straw that broke the camel's back". And if there had, in fact, been slight pulmonary edema from minimal left ventricular failure prior to the administration of these antibiotics, this pulmonary edema would have become more severe by the administration of these specific drugs. A perfectly functioning prosthetic valve would greatly assist in clearing the lungs of fluid while the kidney function was slowly improving.

What is known with certainty from the medical records is that, with the switch to ampicillin, the renal picture improved dramatically over a period of several days. BUN dropped from 55 to 28 mg/dl and creatinine from 7.3 to 1.3 mg/dl or just below the upper limits of normal. However, the pulmonary edema did not resolve and left ventricular failure continued. Ampicillin is one of the many semi-synthetic penicillins developed because of the inadequacies of pen G, "its instability in the acidic gastric contents, rapid renal excretion, susceptibility to inactivation by penicillinase" and "limited antibacterial spectrum with particular reference to gram-negative bacteria".[21] Ampicillin is recommended as the drug of choice if gram negative infection and renal impairment are suspected, and, in doubtful cases, it is preferred because of its effectiveness against both types of microorganisms. Unlike pen G, the semi-synthetic penicillins, such as ampicillin, are not rapidly excreted through the kidneys and hence can be given in much higher doses than pen G and gentamycin.[22] As much as 12 gm. and even 18 gm. per day of this drug have been used safely and successfully in cases of life threatening disease, specifically IE caused by gram-negative species of the haemophilus variety.[23] Once the gram negative bacteria was grown from Margo's blood, her doctors switched to ampicillin.

The microorganism causing Margo's IE could not be cultured in the hospital's laboratory. Moraxella or M[6] is a haemophilus species which normally inhabits the mouth and has been implicated specifically in cases of IE and MVP in the medical literature. This microorganism is not difficult to grow in the proper medium, yet Margo's blood samples had to be sent to the Bacteriology Section of the Atlanta, Georgia Center for Disease Control in the U.S. Why could this microorganism not be cultured in a sophisticated laboratory of a Toronto hospital?

Margo was never told what microorganism caused her IE. She had to learn this by calling the Atlanta Center herself. It was this centre which then directed her to the article which had been written about her in the *Journal of Microbiology*. This article would, of course, also have remained unknown to her. When we consider how many people have MVP, it is safe to assume that the events in Margo's and my life are likely happening frequently to other individuals with MVP. Only a few cases of IE are described in the medical literature. Most go undocumented, and, like mine, unidentified, because oral antibiotics have been used and immediate valve replacement or death is prevented. Rarer still are those cases in which admission of error is made. One such case was described in *The New England Journal of Medicine*[24]. The sequence of events in this case is similar to Margo's.

The patient, a male, referred to as Case #30 at The Massachusetts General Hospital was "discharged with the diagnosis of the "floppy valve syndrome" and "allowed unrestricted activity."[25] This was his first visit to a cardiologist. Two years later, at the age of 44, he developed a fever of unknown origin (FUO), which according to researchers, Jacoby and Swartz, is caused by IE in 40 percent of cases.[26] However, IE was not suspected in this man's case. The matter of dental manipulation as a precipitating factor was not, therefore, addressed. In fact, the patient does not appear to have been told on his first visit to the cardiologist that there was any connection between his teeth and his heart and that he required protection from IE. In fact, his MVP, though known, was not considered a factor at the time of his admission, even though the case occurred in 1974 when ten years of warnings in hundreds of articles already existed, and Hurst, in his textbook, had included MVP as a condition predisposing the patient to IE.

If MVP had been regarded as a predisposing condition and part of the whole picture, IE would likely have been included in the differential diagnostic process. Instead, this man's illness was diagnosed as rheumatoid arthritis which, as I have pointed out in the previous chapter, can be the mistaken diagnosis in cases of IE. As for the underlying MVP, Dr. Federman summed up by saying, "I don't plan to spend much time on the basic cardiac lesion since I don't consider it intimately relevant to what happened subsequently."[27] However, the failure to identify IE in life is closely related perhaps to the failure to regard MVP as a risk situation. If the risk had been appreciated early in the man's illness, blood tests would likely have been done at that time when it became apparent the patient's fever would not subside and prior to administering oral antibiotics which were likely the cause of the negative cultures. If this case, Margo's and mine and the others referred to in the previous chapter are any example, it would seem that doctors are no more convinced today than they were a hundred years ago that symptoms, ordinarily associated with IE, in a patient with a systolic murmur of MVP indicate IE.

The use of oral antibiotics created confusion in this case as it did in Margo's and mine. For three years, Margo had been using tetracycline for an acne condition. Though there was a record of this, when negative cultures showed up, this did not appear to have been an influencing factor in the diagnostic process. Tetracycline may have confused the picture in another way. This drug is dangerous when renal function is impaired and, in such cases, it can cause liver toxicity, a fact which could explain Margo's elevated liver function tests. By its ability to depress prothrombin activity, or the ability of the blood to clot, tetracycline can lower platelets as well.[28] Before rejecting a diagnosis of SBE in favour of a harmless "flu", the whole picture should have been analyzed.

In my case, numerous dentists and doctors responded to fever and a periodontal abscess, along with change in murmur and enlarged heart, and likely spleen if it had been looked for initially, not by thinking of IE and by doing blood cultures but by prescribing oral antibiotics intermittently over a four month period when it is known in the medical literature that such drug administration is ineffective in sterilizing infection of bone when there is a root abscess. Case #30 from the Massachusetts Hospital had been given a brief five day course of oral penicillin for fever, chills and diarrhea before blood culturing was done. Negative cultures resulted. Slow-growing bacteroides was eventually cultured from his blood samples which were collected just prior to his death. However, despite many signs, this man's IE remained undiagnosed in life.

In all three MVP cases, there were classic symptoms of IE, in particular the changing murmur. Dr. Austin told me personally, at the time of my infection, that my murmur had changed, presumably from late systolic to pansystolic. On admission to TMSC, a second murmur was noted in the medical record. This was called, by different observers, a systolic ejection murmur (SEM) and a mid-systolic murmur (MSM). MSMs are usually associated with aortic or pulmonic valve problems. Likely, however, this second murmur was the murmur of tricuspid regurgitation which I have only recently been told I have. Margo's murmur changed during infection from late systolic to grade III/VI pansystolic and it further changed to IV/VI just prior to treatment. She was also, at different times, said to have a SEM. Case #30 in the Massachusetts study also initially had a grade II/VI radiating systolic murmur of MVP heard at the apex of the heart which some doctors appeared to have called a SEM. During IE, this man's murmur became a III/VI PSM. What this all suggests, once again, is the great confusion that still surrounds the auscultatory signs of MVP.

In addition to the classic presentation of fever and a changing murmur in the patient described in the *NEJM*, there were other signs of IE. Like Margo, this man had myalgias and arthralgias, immune complex nephritis, elevated rheumatoid factor (RF) and ESR, splinter hemorrhages, multiple conjunctival and palatal petechiae, protein, red blood cells and casts in urine, uremia with extremely elevated BUN and creatinine, low serum complement, low platelets and, since, at autopsy, splenitis, likely an enlarged spleen, as I had, throughout his illness.

Because Case #30 was thought to have rheumatoid arthritis, instead of antimicrobial treatment, he received large dosages of aspirin and cortico steroids or immunosuppressive drugs which resulted in his death on the 28th hospital day from a massive cerebral hemorrhage.[29] A sign in his case that fooled his doctors as well as Margo's was the low blood platelets which can lead to a condition called thrombocytopenia. Small hemorrhages occur in the skin, subcutaneous tissues and mucous membranes of any part of the body. For example, purple patches, called purpura (from the Latin for purple, deep-red or dark-red) may appear on the legs. This man's platelets were extremely low, life threatening, at 4,000 [30] and it was this which caused his death from cerebral hemorrhage. The normal range is 200,000 — 350,000 per cu mm. of blood.[31] Administrations of aspirin, an anti-coagulant, would only further reduce his platelets. Margo's had been low at 100,000. My platelets were on the low side at 192,000 during my first hospitalization though this was regarded as entirely normal.

In 1948, Libman referred to "purpura" as a frequent sign of SBE in association with low blood platelets.[32] It is known that the presence of bacteria in the blood stimulates platelet production and, for this reason, in cases of longstanding illness, platelet production eventually becomes exhausted and a condition of thrombocytopenia exists.

At necropsy, one large vegetation was found on the mitral valve of the man in the Massachusetts study as was found in Margo's case. As well, the patient had the swollen "flea bitten" kidneys, exactly fitting the preantibiotic descriptions of Libman and Bell, in association with renal involvement in IE. Modern electrophoresis of this patient's kidney tissues revealed, as in Margo's case, the universally occuring immune complex deposition of IgG in the glomeruli, a subject of many studies before 1974.[33]

Once Margo was admitted to hospital, she at least had the benefit of a thorough laboratory investigation for IE and an attempt at treatment prior to replacement of her valve. However, the patient in *The New England Journal of Medicine* report did not appear to have had an investigation for IE since he was treated for rheumatoid arthritis. And, six years later when I finally had a look at my hospital reports indicating what had been done to rule out IE, I was shocked by the sloppiness of the search for this disease. It could never have been said to be an investigation to "rule out SBE". There was an inadequate number of blood samples collected, three, during my hospital stay and the previous use of oral antibiotics would have made my blood negative, The minimum number recommended by experts in this field is six to eight. In a copy of a letter forwarded to my internist, the Respiratory and Special Pathogens Epidemiology Branch, Division of Bacterial Diseases, at the Atlanta Georgia Center for Disease Control said that, in difficult cases when blood is negative but other symptoms and clinical signs are present, investigation should include six sets of blood cultures, each one from different sites, at least ten minutes apart, and some samples should be taken when the temperature spikes in the afternoon. Blood was not taken from me according to any of these recommendations, and, while one sample was spilled on the bedclothes, the other two were taken in the morning. One other sample had been taken immediately on admission, when penicillin was still in my blood stream. My blood samples were kept for only the time that I was in hospital, which was four days, at which time, they were reported growing nothing. The Atlanta Center recommends that cultures be kept for **four** weeks.

Apart from the sloppiness of the blood culturing procedure, there were other serious deficiencies in my investigation. Out of the list of 29 things the hospital included on its routine laboratory report sheet, only six were looked for, potassium, sodium, chloride, bicarbonate, blood urea nitrogen and creatinine, all of which were said to be normal. All of these tests are routine blood tests for any illness. None are specific for detecting IE. The hematocrit, which is the amount of red blood cells in the total blood composition was low, 34.3 percent (normal in females is 40 — 48 percent)[34] and may have pointed to anemia which occurs in longstanding cases of IE. These few blood tests, being non-specific, provide only a general picture. None of the blood abnormalities, associated with IE, described in the previous chapter, RF, CICs, complement, cryoglobulins, immunoglobulins, for example, were looked for.

Nor was any urinalysis conducted for such basic abnormalities as blood and protein. The reasons were astounding. One sample of urine, which sat on my windowsill from one afternoon until the next was rejected as "not fresh". A second appears to have been discarded because the container was leaking. No other was collected and, despite the objectionable quality of either of these two samples, two mysterious results appeared in the lab records, a pH of 9 and a specific gravity (SG) of 16. Since normal SG is 1.003 to 1.030,[35] a figure of 16, which I thought must mean 1.6 though clearly no period was present between the one and the six, could only mean the urine was solid. A figure of 1.6, of course, would represent a slight elevation which, in fact, would occur if there were protein in the urine and would, along with other tests specific for protein, if such tests had been done, point to glomerulonephritis. The pH of 9 (normal 4.6-8.0),[36] is also an elevation. Elevations are found in glomerulonephritis, but considering that 50 percent of the kidney must be non-functioning before symptoms appear and since glomerulonephritis can only be detected by renal biopsy in many cases of IE according to the medical literature, testing for kidney involvement in this way would not be entirely accurate.

I searched to find a cause for my symptoms which my internist insists are insignificant and typical of the MVP syndrome. For me, surgical repair or replacement of two heart valves carries a grave risk that I cannot even imagine. My internist persists in reassuring me that one more leaky valve means nothing, that tricuspid regurgitation occurs frequently in MVP patients and that I will not require such heroic lifesaving tactics for years. But, since I already have signs of increasing cardiac size, though still within what my internist calls normal limits, and hypertrophy on electrocardiogram, ankle edema, abdominal fluid retention, which is very noticeable at the end of the day, though there is no weight gain anywhere else, and, particularly, fatique, muscle weakness and SOB, I fail to understand how these interventions could be useful. The question of the "tiny" or small heart my internist simply does not accept. It's the old adage of putting new wine into old wineskins. The heart would by then have become so enlarged and the muscle so thickened as a result of the burden put upon it that a heart transplant would seem a more favorable option. My internist's response is that my symptoms are not caused by my heart. I can only infer that my SOB is psychosomatic and that

I have merely gained weight or have hysterical bloating as Alvarez described. However my internist has noted the ankle edema and left ventricular dysfunction, according to wall motion study, among other changes and has given me prescriptions for digoxin to strengthen a failing heart and diuretics to remove fluid. While he has never dismissed cardiac failure and, on occasion, has said there must be a degree of failure, he has never offered any other sound alternative diagnosis. Nor has he ever suggested a psychiatrist for a cardiac neurosis. And, throughout it all, I cannot understand why a specialist would treat a cardiac neurosis with such powerful drugs.

In my case, in Margo's and in the case described in *The New England Journal of Medicine*, there was medical error in association with MVP with varying degrees of catastrophic results. In the discussion that followed the presentation of Case #30 in *The New England Journal of Medicine*, one of the treating doctors closed with a confession. "Always treat for infection first, even if cultures are negative," he said, "before proceeding to treat with immunosuppression . . . I violated that rule in this case."[37] But the doctor's confession is confined to the pages of the medical journal which the public seldom, if ever, sees. Margo was not aware there had been an article written about her in *The Journal of Clinical Microbiology.* Unless patients persist against overwhelming odds, as Margo and I have done, they will never know the true medical facts about themselves, and this then is one of the reasons why I have written this book, to encourage the patient to insist on knowing all the facts and to avail him or herself of the knowledge that is in the medical literature.

In September 1992, Margo underwent a second open heart surgery to replace her bioprosthetic valve, which was deteriorating, with a mechanical valve. Two months later, Margo died suddenly. The autopsy report did not specify the cause of death but stated only that the mechanical valve had not malfunctioned. No emboli were found. In conversation with her brother, who is a physician, it was suggested that, possibly, the scarring, caused from both surgeries, may have interfered with the conduction activity in Margo's heart, precipitating a ventricular arrhythmia that resulted in cardiac arrest. It is of great sadness to me to have lost a dear friend who shared my crusade to spread knowledge about MVP and to live with the knowledge that Margo would be alive today if she had been premedicated with antibiotics before her dental interventions.

18

It Should Never Happen at All

The house officer today has no concept of either the importance or the skill in physical diagnosis of the great clinicians of the past. As residents we agonized over the width of a split second sound and masters of auscultation . . . could call a reversed split of S_2 or time an opening snap of the mitral valve with incredible accuracy . . . And we did have technology!

David B. Carmichael, Medical Director, Cardiovascular Institute, Scripps Memorial Hospitals, La Jolla, California, USA. "Reflections on Medical Heroes and Mitral Valve Prolapse." (Sept. 1987) *The Canadian Journal of Cardiology* 3 (6): 261-262.

The appellation "overdiagnosis" of infective endocarditis is misleading and the advice that intravenous antimicrobial therapy should be started if blood cultures are positive (with the implication that the clinician should wait for the results and not start treatment if they are negative) is dangerous. It is this attitude which contributes to the poor results. Unfortunately it is much more common for endocarditis to be missed than for it to be overdiagnosed. Early antibiotic treatment based on clinical diagnosis or suspicion is vital. Antibiotic treatment can subsequently be modified or stopped on the basis of results of investigations as they become available. This gives the patient a headstart, and general adoption of this policy would do much to reduce the complications and mortality of this badly managed disease.

Celia M. Oakley, Royal Postgraduate Medical School, Hammersmith Hospital, London, England. "Missed Diagnosis of Infective Endocarditis." (July 23, 1988) *The Lancet*: 214.

In the age of antibiotics, IE "should never happen at all."[1] These are the words of Dr. Joan Weyman quoted in the well-known *British Dental Journal*. Such a statement is a powerful indictment of those doctors and dentists whose patients develop IE. But, those who have failed to provide their patients with antibiotic prophylaxis will argue, IE is a rare disease, wiped out with the advent of antibiotics, few patients die if treated, the use of antibiotics on a regular basis with dental procedures will produce resistant bacteria, the benefits of prophylaxis do not outweigh the risks, bacteria can get into the bloodstream merely from chewing food or gum and time consuming sensitivity tests will have to be done for each patient. And, who, they cry out anxiously, will be responsible from a legal point of view?

Research, however, shows these protestations to be invalid, and, once again, little has been learned from the valuable lessons of the past. In one of his famous lectures to his colleagues, the conscientious Osler, who was especially interested in bacterial disease, issued a warning about IE. "It is of use from time to time," he said, "to take stock so to speak of our knowledge of a particular disease, to see exactly where we stand in regard to it, to inquire to what conclusions the accumulated facts seem to point, and to ascertain in what direction we may look for fruitful investigations in the future."[2]

It is now time to take stock, once again, of IE. Medical statistics reveal that many practicing physicians, particularly those who are not involved in research and do not write for medical journals, are not re-examining their knowledge about IE, and, for this reason, this disease is not only happening but happening with disturbing frequency. When so much is known about IE, why is it still "happening" in the eighties?

Incidence

The key word in Osler's address is "conclusions" and, for the technologically sophisticated eighties, they are startling. The "accumulated facts" point to the conclusion that the incidence of IE has not declined since the introduction of preventative antimicrobial drugs in the forties! Speaking at the same institution, the Royal College of Physicians and Surgeons in London, England, where Osler had delivered his preeminent address, British physician, Graham Hayward, took stock of the situation regarding IE, just as his famous predecessor had so wisely done in 1885. Hayward drew upon reports from the Office of the Registrar General which, since 1931, has published the number of deaths each year in England and Wales verified as caused from acute or subacute bacterial endocarditis, a figure around 1000 in the thirties. Using his own case studies and those of others, Hayward concludes that, at the time of his address in 1974, "the total number of cases each year (in England and Wales) is about the same as in 1939."[3] Dentists, writing in *The Dental Practitioner* in 1967, came to the same conclusion as Hayward, that the number of cases per year was "disappointingly similar to that found in the 1930s", prior to the use of antibiotics, and might even be higher, they said, at around 1500.[4]

But that was the sixties and seventies! What about the eighties, when medicine has, supposedly, made so many advances? After all, doctors can transplant almost any organ and are even working on transplanting the human brain. Our society tends to measure the significance of new knowledge in terms of decades. Once again, The Royal College of Physicians and Surgeons in London, England has published the facts about IE. Its recent 1983 study of 544 cases of IE occurring in 1981 and 1982 offered the same stunning conclusion as Hayward, that the number of cases a year in England and Wales is the same in the eighties, if not more than, it was back in Libman, Horder and Osler's time, seventy or so years ago. Nothing had changed in a decade.[5]

North American statistics do not differ from the British. In 1971, Cherubin and Neu at the Columbia Presbyterian Medical Centre in New York reported on the incidence of IE from 1938 to 1967 and found only a small decline in the number of cases over the thirty years which span both pre and post antibiotic periods.[6] In his textbook on IE, Lawrence Freedman, a prominent specialist in infectious diseases, cited American and French studies of 1977 and 1978 which indicate that there is a varying incidence of IE from 11 to 50 cases per million people per year.[7] In the United States that would mean 2,750 to 12,500 individuals. In fact, a national survey of hospital discharges showed there were 13,000 cases of IE in 1979 in the United States.[8] Therefore, the upper figure of 50 cases per million people is more correct. Given these figures, the number of cases in the British Isles is, likely, greater than reported.

In Canada, no epidemiological studies of the incidence of IE have been undertaken. However, if we apply Freedman's formula, there would be 250 to 2,750 cases per year in Canada based on a population of 25,000,000. Statistics Canada for 1986 showed 187 deaths from IE.[9] According to a well-known heart textbook, IE is "not a reportable disease" and, therefore, "the overall incidence cannot be accurately estimated."[10] This means that IE, unlike syphillis, for example, does not have to be reported to the Bureau of Statistics in the U.S. and likely not in Canada. It would also be impossible, therefore, to determine the number of valvular replacements occasioned by IE. It follows that no statistics would exist for cases of endocarditis that heal spontaneously, such as mine, which Libman and his contemporaries have described. Late deaths in such cases would be attributed to heart and/or kidney failure, the cause of which would inevitably remain obscure. Even after the introduction of antibiotics, there have been reports, such as that from the Mayo Clinic in 1956,[11] which have described, like Libman's, the revelation at autopsy of healed endocarditis in individuals who were never suspected of having IE and who had received no treatment. In older persons especially, there may be a confusing complexity of illnesses that masks an IE. As well, autopsies are done less frequently than they were in the pre-antibiotic, and this fact contributes to the complexity of the problem of establishing the true incidence of IE. The rate of autopsies in hospitals in the United States has steadily declined, falling from "50 percent in the 1940s to 41 percent in 1964, 35 percent in 1972, 22 percent in 1975 and an estimated 10-15 percent in 1985."[12]

According to Lawrence Freedman, in his text on IE, the incidence may be altered by different criteria within the medical profession for diagnosing IE and by the particular population group being studied; for instance, IE is more prevalent among people with MVP than among those with other cardiac abnormalities. Freedman also pointed out that the use of hemodialysis in patients with associated glomerulonephritis and intravenous drugs, which greatly increase the risk of IE, can confuse the picture.[13]

Stroke and other cerebral disasters may, in reality, be due to unsuspected

IE, bacteria either not being sought at autopsy or no longer recoverable. As I have pointed out, it is well known that cerebral catastrophes can take place two to five years after IE, even with treatment, and, in cases of inadvertent cure with oral antibiotics, a past IE would never be suspected. Death attributed to myocardial infarction, if there is no autopsy, may, in fact, have been caused by IE as in the case of the athlete, cited at the beginning of this book. Libman convincingly proved that patients who had IE, which healed spontaneously, later died from heart and/or kidney failure with no longer any trace of active infection, only the pathological signs of old vegetations. Modern researchers concede that there are patients, like Libman's, who recover but eventually die after a long, "chronic illness sometimes lasting decades associated with massive splenomegaly, lymphadenopathy (enlargement of the lymph nodes) and profound anemia."[14] Such patients, Morel-Maroger and workers suggested, as did Freedman, are the modern hemodialysis patients whose kidneys have at last failed after years of increasing renal insufficiency.[15] Morel-Maroger et al discussed other studies which showed that in IE patients who were untreated, 33 percent were found at autopsy to have a diffuse GN and 48 percent a focal GN while, in treated patients there was no diffuse GN and only a 24 percent incidence of focal GN. In 1986, there were 1778 deaths in Canada from kidney disease.[16] How many of these resulted from an undiagnosed IE much earlier in the patient's life?

Mortality

With antimicrobial drugs, improved laboratory techniques and diagnostic equipment and the accumulated knowledge of almost a century about how to recognize IE, it would be expected that, while individuals might still contract this disease, they would never die of it. However, this is not the case, and the facts on the mortality rate are equally as disturbing as the revelations about the incidence of IE. Once the shine has worn off any new discovery, a kind of careless indifference creeps in. This is human nature, and doctors are no exception. Their belief that penicillin has transformed bacterial endocarditis into a disease of the past has made doctors quite complacent, but, if this disease is neither being prevented nor diagnosed, then penicillin, or any other anti-microbial, is useless. It becomes just another dinosaur of the past, once all powerful but now totally unadaptable to a new environment. Bacterial infections, specifically infections of the heart, no longer excite fear in the public. The talk is all about cancer or heart attack or just the undefined, generic entity of heart disease. Every doctor to whom I addressed the question of IE said it was an extremely rare disease, really only a disease of the pre-antibiotic era. "You don't see it much anymore," they told me. However, the true facts are startling. Lawrence Freedman, writing in 1983, said:

> I have the impression that in a general university-hospital patient population about as many cases of endocarditis are diagnosed for the first time at autopsy

as are diagnosed clinically. In Nigeria, 44 percent of 90 cases were first diagnosed at autopsy. In patients over 60 years of age, the diagnosis is often missed clinically. In a recent series of patients diagnosed at autopsy, the diagnosis of IE was not suspected clinically in 60 percent of patients. In the absence of a heart murmur, IE was suspected in only 9 percent of patients.[17]

As age increases, other illnesses confuse the picture. The Registrar General's reports for England and Wales showed, for example, that the number of deaths from bacterial endocarditis in patients over fifty years was the same in 1958 as in 1939.[18] Twenty years of antibiotics, it appears, has made absolutely no difference.

In 1966, *The Archives of Environmental Health* published an editorial reviewing the medical profession's progress in the war with the microbes. Its author, Dr. H. A. Reimann of Hahnemann Medical College in Philadelphia summed up the situation in one shocking sentence: "Surprisingly the mortality from bacterial infections in hospitals is about the same as it was in 1930."[19] Though Reimann does not specifically refer to IE, his statement, when taken with others on the mortality rate in IE, suggests that many of these bacterial infections must have involved the heart since death is then more likely. Reimann's contemporaries, Uwaydah and Weinberg, assessing a period of twenty years since the introduction of antibiotics, concluded virtually the same thing, that, "In spite of all the advances in chemotherapy, the survival rate for bacterial endocarditis in our hospital (Massachusetts General Hospital) improved only slightly, if at all, during the past twenty years."[20] Once again, these researchers say that the poorest prognosis is in the elderly.

According to investigators, the mortality rate is said to be somewhere around 30 percent.[21] In Britain, for example, one group of researchers, Shinebourne et al, reported in 1969 that 31 percent of their patients with acute IE died after six months and 40 percent were dead after two years. The mortality statistics varied only slightly for subacute or chronic endocarditis, 25 percent of patients dying at six months and 32 percent at two years.[22]

The mortality rate in the United States is similar. In children the mortality rate appears to be higher than in adults. A review of 266 cases of IE in children showed that mortality has been as high as 40 percent, though other studies would put it closer to 20-25 percent. In newborns, the mitral valve is the most common site as it is said to be in adults. Curiously, 8-10 percent of the reported cases of IE in children do not have any predisposing heart condition. This suggests IE can be imposed on a normal valve.[23] MVP has been documented in infants aged two months,[24] and one would wonder how many of these infants who die with IE had an unidentified MVP of only histological significance.

There is evidence, however, to suggest that the immediate and early mortality rate may be much higher than 30 percent. In 1978, the University of Mississippi Medical Centre reported very bleak results from a study of 102 patients treated for IE. 26 died within 30 days of admission to hospital and an additional 32 died within the first year after the commencement of their illness, giving a total of 58 patients or 56 percent dying in the first 365 days, or a survival rate of only 44 percent. After 11 years, only 36 percent of the patients who had had strep. viridans IE were alive.[25] In that same year, the Columbia Presbyterian Medical Centre which sees, on average, 23 cases of IE a year, presented similarly frightening results of a six year study. The mortality rate for 101 of their patients with natural valves, as opposed to prosthetic devices made from calf or porcine tissue, was extremely high. 34 percent died in hospital and 46 percent within two years after the onset of the infection. By the end of the six year review, 51 percent of the original patients had died.[26]

Treatment does not guarantee the patient a normal lifespan. The results of a long term study from New Zealand, published in 1981, showed that 13 years after infection and treatment, only 47 percent of the patients remained alive. These authors concluded that early and late death from IE "remain distressingly high" in spite of the availability of treatment.[27] A review from The New York University Medical Center in 1976 showed extreme variation in the survival rate as low as 47 and as high as 82 percent.[28] This discrepancy suggests, once again, that the chances of survival may depend upon the institution to which one is admitted. When we talk about mortality or valve replacement in these studies, it must be remembered that these are cases that come to the attention of a doctor and that there are all those "unreportable" cases of IE that all the giants of the pre-antibiotic era, Horder, Libman, Grant, Osler and others talked about, cases such as mine, that progress to severe regurgitation, involving one or more valves once the heart is enlarged, and terminate, ultimately in heart failure long after the precipitating febrile illness has passed.

Endocarditis Prophylaxis Failures — Do they exist?

Naturally with such disappointing statistics, it will be assumed that antibiotics, the wonder drugs, have failed us. It is always easier to blame something other than human error. The unproven efficacy of antibiotic prophylaxis is an argument doctors use frequently to justify their neglect to provide preventative medicine. It was used with Margo and myself. We were told that no proof existed of the success of antibiotics in preventing bacterial endocarditis during dental or surgical interventions, yet neither of us was provided with this protection and both of us contracted this disease.

In 1955, the American Heart Association's Committee for the Prevention of Rheumatic Fever and Infective Endocarditis published its first recommendations on the prevention of IE in the medical journal, *Circulation*.[29] This Committee identifies patients at risk and establishes the most effective antibiotic regimens for them during bacteremic situations. Periodically, it updates its recommendations in accordance with new research. The Committee's guidelines are based on studies, including experimental animal research, on the treatment and prevention of IE, much of which has been done by David

Durack, one of the members of the Prevention Committee. The AHA's guidelines are used by doctors and dentists in Canada and the United States.

Members of that Committee also set up a registry in 1979 to record endocarditis prophylaxis failures. Up until 1978, according to this registry, there had been about 30 known cases of antibiotic prophylaxis failure in the entire medical literature since the introduction of antibiotics, and the proof of failure was said to be inconclusive [30]. As well, there is much documented experimental evidence, using the rabbit model, of the efficacy of antibiotics in preventing IE [31], most recently that of Drake and Sande of California in 1986.[32]

In 1983, some members of the AHA's Prevention Committee, Durack, Bisno and Kaplan who established the registry, wrote a paper on 52 cases in which antibiotic prophylaxis appeared not to have worked. In 92 percent of these cases IE occurred in association with a dental procedure. Only 6, or 12 percent, of the 52 patients who had penicillin prophylaxis were given the regimen most recently recommended by the AHA's Committee on Prevention of IE. There were errors in the timing of the drug administration, which must be given preoperatively, the amount of the loading dose, the duration of the preventative treatment and in the choice of patient to be protected. MVP proved to be, once again, the most common predisposing condition present in 33 percent or possibly more, according to the authors, of the cases. Just what this fact means remains undetermined but suggests perhaps that these patients' regimens were less adequate than those of others. The group concluded that while "advisory statements", such as that of the AHA are "widely known", they are "seldom followed". The authors also believe that the actual rate of failure of antibiotics to prevent an IE is unknown but that the incidence of IE would decline if the AHA recommendations were followed with susceptible patients.[33]

This study of Durack et al, like others, raises a very important issue, that of the uniquely iatrogenic nature of a disease that "should never happen at all." Impressive evidence has accumulated in the medical and dental literature to confirm that doctors and dentists are not practicing prevention and that little has changed in their understanding regarding the protection of susceptible patients since the introduction of antibiotics in 1944 and the first warnings that followed. It is the failure of the medical profession that is the major cause for the unchanging incidence of IE since the introduction of antibiotics.

Prevention — medical failure

As already pointed out, in numerous studies, it is MVP that is generally the underlying cardiac lesion upon which an IE is superimposed. Obviously these people are not being protected. It should not come as a surprise that Barlow's warning of 1963 was, in fact, not the first regarding the risky nature of the LSM that accompanies the click of MVP. It was W. Proctor Harvey in 1949, who, at a time when mitral regurgitation was being downgraded in importance, specified in his book, *Clinical Auscultation of the Heart,* that the innocent, apical LSM, now known to be the typical murmur of MVP, required "the same precautions against bacterial endocarditis as would be employed in cases of rheumatic mitral insufficiency."[34]

Harvey bravely took a stand in that great debate, encouraged by Evans, Lewis and others, over the significance of extra systolic sounds and mitral incompetence and even went beyond by casting the entity now known as MVP in the same league as RHD with respect to the risk of bacterial endocarditis. We are reminded of the pathological studies at the turn of the century which revealed abnormalities that more closely resembled prolapsed rather than stenosed valves in the presence of the vegetations of IE. Tragically, a superior clinician and researcher like Harvey was unable to persuade doctors still influenced by the tradition of Gallavardin, Lewis, McKenzie and Evans. The wonder drugs were thus ignored for almost another twenty years until Barlow would again raise the issue, settling it once and for all with his indisputable evidence in 1963 of the necessity for such protection. Writers, Hobson and Juel-Jenson from the Radcliffe Infirmary at Oxford, reviewing the situation in 1956 for the dozen years following the introduction of antibiotics, lamented that antibiotic cover, even for RHD patients, long recognized as susceptible, was "casual and inconsequent" or, worse, "frequently ignored."[35]

There have been many attempts to define the patient at risk in order to assist doctors and dentists in adopting preventative procedures. At the Queen's University in Belfast, Ireland, McGowan and Tuohy made such an assessment. Naturally, in their view, patients with RHD were at the top of the list, followed by those with congenital cardiac anomalies, a history of rheumatic fever and, finally, "a history of a murmur", described as functional or "harmless."[36] This last group would have included the late systolic murmur of MVP since it has been called harmless, innocent or functional by so many writers. This work published in 1968, five years after Barlow makes no reference to his studies, once again, suggesting the slow speed at which medical news travels, even to other researchers. The two authors from the Dentistry Faculty of the University of Belfast found that 77 percent of 424 procedures, extractions, scalings and root canal treatments, involving 113 individuals at risk, were not done under antibiotic cover, and, in 64 percent of these cases, no inquiry as to heart murmur had even been made by the dentists. 81 percent of the patients had never been warned by their medical doctor of the risks of their condition. Of the 19 who had, 11 percent had been warned by their own physician and 8 percent incidentally by a physician in a hospital. This study shows that there has been consistent disregard for the benefits of antibiotics.

Nor has the antibiotic revolution taken place in the United States. Studies done in the early sixties and seventies, twenty and thirty years after the introduction of antibiotics, showed that dental practitioners did not completely understand how their interventions could produce a bacteremia and thus the risk of IE in susceptible patients. In the early sixties, W. Proctor Harvey continuing his research into IE and the question of prevention, published a report with his colleague, Maurice Capone, from Georgetown University Hospital in Washington, DC.[37] The number of patients knowing they required cover varied greatly with the type of cardiac abnormality and the type of manipulation. Extraction commanded the most attention while the dentists held cleaning and filling to be of little danger. Likewise, Margo was told in the 1980s that root canal and abortion were the only two dangerous situations when in fact it was dental cleaning which was implicated in her IE. Harvey and Capone also point out the danger from an endodontal infection such as I had. Dentists in the Georgetown study, following tradition unquestioningly, placed the RHD patients in the highest risk category followed by congenital abnormalities while the least informed of their patients were those with the "functional or harmless" murmur, the murmur which McGowan and Tuohy of Belfast listed and which now is considered to be MVP. Of the 258 patients in the study, only 56 or 21.7 percent were familiar with precautions about extractions and 7.7 percent, or 20 patients, about cleaning and filling.

The passage of time has not improved the situation, and it is easy to see why people are still developing endocarditis in 1989. There is something seriously wrong when patients suffer two and three episodes of IE related to dental procedures because their physicians and dentists have continued to fail to provide them with antibiotics for interventions that draw blood. A study done in Britain in 1971 [38] revealed that almost 25 percent of the patients admitted to hospital for a second time with Strep Viridans endocarditis were still not aware of the need for antibiotic cover with extractions, considered one of the most dangerous of procedures, and, in 40 percent of these patients, the first attack was associated with dental procedures.

Nothing had changed by the late seventies and eighties even in the large, metropolitan centres. The known dangers of specific dental and surgical interventions made little difference. The American researchers, Petersdorf and Pelletier, reporting in 1977 revealed that 82 percent of a group of patients within a certain series at the University of Washington Hospitals had developed IE from dental extractions or cleaning without antibiotic prophylaxis.[39] It is astonishing that a dentist would not protect a patient with a heart murmur during extraction of a tooth, one of the most dangerous procedures because the bloodstream is showered with bacteria. A recent 1986 British survey showed that less than one fifth of patients in the study knew it was important to have antibiotic coverage during certain procedures and for one half of the patients responding, there was no hospital record of the necessity of antibiotic prophylaxis.[40]

In the city of Toronto, where I was receiving my medical care, ABP was a well established subject among professionals. According to the Heart and Stroke Foundation, Toronto doctors officially follow the American Heart Association recommendations. The 1977 guidelines had been published one year before my MVP was diagnosed. Those guidelines, now superceded by the 1984 update, contained the recommendation that MVP with mitral insufficiency (regurgitation) should be protected during dental and surgical procedures. My cardiologist and dentists could not help but be aware of the opinions of their colleagues. But they, like other physicians and dentists, were not following these recommendations, even though there was no equivalent Canadian standard to replace them, and this concern was vocalized in the medical literature by local specialists. Two years before my cardiologist had identified my MVP, Toronto researchers, Monroe and Lazarus, published an article warning Toronto doctors and dentists that "a high percentage of patients who are at risk of developing a disease with very serious consequences are being treated without adequate protection."[41] This complaint mimics others repeated year after year in the dental and medical literature ever since the introduction of antibiotics. The Toronto researchers, in words stronger than those of many articles, lay the blame at the doorstep of the physician and the dentist. Failure to provide protection for susceptible patients, is, in their words, "totally unjustified considering the little time it takes to determine if a patient is at risk and to administer appropriate prophylactic measures. It is the physician's responsibility to ensure his patient is aware of his medical condition and the need for antibiotic coverage during certain dental procedures. The dentist on the other hand must be prepared to elicit this information by taking a careful history and consulting with the physician if necessary."[42] The onus is **not** on the patient to offer the information, but on the dentist to obtain it by means of direct questioning in a written information form for the permanent record. Members of the AHA Committee for the prevention of IE have also spoken sternly to physicians and dentists about communicating with one another. "For the physician to ignore the dentist, or vice versa, is unacceptable,"[43] they said.

The most troubling aspect of the whole battle to prevent IE is the refusal of both doctors and dentists to accept new medical evidence that the syndrome of click and late systolic murmur, or MVP, poses more risk than mitral stenosis from rheumatic fever. The authors of the Toronto report still held the view, in 1976, that the latter was more susceptible to IE, a view that was being challenged by new research for some time prior to their report. There is much evidence of this dramatic change in medical perspective regarding these two conditions that have been discussed and compared for over a century. The revelations, like those regarding extra systolic sounds and murmurs, are not recent as many doctors, and therefore their patients, might suppose. Current studies confirm the opinions of Samuel Levine way back in 1928 that individuals with "a mitral systolic murmur without evidence of mitral stenosis", which results from RHD, were the most vulnerable to IE,[44] and Harvey, of course, repeated this warning in 1949 when antibiotics were readily available. Rodbard's studies, previously discussed,[45] and Buchbinder's [46] of the seventies, like these earlier writers, showed that mitral insufficiency, not mitral stenosis is more frequently found in the presence of IE. This argument was strengthened in 1977 when Kaplan of the AHA Prevention Committee pointed out that the number of patients with underlying congenital heart disease had risen from 56 percent of the total cases of IE in the years 1933-42 to over 90 percent of cases in the sixties while the percent of children with RHD, as the underlying cause, had declined.[47] It is not known from this study how many MVP cases would make up the 90 percent, but this condition is regarded by most researchers as a congenital disorder of the mesenchymal tissue [48], and MVP has been reported in over 30 percent, and possibly many more, of IE cases. This fact would explain the shift away from mitral stenosis of RHD as a risk factor. Others have reported that a "murmur of unknown etiology" has replaced RHD as the underlying feature in cases of IE.[49] This viewpoint was expressed in 1971, and most murmurs that could not be defined, i.e. of "unknown etiology", have subsequently been identified as MVP.

Currently, the situation does not appear to be improving in any of the developed nations of the world that have produced extensive research on the association between IE and cardiac abnormalities, with the aid, one should add, of thousands of tax dollars. If dentists are not giving patients at most risk, specifically those with prosthetic valves, the maximum protection, it is certain that supposedly "harmless murmurs", as MVP is still being called, are going unprotected. In 1981, an American survey revealed that of 359 dentists, only 15 percent followed the AHA recommendations regarding the use of ABP for at risk patients.[50]

The latest research, in 1988, from the Department of Dentistry, Albert Einstein College of Medicine in New York, provides us with some frightening facts.[51] The authors, Sadowsky and Kunzel, wished to ascertain if dentists were following the latest 1984 AHA guidelines regarding the antibiotic regimens for at risk patients. 460 general dentists were contacted and asked to provide the actual prescriptions they would use with their patients during certain procedures. The same problems arose as in all the other studies. The dentists were uncertain and frequently mistaken in their understanding about which cardiac problems posed a danger. For instance, 20 percent said they would provide ABP for patients who had had a heart attack and 40 percent said they would for patients who had had coronary artery by-pass surgery, neither of which requires antibiotic coverage for any procedures. Yet, one-third of the dentists did not know that congenital heart disease posed a risk, and nothing was said of MVP. A single respondent was correct about the regimen for prosthetic heart valve patients. Compliance with AHA recommendations was in general very low. Of those who did use the guidelines, 55-93 percent prescribed loading and 37 to 90 percent postoperative doses half or less than suggested in the guidelines, and, once again, patients with RHD or a history of rheumatic fever received the most attention. The timing of administration of doses was also incorrect; there was both over-medication and undermedication. While 90 percent claimed they were familiar with the AHA guidelines, of the 12.5 percent who said they consulted them during the survey, 40 percent could not answer all the questions correctly. The authors of the survey concluded that dentists have difficulty identifying patients at risk for IE and do not fully understand how to use antibiotics as a preventative measure. The authors also concluded that their results will help to explain the antibiotic failures reported by Durack, Bisno and Kaplan of the AHA Prevention Committee. From this and other studies, it is clear that the understanding of how and when to use antibiotics has not greatly improved since these drugs were first introduced in the 1940s.

Cause of High Mortality in the Antibiotic Era

While the unchanging incidence of IE is related to the lack of prevention, persistent high mortality rates can be attributed to two main factors: the misuse of antibiotics and the inability to diagnose IE because the physician is not familiar with all the physical signs and symptoms, and the particular laboratory tests, discussed in Chapter Four, that might uncover an elusive IE. If the IE is mild, there may be spontaneous cure, with or without valvular damage, as Libman described, or less virulent, acutely sensitive microorganisms, as mine appears to have been (possibly because I had never used antibiotics prior to my endodontal infection) are suppressed with less than the expected curative doses of penicillin. My case may be the first to be documented from its inception with a root canal inflammation, dental intervention and a root abscess, to serious valvular damage and seems to verify Libman's observations.

In support of my contention in this book that I had IE, the modern medical literature respects the opinions of Libman and others with regard to self-healing which leaves the patient with further valvular damage and eventual death. In the ten years following the introduction of penicillin, researchers from the Mayo Clinic, Hepper, Burchell and Edwards,[52] observed at autopsy cases of healed IE of the mitral valve. They speculated that these patients were likely to have been given oral antibiotics early in their illness which repressed the infection. They concluded that "it is logical to assume that with the widespread use of antibiotics in cases of a febrile illness without diagnosis, the number of cases of unrecognized, healed, subacute bacterial endocarditis will be greater than in the period before the use of antibiotics" and that healed, unrecognized endocarditis should be considered as a possible cause of mitral insufficiency which would, ultimately, lead to congestive heart failure.

Once again, whether prolapsed valves are actually caused or become more prolapsed and, therefore, more insufficient with greater leakage of blood, because of IE, is a real issue, that is, whether the IE itself is the injurious agent that causes the valvular tissue to change in response. It is known that "hemodynamically important mitral regurgitation", that is regurgitation that causes left ventricular dysfunction, is the most common complication in the MVP syndrome.[53] In 1980, Guy and co-workers of Victoria General Hospital and Dalhousie University in Nova Scotia published their observations that MVP is responsible in **fifty percent** of cases for serious regurgitation requiring mitral valve replacement.[54] And, in 1982, Waller et al[55] indicated that of 97 patients requiring MVR, 60 or 62 percent had MVP and only 3 patients of the 97 had regurgitation resulting from rheumatic heart disease. This goes a long way toward finally squashing the verdict that the systolic regurgitation of MVP, whether late or holosystolic, is of no importance compared to the regurgitation of mitral stenosis and that the term, mitral insufficiency, itself, ought to be struck from the medical record as Evans claimed. I now have severe mitral regurgitation and unquantitated tricuspid regurgitation as well as signs of early heart failure in what is called a benign syndrome, and I am tempted to ask how many of Guy et al's patients have shared my fate, suffering from an earlier unrecognized IE that healed spontaneously or inadvertently with oral antibiotics for some other flu-like illness. In Ontario alone in, for example 1981-82, there were 397 valve replacements.[56] How many of these patients had underlying MVP? How many had IE?

Misuse of antibiotics as a cause of continuing high mortality

Although it has been said that "probably 90 percent of antibiotics are applied unnecessarily,"[57] it would be more correct to say improperly and dangerously, without benefit of diagnosis. There are many articles in the medical literature testifying to the misuse of antibiotics prior to blood culturing, especially in cases of unexplained fever in the presence of a murmur. "Articles concerning antibiotics tend to have a certain sameness about them," wrote Dr. John Tarsitano in 1970, one of the many critics of imcorrect antibiotic treatment. "The overuse and misuse of the antibiotic agents are decried," he said, and "the dangers of uncontrolled therapy are enumerated; a few catastrophic cases histories are cited and we are urged to put our houses in order. The sad thing is that these articles are for the most part telling it like it is."[58]

Even if IE is diagnosed, the choice of drug treatment may be "both inappropriate and ineffective" according to Pelletier and Petersdorf [59]. Margo's treatment was questionable. These workers describe the case of a woman treated in 1977 for only two weeks with IV penicillin for S. viridans endocarditis and then released from hospital. This woman's case is similar to that of Doug, described in the previous chapter, who had been admitted to his local hospital with diagnosed IE, but was, unfortunately, treated for only two weeks. He was released and promptly suffered an embolism in his arm and severe one-sided headache which was likely a cerebral embolism. Because of persistent fever, the woman's GP treated her with oral oxacillin for another two months after discharge, in spite of neuropsychiatric symptoms, forgetfulness and inco-ordination which pointed to an ineradicated IE. The patient eventually died of CHF as a result of this improper treatment. Correct treatment for IE consists of immediate administration of bactericidal antibiotics parenterally for lengthy periods of time, usually 4-6 weeks.

Much has been written about the dangers of misusing oral antibiotics. The nature of this misuse, however, must be explained because it is often misinterpreted by dentists and doctors. Their primary concern is to challenge the efficacy of ABP largely because of the extra burden of time and anxiety it imposes on them and, inevitably, because of the legal implications of failing to provide it. To provide ABP, they protest, is to overuse it and run the risk of producing resistant strains of common bacteria. Therefore, the risk, they complain, of providing protection far outweighs the benefits. David Durack who is on the AHA Committee for Prevention of IE corrected this misperception. "It should be noted," he said, "that the use of antibiotics for prophylaxis of endocarditis is infrequent in comparison with the frequent, needless use of these drugs to treat minor upper respiratory infections." Durack also adds that the life of bacteria entering the bloodstream from dental manipulations is short and the duration of the course of antibiotics is short. Therefore there is not much likelihood of fostering the growth of untreatable microorganisms.[60]

It is precisely the problem identified by Durack and others that should be addressed if mortality from IE, indeed, if IE itself is to be wiped out. Frequent treating of minor illnesses such as flu, sore throat without culturing for bacteria, and colds with penicillin, apart from being ineffective, may produce unusual microorganisms resistant to treatment, but there appears to be no danger if the patient does not have a cardiac abnormality. However, treating an unexplained fever with oral antibiotics, before culturing the blood, in patients with murmurs and other susceptible heart conditions has been proven, many times over, to be hazardous. The chief problem with oral antibiotics is that they can delay diagnosis of IE as long as seven to ten months. The antibiotics kill the bacteria and control the disease without eradicating it. Negative cultures fool physicians who have overlooked symptoms related by the patient or clinical signs such as murmurs, enlarged spleen, clubbing of fingernails etc. The longer the delay in diagnosis, the more significant the valvular damage and the greater the likelihood of valve replacement or death. In the 1980s, doctors have said that brief treatment of a febrile illness with oral antibiotics is "the most important explanation for the failure to isolate microorganisms from the blood of patients with IE and clinical manifestations."[61] Pesanti and Smith from the University of Iowa Hospital and Clinics reported that 63 percent of the patients coming to them with culture negative endocarditis had been given oral antibiotics before any blood sample was collected for culturing of bacteria.[62] Such results demonstrate that the problem is not the antibiotics themselves, as has been claimed, but those who administer them.

Pelletier and Petersdorf state frankly that the use of oral antibiotics is the direct cause of death. They found that 48 percent of their IE patients had been given oral antibiotics prior to a diagnosis. "Suppressive but not curative drug therapy in undiagnosed patients," they said, "was clearly related to subsequent morbidity and mortality due to valve destruction, rupture of mycotic aneurysm, or fatal embolism."[63] The mortality in their series of patients was high at 38 percent. The number of deaths among the patients who received antibiotic therapy prior to diagnosis was, however, less than in the group which had not received any prior therapy. Those who received oral antibiotics likely had developed resistant microorganisms while those who received no antibiotics would die from acute infection if no treatment, whatsoever, was given. Patients in Pelletier and Petersdorf's study "who received antibiotics without a specific diagnosis of IE either failed to demonstrate any clinical response or experienced remission of symptoms while receiving antibiotics only to relapse after cessation."[64] Generally, according to Dr. VanScoy of the Mayo Clinic, patients with culture negative endocarditis, usually resulting from prior use of oral antibiotics, do not do as well as those with culture positive endocarditis since they suffer from major emboli and CHF twice as frequently and their mortality within the first three weeks of treatment approaches that of patients with endocarditis of the prosthetic valve which is unanimously considered the most risky of the susceptible situations. Half of the patients in VanScoy's study with culture negative IE who still had fever after one week of therapy died.[65] The automatic prescription for an undiagnosed febrile illness can thus be a death sentence.

Dr. Petersdorf maintains that the events of IE should be known by every *third year medical student* and that taking a blood sample from a patient with a fever and "known heart disease", which means a murmur, for culturing should be a "reflex action".[66] Handing out a prescription for oral antibiotics should not. Petersdorf's advice about culturing the blood immediately is the same given by Libman and others at the turn of the century, and the importance Petersdorf places on familiarity with this disease implies that IE is far more common than many doctors suppose. Not to order a blood test for bacteria is a manifestation of the complacency that misunderstanding of the purpose of antibiotics has engendered.

The misuse of these lifesaving drugs has resulted in a tough, ongoing battle with more and more powerful microbes whose mutations have gone, in some instances, beyond human control. But rather than address the real cause, iatrogenic production of untreatable strains, scientists keep searching for bigger and better weapons, as, metaphorically speaking, the name of the antimicrobial, Pondocillin, suggests. Certain common microorganisms, for instance the fragilus convexis group of "bacteroides", which are very slow-growing organisms, have now become resistant to a whole host of antimicrobials such as benzypenicillin, ampicillin, methicillin and cloxacillin.[67] It is known that 40 percent of the enterococci species are resistant in vitro to combination penicillin and streptomycin and, for this reason, alert physicians, like Petersdorf,[68] recommend penicillin or ampicillin and gentamycin, ampicillin being the drug of choice according to Goodman and Gilman.[69] Yet, a 1978 report on IE over the years 1960-1974, described, among other patients, a 37 year old woman with enterococcal endocarditis who died after treatment for an extremely long period of time, 142 days, with pen G, vancomycin, ristocetin, streptomycin, erythromycin, tetracycline and chloramphenicol in a variety of combinations. Though ampicillin and gentamycin were available in the early sixties, neither appeared to have been used in her case.[70]

It is horrifying to learn that there are microorganisms resistant to every known antimicrobial agent. The futility of this iatrogenically induced microbial war comes shockingly to life in such cases as that described in 1965 in *The American Journal of Medicine*[71]. One can only conclude that "inappropriate and ineffective" treatment, to use the words of Petersdorf and Pelletier,[72] with either oral or parenteral antibiotics had been used at some time during the patient's illness. This patient's IE was caused by streptococcus viridans, one of the most common microorganisms, acutely sensitive to penicillin. He was treated with varying combinations of drugs for two years. The administrative route was not indicated, though there is some suggestion that the drugs were administered orally. The microorganism was briefly suppressed at times but never eradicated although negative cultures were intermittently obtained. Over the two years, the patient had 48 positive and 33 negative blood cultures, a little less than the 100 cultures cited in a similar case described by Graham Hayward in 1960.[73] The strain of S. viridans that developed ultimately became resistant to almost every known antibiotic in spite of the fact that the patient had received in the two years, 2,398,000,000 units of penicillin, 62 gm. of chloramphenicol, 7 gm. streptomycin, 19 gm. vancomycin, 27 gm. restocetin, 40 gm. of kanamycin, 3,750,000 units of bacitracin and 655 gm. erythromycin. His cultures remained positive and he died suddenly at home. Probably from toxicity!

Other Causes of High Mortality

Most researchers agree that there is a greater mortality rate in cases of negative blood cultures because they influence the doctor to reject a diagnosis of IE. This happened in Margo's case. As I pointed out in Chapter 4 on symptoms, if the physician is not familiar with the clinical signs and symptoms of IE or does not know what tests to order, the uninformed patient will not have as good a chance of surviving or saving his or her natural valve. Prominent researchers say that IE is often overlooked when what doctors regard as atypical signs are present such as arthritis, arthralgia or myalgia. Part of the problem is that these clinical signs are poorly described or omitted altogether from textbooks on medicine and rheumatology and even from some important clinical reviews in the medical journals.[74]

Other Causes of Negative Cultures

While the prior use of oral antibiotics is the most common cause of negative cultures, there are other important causes. These are endocarditis involving only the right side of the heart and the tricuspid or pulmonic valves[75], which is frequently found in drug addicts and often manifests solely as pneumonia with embolism to the lungs, or acute meningitis[76], CHF, mural endocarditis, without valvular involvement, which has been found in a case of IE and MVP discussed earlier, and uremia as a result of kidney involvement, specifically glomerulonephritis.[77]

Laboratory Difficulties

A frequent cause of negative cultures is simply laboratory error. Accuracy in culturing blood depends solely on the skill of the technicians. Negative cultures turn up more frequently in the inadequately equipped, mediocre laboratory staffed with careless technicians.[78] Experts on IE believe that positive cultures can be obtained in almost 100 percent of cases if the laboratory's bacteriological techniques are first rate. For instance, in the New York Hospital, where there has been a longstanding interest in IE and thus an excellent record in culturing the blood, only about 3 percent of patients ever have negative cultures.[79]

Frequently not enough blood cultures are done. This is the fault, not of the lab technician but the physician who orders the tests. Most researchers agree that five to six cultures will be sufficient but it may be necessary to do many more if a positive culture cannot be obtained. Cultures should be kept for as long as two to three weeks but, in cases of negative cultures, Robert Van Scoy of the Mayo Clinic suggests the cultures be kept three to four weeks to encourage the slower growing microorganisms.[80] Bone marrow cultures should also be done, and it may be necessary to culture an Osler's node or the fluid from an inflamed and swollen joint, especially if that happens to be the only sign of illness as in the case of the young girl with the swollen ankle. Naturally treatment should be begun on the basis of clinical signs and symptoms and, once the microorganism is identified, and its sensitivity known, the drug regimen can be altered. If a patient has been taking oral antibiotics, the cultures may remain negative for long periods of time. Lawrence Freedman has observed that a patient who had taken only three capsules of vibramycin 24 hours before coming to the hospital had negative cultures for twelve days in spite of fever.[81] An antibiotic removal device, such as penicillinase is helpful in certain circumstances. In my case, only four samples of blood were taken at TMSC, all within a 48 hour period after the termination of four months of intermittent use of oral antibiotics and, since nothing was grown in 3-4 days, the cultures were discarded. Nor was penicillinase used despite prior use of oral antibiotics..

Inferior laboratories may not have the special media necessary for culturing the slow-growing or fastidious microorganisms such as gram negative bacilli. In Margo's case this was a problem. In infection with such microorganisms, including fungi and staphylococci, the mortality rate may range from 50-80 percent [82]

There are microorganisms which some laboratories discard as "contaminating normal flora or harmless bystanders", according to a recent Toronto study.[83] One such example is the unusual Group F streptococci, a normal inhabitant of the upper respiratory, alimentary tracts and vagina. These microorganisms are rejected because doctors order lab technicians to look for the more common streptococci that have Lancefield antigens, such as the pneumococci or enterococci. S. Milleri is another uncommon, frequently discarded microorganism. It is found in dental abscesses and was isolated from the patient's blood in this Toronto study. This pathogen was isolated from the granulatomous material attached to my extracted tooth. However, no effort was made to culture this microorganism from my blood samples. As well, these authors say, nutritionally deficient satelite streptococci are often overlooked since, as their name suggests, they grow only around other bacteria.

Researchers recommend that all hospital laboratories have carbon dioxide incubators as standard equipment though many do not.[84] The slow-growing, fastidious gram negative microorganisms, like that which Margo had, as well as cardiobacterium hominis, actinobacillus, actinomycetamcomitans, the haemophili (aprophilus, parainfluenzae and paraprophilus) have special requirements. They grow best on a solid medium in the presence of carbon dioxide and they need up to three weeks' incubation according to a group of prominent researchers.[85] If grown in broth rather than on solid medium, these workers warn, the lab technicians must look for the granular colonies which stick to the glass at the blood broth interface or on top of the blood sediment. This can be accomplished by tilting the glass at regular intervals. Otherwise, the bacteria may be missed. A careless lab technician may simply overlook these tedious procedures and, thus, negative cultures result.

Bacteroides, a slow growing anaerobic, gram negative microorganism, associated with high morbidity, as in the case discussed earlier of the MVP patient at The Massachusetts General Hospital, presents difficulties to unskillful laboratories. Bacteroides is found on the skin and in the upper respiratory, gastrointestinal and genitourinary tracts. Mortality from this microorganism varies from 32 percent in one study up to 70 percent. Bacteroides have a propensity for forming abscesses in other parts of the body distant from the heart.[86]

The "L" forms of cell wall defective microorganisms, which are strains often produced by short courses of oral antibiotics before blood culturing, can also stump an inferior lab. For instance, "L" forms of strep. faecalis and cornebacteria, according to Lerner in 1974, in addition to candida type fungi, may not be cultured "unless the blood has been incubated in appropriate hypertonic media"[87], a solution which has a higher osmotic pressure than that of a physiologic salt solution or the solution used as a standard. One researcher reported that "the frequency with which we fail to recover fungi from the blood of patients with autopsy-proven disseminated infection is disconcerting."[88] It must be remembered, too, that fungal infections cannot be considered successfully treated until several years have passed without reinfection.[89]

Unusual slow-growing microorganisms take a long time to wreak havoc on the body, as long as eighteen months.[90] Reports in the medical literature describe patients with very high temperatures and pulse rates who do not look ill. At St. Francis Hospital in Connecticut, a woman with MVP had a temperature of 105° F and a pulse rate of 140 but did not "appear acutely ill."[91] And another case described a patient with a temperature of 104° F as "a healthy appearing woman in no acute distress."[92] These were the same descriptions applied to myself and Margo in our medical records, even though Margo was dying. If the physician is not aware of all the signs of IE or ignores the patient's underlying predisposing cardiac condition, he is not likely to diagnose the disease.

Delays in Diagnosis

Delays in diagnosis and hence treatment usually result in surgery to replace valves, either immediately or at some future date as a result of CHF, or in death from one of the many complications in IE. CHF is considered to be the major cause of death from IE in the antibiotic era and reflects the fact that the disease is not being treated early. In cases of unexplained heart failure in a MVP patient, as I have already pointed out, there is almost always a history, diagnosed or undiagnosed, of IE. In cases of IE with severe CHF, involving the aortic valve, mortality can range from 40-93 percent and, with the mitral valve, from 17-66 percent.[93] In one series, aortic valve endocarditis with moderate or severe CHF resulted in 100 percent mortality.[94]

But surgery, itself, also contributes to the high mortality, about 10-22 percent at operation, and varies according to the degree of CHF present, being higher with the aortic than the mitral valve.[95] The cases of Margo and Doug, described earlier, raise the question of whether doctors are relying on replacement of the natural valve with a prosthetic device as a treatment for IE instead of the more difficult, and more risky route, from a legal point of view, of identifying the bacteria and treating with an appropriate antimicrobial. It is known within the medical profession that the individual doctor's diagnostic skills have declined with the advent of technology. For instance, in the diagnosis of MVP the echocardiogram has replaced the stethoscope, though the stethoscope is unanimously regarded by researchers as the "most specific and sensitive method" of diagnosing prolapsed valves.[96] The same thing is happening, as I have already discussed, in diagnosing IE; the "machine" has replaced the human brain.

There are many serious complications of prosthetic or artifical valves. The percentage of patients requiring a second operation is as high as the percentage of medically treated patients requiring a first valve at a later date. Acute CHF can develop if the valve comes away from its moorings so to speak (dehiscence). Leaks may develop, especially in MVP patients, since the mitral ring is likely stretched from myxomatous tissue. A patient with a prosthetic valve runs a very high risk of IE, and mortality can reach 70 percent.[97] The threat of cerebral or coronary embolism is substantial and is higher with mechanical than with tissue valves, but both types of valves require anti-coagulants which do not always prevent thromboembolic catastrophes. There is also the risk of anti-coagulant-related hemorrhage.[98]

Two recent studies in 1978 and 1979, which Lawrence Freedman refers to, provide some statistics on long term survival with prosthetic valves. Patients whose valves were replaced during the infection, a necessity if the patient is dying from CHF as Margo was, did not have as good a five year survival rate as those whose valves were replaced after antimicrobial treatment when healing had taken place, 66 percent compared with 72 percent. However, other studies showed that of five year survivors in both categories, 15 percent develop Class III and IV CHF. In one quarter of these people, there were paravalvular leaks, one quarter of which required re-operation.[99] Since the 5 year survival rate with replacement of severely prolapsed valves without IE can be as low as fifty percent, it is not difficult to imagine how serious the mortality risk is in an MVP patient when IE is present.[100]

"It should never happen at all" should be the motto of every physician vis à vis this totally preventable disease. But how can the public be assured that all doctors will be up to date about patients at risk or on how to recognize endocarditis? Osler wrote his own textbook on medicine precisely because he believed most of the textbooks of his day were out of date especially in the matter of the bacterial etiology of disease. Heart textbooks did not include MVP until ten years after Barlow's important observations. The medical colleges which license the doctors are supposed to set the standards, presumably in keeping with other countries of their economic status, and assure that the doctors follow them. But, in reality, doctors are accountable to no one but themselves. Doctors set their own personal standards and govern themselves. The specialists we see in the offices and the hospitals are also the professors at the colleges which licence, criticize and correct and, ultimately, remove such licenses. Finding a doctor who keeps abreast of the research in the medical journals is a hit and miss endeavor, mostly miss in mine and many other cases.

But do cardiologists not read *Heart, The American Heart Journal* or *Progress in Cardiovascular Disease*, internists, *Annals of Internal Medicine*, infectious disease consultants, *Infection and Immunology*? The public believes they do and that even GPs do. But doctors do not have to up date themselves with exams any more than a person must up date his driving skills. And how much can a GP have learned in the few weeks devoted to a study of the heart in medical school? I once asked my GP to explain MVP. He drew a very poor diagram, a box divided into four compartments. He pointed out the location of the mitral and tricuspid valves and said unashamedly that this was all he could tell me. I'd have to ask a specialist anything else. And how could this man who knew nothing of my condition protect me from IE when the specialist could not?

The medical journals, it seems, are written largely for debate and competition among researchers. Who will be the first to report on a particular aspect of a disease? Is it common or uncommon? The medical journals are repetitive, the same pathological studies of prolapsed valves, the same reports on IE, the same reviews of clinical signs, the same histories of MVP or its complications, the same warnings about the risks. Repetition can be the classic response to indifference; this is certainly true in the matter of ABP. But repetition means hemorrhage of valuable tax dollars with little benefit to the public because the information has not yet filtered down to the average physician. All the physicians I talked with in Toronto insisted IE is rare, as rare, they said to me, as leprosy and almost never seen in the antibiotic era. In their opinion, I could never have had it, especially since I escaped with my life. They made the same mistakes as their predecessors and they have not learned from the past. IE, Libman once said, followed in frequency arteriosclerotic, hypertensive and rheumatic heart disease.[101] We now know that MVP is more common than any other heart disease.

Through carelessness in the use of the "miracle drugs", the antibiotics, physicians have been lulled into a false sense of security regarding this disease as they are with many other diseases. It is believed, for example, that rheumatic fever is rarely seen, especially in adults. Yet, it caused 12,930 deaths in 1975 in the United States. Astounding facts for a disease believed to be virtually wiped out and now said to appear in only one to two percent of the childhood population![102] And, if RHD can cause that many deaths, how many are caused by MVP which is regarded by many researchers as a much riskier form of heart disease?

According to an article in *The Toronto Globe and Mail*, tuberculosis is also very much alive though doctors like to believe that their efforts have resulted in its having "dropped out of the public consciousness", but, again, 3000 Canadians a year contract TB and 150 die.[103] Miracle drugs have supposedly conquered typhoid fever, but recent statistics reveal one new case a month.[104]

What was said in a report on typhoid fever in the media could be said, ironically, of IE, "a disease to be dreaded at the turn of the century" but "now easily treated with antibiotics" and, like IE, "there are other cases of typhoid which go undiagnosed and therefore unreported."[105] However, no such article on IE would appear in the media because most people have likely never heard of this disease or, if they contracted it, no fuss would be made about a disease most physicians and dentists, who are not involved in research, regard as rare. One case of typhoid a month cannot compare with the hundreds of cases of IE, a disease that "should never happen at all".

One might say that IE can have the deadliness of the plague which recent reports indicate periodically enjoys a revival in Asian countries such as China and that there is still a five percent mortality. The West, we are warned, must be on the alert because rats, coming in ships from China, are bringing the disease to North America and Europe.[106] But, if the plague truly comes to the west, will there be doctors able to spot it? If they can't diagnose IE with all that's been written about it, how can they diagnose a disease that has truly rarely been seen, in North America since 1900.

19

The Giants on Whose Shoulders
We Now Stand[1]

Doctors should stop scaring patients half to death with casual comments about "clicky" heart valves. Evidence indicates that the noise of the heart isn't important. Yet patients who've been given this diagnosis-formally called mitral valve prolapse and informally "mitral click" — write anxious letters to me. They're convinced they're destined for an early demise . . . A floppy mitral valve is like the swinging door of a western saloon with hinges that are a little too long . . . Aside from the machines' identification of the source of heart clicking, doctors became concerned because some patients with it complained of chest pain, heart palpitations, shortness of breath and fatigue . . . However, often the symptoms didn't appear until after the patient was told about the click. This shouldn't surprise anyone. We know some patients become "cardiac cripples" if they're told of an unimportant heart murmur. The diagnosis, mitral valve prolapse, sounds even more ominous . . . don't start preparing your will if someone informs you of a mitral click . . . I have another suggestion for doctors; listen to the interesting sound, make a note of it on the patient's chart, but please omit telling the patient. Otherwise, you might as well tell him that his crooked legs or deviated nasal septum will shorten his life.[2]

The above quotation by the well-known medical columnist and author of popular health books, Dr. W. Gifford Jones, was printed in *The Toronto Globe and Mail*, April 21, 1983, twenty years after Barlow's definitive publication on the MSC and the LSM. Jones' piece is ambiguous. He offers no advice on antibiotic prophylaxis although he talks about "unimportant heart murmurs", and it's to be inferred he means the murmur of MVP since that is the subject of his column and since the late systolic murmur of MVP has been regarded as the classic "innocent" murmur, likely since the term, "innocent", was first introduced by William Evans in 1943.[3] What are we to infer from Jones' statements? That, as late as 1983, he subscribed to the belief that MVP with or without a murmur is no more harmful than "crooked legs" or "a deviated nasal septum" and, therefore, MVP patients do not require antibiotic coverage during surgical or dental interventions? If he was advising colleagues not to tell patients they have MVP, an "ominous" sounding label he says, or an "unimportant heart murmur", since knowledge creates a "cardiac cripple", how would he, or the colleagues he is advising, then handle the issue of antibiotic prophylaxis? How can a drug be prescribed without any explanation for its use? Unless it's to be assumed that a patient will not question the doctor. And, if an explanation is given, the patient must then be informed of a murmur. Jones' advice is based on the conviction of the medical profession that knowledge will make the patient a cardiac cripple; the converse is never considered: that ignorance can kill.

Fifty percent of the people with MVP, most of whom were women, who responded to my questionnaire in the 1983 *Healthsharing* article, had been told, when they complained of chest pain, SOB, irregularities in the heartbeat and fatigue, that they were neurotic or had anxious personalities. Gail's GP called her "emotionally labile", and sent her to a psychiatrist who, once he knew of her MVP and CHF, said she did not need his services. When Margo was very ill and complained of chest pain, she was told that she was being hysterical. And, at the time of my abscessed tooth, fever, enlarged spleen and heart, rapid heartbeat and chest pain, Dr. Austin wrote in his letters to my GP that I had pathological anxiety and that I was emotionally labile. The two terms imply hysteria and possibly even the need for institutionalization. It was, in fact, the label of cardiac neurosis that was largely responsible for Margo's delayed diagnosis and treatment and the reason why I never had a diagnosis at all.

The Neurotic Female

Historically, doctors have always regarded women as neurotic, and this view is, somehow, intimately connected with the distorted male perception that the female reproductive organs, specifically the womb, (Greek, hystera), are responsible for the unstable character of the sex, Dr. Austin's "emotional lability". Women, in short, are victims of their biology. Hence there sprung up a literature, both medical and fictional, attacking the womb, one of the most excoriating being that of the famous, fictional Dr. Rondibilis in François Rabelais' *Pantagruel*. Holding forth on the cause of women's emotional and mental instability, he described that secretive, inner organ, the uterus, from which issue "fluids that are foul, nitrous, sulphuric, sharply corrosive, stabbing and bitterly offensive to the nose" . . . "and, unfortunately, any stimulus, via the orifice of this organ, which is acutely nervous and morbidly sensitive, will cause a woman's entire system to be utterly overwhelmed."[4]

But do modern doctors really believe that the majority of female aches and pains are the product of an overactive female imagination, a propensity for hysteria by virtue of the sex itself? The following passage, written by a physician, is the typical inspiration for modern medical thinkng.

The fact that the patient is a woman will, of course, suggest a neurosis, because women are perhaps ten times as subject to neuroses as men are. Some women, like spinsters, divorcees, and broken-down music teachers, are even more likely to have a neurosis . . . commonly the doctor's receptionist recognizes a bad neurosis when the patient, often a woman, keeps coming to the desk every few minutes to ask why she cannot go right in. Soon she may get unreasonable and abusive. She cannot sit still. She may keep going to the toilet or she may be in the hall much of the time smoking one cigarette after another. Sometimes in desperation, the harried receptionist will beg the physician to take the woman right in before she drives everyone in the anteroom crazy.[5]

The above excerpt would appear to belong to one of those funny books about doctors and their patients in which laughter is directed at both parties. However, the book from which this passage is taken, *The Neuroses*, is in no way humorous. The humour is a matter of style only; the content is deadly serious. The author, Dr. Walter Alvarez, is an experienced physician who considered his advice to be the culminating wisdom of forty-five years of practice. His purpose was to pass these pearls on to young physicians to assist them in differentiating between similar symptoms, produced, on the one hand, by genuine organic disease and, on the other, by nervous, neurotic or psychotic conditions, including cardiac neurosis, the hardest, Alvarez said, to get rid of.[6]

Although Alvarez expressed the belief that he spoke "truly and kindly and humbly"[7], and without bias, the majority of his anecdotes demonstrating feigned illnesses involved women. Scarcely a page is free of disparaging remarks about the female sex while one is hard pressed to find similar comments about men. The litany is endless. There is the "tartar and a nuisance and an ingrate"[8] because an operation has not cured her, the "fluttery-looking woman"[9] with "the disorganized brain" of a "psychotic"[10] who cannot give a direct answer to the frustrated doctor's simple questions, the "asthenic, somewhat psychopathic woman" with "small, tender breasts"[11], today's flat-chested female with MVP, and the highly educated, tightly controlled, well-dressed woman with migraine who has a pathological fear of dust and keeps cellophane covers over every object in her home or the weak, migrainous woman who is always complaining and taking to her bed while the migrainous men are strong and stoical, taking aspirin and going on with their work.

Alvarez attributed female complaints to female sexuality, just as his fictional counterpart, Dr. Rondibilis, had done. The over-protected, emotionally disturbed girl with painful menses should be "taught some stoicism and self-control" early in life," he advised.[12] In fact, Alvarez viewed women as biologically closer to savages or beasts than men. Thus he described at considerable length, the woman who repeatedly washes and disinfects her hands before serving food. She reminds him of some ritualistic "savage" preparing for a hunt.[13] And the women whose menses drive them to obsessive cleaning behave like rats during oestrus when the hormones make them "run for miles".[14] Women are obsessed with purification, according to Alvarez, because they are victims of their hormones or their sexuality. Obviously Alvarez had never read Dickens or he would have encountered the male compulsive-neurotic, Jaggers, who was continuously washing his hands. From this belief in a subconscious desire, unique to the female, to rid the body of contaminants arose Alvarez' view that women fanatically seek out the surgeon's knife, whether it be menstral blood or disease they wish to have excised. "All surgeons," Alvarez said, "know that many a psychopathic woman loves operations".[15] This is equivalent to saying women like rape. Rape and surgery have something in common; they are both acts of violation.

But Alvarez would not likely have held this view of women if he had not had scorn, even repugnance, for the sick in general, especially the ugly and the deformed. His 617 page gargantuan work of advice to young doctors is a monument to all the glaring faults the public has ever ascribed to members of the medical profession: insensitivity, callousness, snobbery, arrogance, condescension and complacency. Patients are not human, especially females; they are insentient beasts or disposable, assembly-line products with varying degrees of quality, like the woman with remarkable absence of stretch marks after childbirth whom Alvarez said had "good rubber in her".[16] His picture of the woman "whose brain has been hit pretty hard" with "a little stroke" can only be described as exceptionally callous.[17] His advice to colleagues was to size up illness in people the way "any good farmer, cattleman, shepherd or poultry-raiser" would his stock.[18]

To this ardent defender of society's conventions, all persons not married by the age of thirty-five, especially women, are neurotic.[19] The unconscious arrogance of his profession comes through in his descriptions of "poor, little" salesgirls [20] and the neurotic woman who wears "a dress her cook would not want to be seen in" or has a husband she could not "trust to leave at home with the maid."[21] From his citadel of affluence, Alvarez assumes that everyone has a cook and a maid, and to him doctoring is decidedly a business. With unabashed greed, he declares, "I know of no surer way to build a big practice than to like people."[22] It is clear that, with Alvarez's loathing for the sick, the poor and women, his friendliness and concern were nothing more than tools of his trade to assure himself a lucrative income.

The Psychological Assessment

Long before psychiatry became a specialty of medicine, psychological counselling was an inevitable part of the doctor's treatment. The practice of including a psychiatric assessment of the patient in the medical record, as Dr. Austin did in my case, owes much to Alvarez, to what he called his "pen picture of the patient as a human being."[23] Few patients are aware that doctors are evaluating their mental as well as their physical health. Ironically, there is nothing "human" nor "humane" in these offensive, often brutal portraits. In detailing his thoughts on the unattractive person, Alvarez's psychoanalytical skills are frankly impoverished. A stout, unattractive middle-aged Dakota farm widow suffering from sexual deprivation moved him to record "because of her age and unattractiveness it never occurred to me she could have a sexual problem."[24] Ergo, unattractive people, especially older women, are not supposed to feel sexual desire, and, if they do, they are neurotic, while the sexual appetites of beautiful people are normal.

The ugly or deformed individual is not only neurotic or psychotic but of inferior intellect according to Alvarez. "The hand of the potter slipped and the body was botched. Poor materials went into it, and it may look as if it were made up of odd parts. The abdomen, buttocks, thighs or breasts may be too large for the rest of the body. Poor physique is seen often in schizoid persons, in persons with a poor nervous heredity and in persons with a low intelligence." The sick inspire revulsion, and illness, itself, is a deformity. These "botched persons" belong in the lowest economic and social strata Alvarez declared. They are the messenger boys, "the peanut butchers", the newsboys and busboys. As proof that God heartily approves, Alvarez referred to that much maligned book, the Bible, and with the same species of argument which advocates use to keep women subject to men and blacks subject to whites, Alvarez claimed "as the Bible says these sad persons were doomed by Nature to be hewers of wood and drawers of water."[25]

Doctors who insist that the medical profession is enlightened and unbiased will quickly point out that Alvarez's book was last printed in 1955. But six printings in four years indicate that *The Neuroses* was a very popular manifesto. But the fame of its creator and the effects of his teachings throughout a long career of almost 50 years would far outlast his creation. A physician of extraordinary influence, Dr. Alvarez had published many articles in the medical journals, and, at the time his book was first published in 1951, he was a prominent internist with the impressive title of Emeritus Consultant in Internal Medicine, at no less a distinguished institution than The Mayo Clinic, and Professor of Medicine at The University of Minnesota. His scope for molding the opinions of the young doctors as they were ground through the medical mill was far-reaching.

The arrogance and disrespect of Alvarez for the patient are very much alive today in the recent opinion expressed by Dr. Geoff Issac, former head of the Ontario Medical Association, "Because you are a carefully selected group with IQs and memory capacity in the top one percent of the population, you will spend your days not with your peers but with patients who are your intellectual subordinates."[26] Alvarez's opinion of women in particular rears its ugly head in the "disrespect", "paternalism" and "authoritarianism" that doctors still demonstrate, according to Dr. Susan Sherwin of Dalhousie University, toward women whom they regard as "weak, illogical, dependent and not fully rational".[27] Dr. Austin used Alvarez's technique in his corrosive, pen-picture of me as the neurotic "broken-down music teacher"[28] with "labile mentality" and "pathological anxiety" and, when, in the effort to get a second opinion on my illness, I had to drag out these reports in which the results of medical tests were mixed indiscriminately with these damaging "pen pictures" of my psychology, doctors likely believed they could, in Alvarez's phrase, "smell out the offending witch", [29] the neurotic female obsessed with her health who can only cause trouble for the doctor.

Cardiac Neurosis

It is not difficult to imagine how the MVP patient might fit into this category of botched persons. "Constitutional inadequacy", Alvarez said, was at the basis of nervous disorders such as cardiac neurosis and was recognizable in poor physical development. The neurotic women, he said, could be identified by "small nodular breasts, a long thorax, a flat simian type of pelvis, a male type of thin legs and an infantile uterus"[30] and, males, by a narrow, thin chest and lack of muscular development, though I hasten to add that most MVP people, including myself, look like people without prolapse. A physician of Alvarez's scope and influence could easily have reinforced the idea proposed by Da Costa, Lewis, MacKenzie and others that a systolic murmur and a set of related symptoms, chest pain, fatigue, tachycardia, did not indicate disease but rather cardiac neurosis with its particular affinity for women. The longstanding debate over how the symptoms are produced or from where the extra systolic sounds come, inside or outside the heart, is of no further importance to doctors like Alvarez. The discovery of a label, cardiac neurosis, resolves the matter promptly.

The concept of cardiac neurosis has had a significant impact on the interpretation of patient symptomatology, especially with regard to MVP, and has opened up the whole area of emotionally inspired or psychosomatic illness. Alvarez's book was one of the important reference works in this regard and its influence can be felt in the writings of his contemporary, Paul Wood, who defined cardiac neurosis and its symptoms:

> The cardiovascular system may be profoundly influenced by psychological or psychiatric states through the medium of the autonomic nervous system. The stimulus is emotional and appears to act on the central vegetative nuclei in the region of the hypothalamus. We are all familiar with the uncomfortable thudding of our hearts during moments of fear, and most of us have witnessed a fainting attack provoked by the sight of something that is at once queer and frightening. The physiological basis for such phenomena is relatively simple; sympathetic or adrenergic activity may cause palpitations by accelerating the pulse, elevating the blood pressure and strengthening the heartbeat; parasympathetic or cholinergic activity may induce syncope by retarding the pulse, lowering the blood pressure and weakening the heartbeat. Cardiovascular upsets of this kind, sufficient to bring the patient to seek medical advice almost invariably indicate psychiatric disorder.[31]

Paul Wood succinctly described a set of symptoms which gave the doctor the clue to a cardiac neurosis. They are exactly those of MVP: breathlessness, palpitations, fatigue, left inframammary pain, dizziness and syncope or fainting. In his definition, he clearly stated that these symptoms did not arise from any disease of the heart but from excesses of adrenalin produced by powerful emotions such as anxiety or fear. Curiously his well known textbook, *Diseases of the Heart and the Circulation*, from which this excerpt is taken, was reprinted in 1968 but was not revised to accommodate the new medical findings on MVP as a valvular disease. In fact, Wood did not refer to MVP though it is obvious he had encountered this entity under a host of other names and included it in the category of cardiac neurosis.

In his inimitable style, Alvarez described at length how the patient, female, of course, reacted to these cardiac related symptoms. The worst cases, he vowed, were found in "mildly psychotic" persons who had been told of "a little murmur". [32] Though he was less direct than W. Gifford Jones, Alvarez implied these people should not be told they have a murmur because cardiac neurosis was the hardest of all the neuroses, in his opinion, to get rid of and, if the physician tried to take heart disease from the patient, she, for it is always a woman in Alvarez's view, would only go from doctor to doctor for another opinion.[33]

"Palpitation," Alvarez said, "with a fast, pounding beat" or the extrasystole is the commonest sign of a cardiac neurosis. I stress that a disorder of the heart beat, either in rate or regularity, is the most common symptom of MVP and likely is the first sign which brings an otherwise well patient to the doctor. I also stress that doctors do not make distinctions for patients between different rates of rapid heart beat and a few extra beats, or a pounding rhythm from exercise or fear. Every kind of disorder in the heartbeat becomes a few palpitations to the doctor dealing with MVP. Thus Dr. Austin translated the paroxysmal atrial tachycardia I experienced into a few, benign palpitations of the sort that might arise from fear. Sudden rapid heart action such as that I had may, in fact, be the first sign that the patient has mitral regurgitation and may be associated with extremely exhausting physical work or exercise, as in my case. Alvarez said, "a neurotic woman sometimes wakes at night, perhaps with a big thumping extrasystole, and gets panicky with the idea that she is about to die with a heart attack. What with air hunger, hyperventilation, and some hysteria, she is soon putting on a good show. Perhaps several physicians are called."[34] To Alvarez, women over-dramatize, exaggerate, "put on a good show". This suggests that there are a lot of individuals, male and female, like myself, who are first made aware of their hearts during sleeping or just as they are falling to sleep. After my exhausting routine of removing six layers of wallpaper from twelve foot walls with a steamer that weighed between 30 to 40 pounds, I felt the rapid heartbeat not immediately but only later when I was lying down and falling to sleep.

Fear of death is the major emotional response, Alvarez said, of the cardiac neurotic and it is this that produces the symptoms. The sudden death of a relative, especially one under 50, usually deepens a cardiac neurosis he claimed.[35] My report on my first visit, upon questioning from Dr. Austin, of the three sudden deaths among my relatives, all under fifty, lead him to create a pen-picture of me as a cardiac neurotic. Thus when I complained of symptoms of chest pain, rapid heart beat at night with SOB, fever etc. in the presence of a dental abscess, he was not prepared to see these new symptoms in a different light.

Alvarez did not know he was describing MVP in his discussion of cardiac neurosis in association with little murmurs, palpitations and extra systoles.

The belief, that the set of symptoms now associated with MVP is evidence of neurosis, could not have emerged from anything but the old hypothesis of Gallavardin, the pleuro-pericardial adhesion theory, that the extra sounds, the clicks and murmurs, heard in systole, came from outside the heart, and thus indicated there was no organic disease of the heart or its valves. In the absence of heart disease, the symptoms must be all in the head. Thus, for those doctors who rejected the disease theory, neurosis offered a suitable explanation; knowledge of a heart murmur produced a fear of death and, therefore, symptoms of a cardiac nature. The only effective medicine was to avoid telling the patient of a heart murmur. This is why MacKenzie and Evans argued that the concept of mitral regurgitation be struck from the medical vocabulary. It only stands to reason that, if doctors regard the clinical signs as unimportant, the clicks and murmurs, the patient's complaints of chest pain, rapid heart etc. must also be insignificant and, ergo, brought about by their emotions.

The Neurotic Male — Da Costa, Lewis and War

The association of the symptoms of MVP with neurosis is as old as the discussion of the extra systolic sounds themselves. Medicine progresses at a snail's pace, and, to truly appreciate what effect this fact has had on the care given to patients with MVP, it is necessary to go back further than Alvarez or Wood. It all began with Da Costa, Lewis and war, and, therefore, with men, not women. This is the great irony, that the first application of the term, cardiac neurosis, in association with the clinical findings and reported symptoms, was to men. That the early prototype was a male, not a female, is confirmed in Ian Tillarc's life-size portrait of a dejected looking man with drooping shoulders, said to be an example of Lewis' Effort Syndrome, that hung for many years in the museum of the Royal Postgraduate Medical School in London, England.

Da Costa pointed out that, even before the American Civil War, the same cardiac complaints had been noted in men in other wars,[36] but he was likely the first to attach great importance to the neurotic element in these symptoms. His "report on the official history of the war"[37] in the United States would be incomplete, he said, without including, in addition to clinical evidence of murmurs, extra beats and rapid heart beat, the soldiers' complaints of a highly neurotic nature: headache, disturbed sleep, dizziness, dreams of falling from high buildings, (possibly visual imagery inspired by nocturnal tachycardia), itching of the skin, excessive perspiration, inordinate sweating of the hand, indigestion and abdominal bloating. Alvarez had sought these same symptoms in people he supposed were neurotic. Abdominal bloating he regarded as evidence of hysteria in women who desired but were unable to conceive.

Although many of the cardiac findings Da Costa described first appeared during a prolonged febrile illness, with rheumatism and diarrhea, that resembled a mild IE of the kind Libman described, Da Costa was, in fact, more interested in disease of the psyche than the body. The opponents of the evolutionary theories of Darwin clung to blind faith, even superstition, and, certainly, on the subject of a neurosis manifesting as cardiac symptoms, Da Costa, a good Victorian, and likely other doctors of his time, lacked a certain scientific judgement. Given to moralizing on sin and punishment, Da Costa argued that, although excessive sensuality, nocturnal emissions and mastur-bation were not likely to have caused the cardiac symptoms, they certainly predisposed the patient towards them and even perpetuated them. This is just another version of the old superstition that masturbation grows hair on the hands, a kind of unacknowledged concession to Darwin.

The idea of a cardiac neurosis would not have replaced the concept of heart disease without the economic factor. As a medical officer for the Northern army, Da Costa's job was to minimize the government's losses, both economic and political. Men with cardiac symptoms that kept them off the battle field were a liability in the war effort. Rather than weed out these men, Da Costa regarded their symptoms as evidence of anxiety neurosis and refused to approve their medical exemption. Early discharge, he said, was not economically sound. While the worst with treatment and no improvement might be let go, he advised, others should be consigned to reserve batallions, guard duty or hospital service because "to discharge the large number of cases of functional disorder of the heart, which must exist in every army during the war, would . . . deplete it . . . and have on many a soldier, seeing the ease with which a discharge can be obtained, a demoralizing effect."[38] Mollycoddling encouraged cardiac neurosis and might, Da Costa warned, provoke an epidemic of feigned cardiac illness in cowardly men. "It is impossible," he said cynically, "to discuss any malady to which soldiers are liable without discussing its being feigned."[39]

The term Da Costa chose to identify this condition, "Irritable Heart Syndrome", finalized his opinion of the neurotic element in the cardiac findings and symptoms. "Irritable" is a word commonly reserved for personality or nervous disorders, rather than physical manifestations. It suggests crankiness, nastiness or unpleasantness of an unpredictable, transient nature, as though the heart itself were neurotic or in bad temper rather than diseased.

Sir Thomas Lewis, familiar with Da Costa's work, simply picked up where he left off, but the conflict was now the First World War. Lewis strengthened the connection between extra systolic sounds, cardiac symptoms and nervous disorders. Without war, the association might never have been made, and Griffith and Hall's theory of regurgitation of blood backwards from the left ventricle into the left auricle because of an underlying organic disease might then have taken hold of the medical imagination, thus sparing a lot of people disability and death. Lewis, like Da Costa, was a medical officer, but his fame was far greater. In fact, he was knighted for his efforts to separate the wheat from the chaff, the brave from the cowards.

Being responsible for recruitment, training and discharge of soldiers, Lewis was able to observe his theory firsthand. He renamed the condition Effort Syndrome or Soldier's Heart. This allowed him to lay stress on the idea that these men did not have heart disease but were simply out of shape. Rigorous training would save them from costly discharge. Men snatched unexpectedly from peaceful, sedentary jobs are unfit for the mental and physical stress of combat Lewis reasoned.

At the close of the First World War, Lewis published a book called *The Soldier's Heart and The Effort Syndrome*, which he reprinted in 1940 at the beginning of the Second World War, in order to prevent the economic disasters that he felt had taken place in the first war as a result of the syndrome we now know as MVP. As moralist and guardian of the public purse, Lewis reminded medical army officers of the hard earned lessons of the first great conflict. Effort Syndrome or Soldier's Heart cost the government billions of pounds in disability pensions, he said, and wasted training on men who could or would not conform. Lewis, appalled by the statistics, stated that, by the summer of 1918, 70,000 soldiers were classified as having a cardiac condition and 44,000 became pensioners. Lewis stressed that for every four cases of wound there was a case of cardiovascular disturbance but, in his view, only one of six of these soldiers actually suffered from disease of the heart. The rest were Irritable Heart or Effort Syndrome cases. However, 43 percent of these soldiers who reported sick had shown symptoms at the time of enlistment,[40] and this suggests that fear of dying in battle was not the cause of their symptoms.

Lewis' reprinted book had guidelines for interpreting "derangements, real or supposed" of the heart, cardiac size and murmurs.[41] At the Military Heart Hospital in Hampstead, training programmes with graded drills and exercises were used to uncover the malingerers or cardiac neurotics. "The surest means," Lewis said, "of gauging physical endurance is to test those suspected of lacking it by putting them to work."[42] He argued that healthy people, on exercising, experienced the same symptoms as "effort syndrome" patients: breathlessness, increases in heart rate and blood pressure, consciousness of the heart beat, giddiness, faintness, fatigue, aching of limbs, tremulousness, exhaustion and even chest pain. The difference, he stressed, is in the lesser amount of exertion required in "effort syndrome" cases to produce the symptoms, but this fact did not suggest to Lewis a physiology compromised by a less than perfectly functioning heart, no more than it did to the moderns in the case of MVP. To Lewis these men were simply out of shape and could be trained to a level of physical fitness suitable to the war effort.

Lewis was fanatical in his conviction that neurosis was the cause of the specific cardiac symptoms and, thus, he contributed significantly to the distorted view that many doctors hold today of the symptoms of MVP. He believed that the success or failure of the war effort was intimately related to cardiac neurosis and admitted to being "dogmatic" and to holding views "tinged with a war purpose"[43]. It was because of these views that Lewis, like Da Costa, ignored the connection between the onset of cardiac complaints and the beginning of a febrile illness usually in association with tonsillitis. He dismissed the apical systolic murmur as insignificant, yet, Grant, who followed up these soldiers five years after the war, found this murmur in over half of the men.

Like Da Costa, Lewis supported his charge that the patient's mind was causing his cardiac symptoms by emphasizing what he believed was the neurotic character of these soldiers. Their family histories, he said, were "tainted with epilepsy or insanity" and, in childhood, these men were "nervous weaklings, bed wetters, sonambulists, or possessed of night terrors" and grew up to be overly sensitive, querulous, apathetic or depressed as a result of overactive imaginations and infantile fantasies.[44] Alvarez also made a case for the psychotic background of people with cardiac neurosis. In fact, much of what Lewis said, Alvarez repeated. Although Lewis didn't use the term "botched souls", he did describe these men as inferior in intellect with defective memory, an inability to concentrate and abnormal sexual tendencies with frequent nocturnal emissions and indulgence in regular masturbation.[45] Breathlessness, he insisted, was clearly of nervous origin and fainting attacks were frankly hysterical in nature.[46] "Abnormal anxiety must be regarded as a real and important contributing cause in given patients"[47] of the increased heart rate and blood pressure and exaggerated breathlessness on effort. It was a mere step from cardiac neurosis to cowardice which was, ultimately, how these men were viewed as the following passage from *The Neuroses* indicated:

> Their trouble was in the brain and, to a large extent, scattered all over a poorly built body. These men were born frail, with poor materials in them. In most cases they developed their symptoms in the induction stations before they had a chance to fight. Then it was found that if they were put to bed and coddled they got worse. They did much better when sent out to play baseball or to raise vegetables for the hospital. Most of them got better when the Armistice was signed.[48]

From Soldier to Civilian

Inevitably, doctors sought Effort Syndrome or cardiac neurosis in the general public. "Much of what I am about to say," Da Costa began his paper back in 1871, "I could duplicate from the experience of private practice."[49] Lewis was intent on "hunting" down cardiac neurosis in the general population and applying the same "prognostic and therapeutic lessons".[50] A zealot, a spokesman for morality and the status quo, Lewis was not content to make merely a contribution to medicine. He cast himself as a sociologist or, in his words, "clinical scientist".[51] As I pointed out earlier, Lewis dismissed the clinical findings of apical systolic murmurs, although, he had found in many soldiers at autopsy stretched, lax valves and crumpled leaflets, which are now accepted pathological features of prolapsed valves, in the presence of bacterial infection. It is disturbing that his views so influenced the rest of the medical establishment when he was not, in fact, a heart specialist but a general physician and one who, according to his colleague, Crighton Bramwell, had "little aptitude" for the "science and art of medicine" and who, ultimately, rejected his practice in 1916 and devoted himself to research.[52]

Lewis was obsessed with the idea of cardiac neurosis and saw himself as a pioneer in social medicine, envisioning the physician's role as that of sublime guardian of public welfare. The following passage from the introduction to the first edition of his work, *The Soldier's Heart and Effort Syndrome*, provides a unique glimpse of Lewis carrying on his own private war against the cardiac neurotic:

> If we are to reap the full benefit of our experiences during this war, these experiences are to be treated on a broader basis; to possess them of permanent value they are to be correlated with the experiences of civilian life . . . if we are to raid more fully that no-man's land, the borderland of disease, which is the hunting ground of the adventuresome, this syndrome will be a foe we shall often encounter . . . but it will be regrettable if in the coming days of peace, we may not find the means to employ similar remedial measures and similar tests of a simple kind upon those manual workers in our midst who in their convalescence in our great civilian hospitals, or while they labour in the factories and workshops, look to our profession to tell them of their fitness or unfitness for their work and to help them towards the former state.[53]

The imagery of combat, the hunt and the harvest is significant. Effort Syndrome or cardiac neurosis is the "foe", the enemy of the people. It must be vanquished or it will eat away the fabric of society as more and more people conceive themselves as "unfit" for the work of their social class. Lewis visualized masses of people, who toiled in the factories and workshops, seizing upon their imagined cardiac illness to revolt against recruitment, not into war, but into the workplace. Clearly he was not talking about the financially independent upper classes of which he was a member, an aristocrat, an educated authority and an officer, but the "manual workers", who form the base of the pyramid. Workers, he feared, would use their heart symptoms, just as the soldiers had, to be exempted from their enslavement in meaningless jobs and to be taken care of by the state. Without realizing, Lewis was predicting the modern conflicts that would arise over job stress and occupational disease, the battles between the workers and industry and the compensation boards and, ultimately, the whole notion of public welfare, of the state's responsibility to care for those who cannot care for themselves. Cardiac symptoms, feigned illness, Lewis warned, must not be used as an excuse to claim "permanent unfitness" for one's role in society, whether fighter or factory worker.

The viewpoint of Lewis was maintained long after and best summed up by Paul Wood in 1968: "It should be understood that there is no essential difference between "effort syndrome" and "cardiac neurosis", they are merely clothed differently, the former in battle dress, the latter in nylon."[54]

Many other medical writers strengthened the causal connection between neurosis and the cardiovascular symptoms that Da Costa and Lewis had described. The disease and non-disease debate was at last solved, and researchers sought a name for a recognizable set of symptoms which has remained unchanged since the time of Da Costa and has lead researchers to make the connection between Irritable Heart, Effort Syndrome, and MVP. However, hasty observations and conclusions replaced in depth scientific analysis, giving birth to a long list of symptoms associated with cardiac disturbances. The name of this medical entity varied over the years reflecting the writer's predilection for a particular theory. Shell shock and combat fatigue were replaced by anxiety neurosis, vasomotor instability and vasomotor neurosis, both of which imply that the nerves, not the heart, are diseased, cardiac neurosis, neurasthenia, hypochrondria, psychoneurosis, somatization reaction general, somatization reaction-psychogenic cardiovascular reaction, somatization reaction-psychogenic asthenic reaction.[55] Doctors tried to outdo each other in naming and defining the syndrome of clinical cardiac findings and "subjective" patient symptoms. A similar contest would take place over the naming of MVP. But the one thing all these names and theories had in common was the rejection of an underlying disease process related to the mitral valve that needed to be protected from deterioration.

Neurocirculatory Asthenia (NCA)

In the United States, during the first world war, Effort Syndrome or Soldier's Heart of the British became Neurocirculatory Asthenia or NCA.[56] The word, asthenia, means muscular weakness or loss of strength and thus retains the connection with its ancestor, the unfitness of Lewis' Effort Syndrome. The prefix, neuro, suggests the emotional, nervous or neurotic origin of the symptoms related to effort. Such a label, NCA, which ignores the association with soldiers and war, suggests the fulfillment of Lewis' dream that the lessons learned in the war would be applied to the civilian population. Yet, remnants of its military origins still exist in the eighties in the tests to uncover the fake. Paul Wood described such a test used on soldiers and civilians alike with NCA. "The effort-tolerance test consists of stepping on and off a chair ten times, and counting the pulse rate before, immediately after, and subsequently at minute intervals until the resting speed is regained. The deceleration time is abnormal (over 2 minutes) in 33 percent of these patients."[57] At one point during my IE when I was experiencing nightly rapid heart beat and SOB that prevented me from sleeping, I went to my local hospital emergency ward. I was requested to perform Lewis and Wood's test of stepping on and off a box. Though doctors may deny the fact that individuals with IE can carry on a normal life, the proof is in the pudding. Doug, whose case I have described, played hockey right up until admission to hospital with a diagnosis of IE. The legacy of Lewis, reinforced by others, prevented me from getting adequate medical investigation at a time of serious complications.

It was Paul White, probably more than any other prominent medical writer, who was responsible for the transition of cardiac neurosis from the soldier-male to the housewife-female. White had been a doubting pigeon in the debate over the origin of extra systolic sounds but he accomplished a volteface when he jumped on the neurosis bandwagon in 1931 in his textbook, *Heart Disease*, in which he devoted a section to NCA and identified the same set of clinical findings and symptoms. White, however, added symptoms of a highly neurotic flavour such as globus hystericus or lump in the throat, choking spells, tremors and flushing.[58] The last two symptoms, tremors and flushing, indicate the connection in doctors' minds between the menopause and neurosis. Alvarez had also included these same symptoms in his book, *The Neuroses*.[59] White defined NCA as a set of "symptoms referable to the cardiovascular system not dependent on any known pathological process of the heart or blood vessels but often associated with a functional nervous disturbance."[60]

White preferred to call this entity, "excitement syndrome"[61] because he perceived these patients as symptomatic specifically when they were emotionally excited. He endeavored to prove that palpitation was one of the chief symptoms of emotional excitement and had a long association with neurosis. Ancient physicians, he declared, like Hippocrates, had maintained that heart palpitations could result from emotion or excitement, and Galen, the ancient Greek physician, considered the influence of the emotions on the heart to be of sufficient magnitude to include in his mammoth work on the pulse.[62]

White, like Lewis, dismissed SOB as "subjective" in the NCA patient, that is, highly coloured by the patient's emotions. SOB has always been considered a classic feature of failure of the myocardium to meet the oxygen demands of the body and thus carry out its workload in a completely efficient manner. SOB, White said, was of no more significance than palpitations and was nothing more than an "unpleasant consciousness of the ordinary respiratory act without much of any evident labour, distress, or rapidity of respiration."[63] SOB then became in many medical minds synonymous with hyperventilation, or sighing, emphasizing its highly psychogenic nature. In fact, the latest name for MVP is "hyperventilation syndrome" according to some doctors.[64] Many doctors today still reject SOB with MVP as entirely insignificant. Despite my two murmurs, cardiac enlargement and evidence on wall motion exercise studies of left ventricular dilatation and lowered cardiac output, my internist, in 1989, tells me that neither my fatigue nor my SOB is related to my heart.

White was a giant in the field of heart disease, as Lewis had been, and his studies, which established the bias that NCA or cardiac neurosis was more prevalent in women than men, were thus all the more important. Later researchers, in particular those doing work on MVP, have likely been influenced by White and others, who made the same observations, to regard the condition as more prevalent in women and to include more women than men in their studies. In one of his reports on 100 cases of NCA, published in 1934, he set down the observation that individuals with NCA were largely female.[65] There were 69 females to 31 males in his study. He commented that 22 percent of the patients with NCA were unmarried and that sexual derangements and unhappy marriages were common in these people. The inference one draws is that people with NCA are on the whole emotionally unstable, reflected in their departure from what is traditionally accepted as normal social behaviour, a happy marriage and a family. White also made the observation that the majority of his patients were housewives whose unstimulating occupation of cleaning house and cooking could lead to a cardiac neurosis. Alvarez came to these same conclusions about neurosis in women many of whom had, in his view, great worries over little murmurs. In a broad, general conclusion, White said that "neurogenic elements" were found in 75-80 percent of NCA patients, or modern day MVP patients, ranging all the way from minimal anxiety to psychoneurosis and insanity which he said had been found in other studies in 23 percent of 100 cases of NCA.[66] This volatile material would be passed on to future generations of doctors who would then use it to reinforce the notion that women with cardiac symptoms were weak, irrational, hysterical and even psychotic about their hearts as Dr. Austin wrote I was.

Like Da Costa and Lewis, White ignored the pathological facts underlying the cardiac symptoms. Although over 50 percent of the patients in his study had systolic murmurs, mostly apical, which White called "functional",[67] he continued in the tradition of Gallavardin rejecting this evidence of organic valvular disease. And, like the other goliaths who threw out the disease theory, White proposed no causal connection between these extra systolic sounds and the febrile illnesses, such as upper respiratory tract infections, which frequently brought these women to his attention. White's contemporary, Grant, who had made the same error regarding his soldier population, even considered infection to be the "predominating causative factor . . . from which the patient had never fully recovered", being left with basal and apical systolic murmurs which we now know are indicative of valvular disease.[68] White and Grant's observations, like the older studies of Libman, support the view that the apical systolic murmur, now one of the characteristics of MVP, could be caused from a mild IE which passes as insignificant. Even Lewis himself said that soldiers with bacterial endocarditis continued on for months, even years, fighting in the trenches. While Libman's work on IE is forgotten, along with Horder and Glynn, the opinions of Da Costa, and especially Lewis, White, Grant or Alvarez are remembered in the literature on MVP.

White, like Grant, also observed that the patient's symptoms and clinical findings persisted long after the resolution of the infection. However, his opinion was that the infection gave birth, not to heart disease, but to a neurosis manifested by continued complaints of precordial pain and SOB. White made this conclusion because his control group of patients with signs of cardiac disease, such as cardiomegaly, hypertension, coronary artery disease or RHD, had the same symptoms. "Anxiety neurosis" and "varied psychic disturbances" that produce "excessive and exaggerated stimuli which reflexly affect the heart" caused, in his opinion, the symptoms of chest pain, SOB and palpitations in the patients with apical systolic murmurs.[69]

The concept of cardiac neurosis as an iatrogenic illness, fostered by frightening patients with knowledge about their hearts, prompted physicians like White to advise colleagues to "take the patient wholly into one's confidence"[70], a phrase used by many of today's physicians. What this means, according to White, is that the doctor should not be shy in telling patients that the mind is causing the cardiac symptoms and that there is no underlying organic heart disease. Treatment, he recommended, should, therefore, consist in changing one's lifestyle. He advocated "normal but quiet work and play . . . with avoidance of late hours, coffee, tea, overindulgence in alcohol and tobacco, strenuous vacations, excitement in general."[71] Omitting alcohol and tobacco from one's diet, it cannot be argued, is beneficial, but the remainder of the recipe would do more to produce a cardiac neurosis than stifle it.

If lifestyle modification did not work, further complaints meant "marked psychoneurosis or a definite constitutional defect", White claimed as Alvarez would after him. "Consultation with a psychiatrist", White advised, was needed to resolve "the emotional conflicts present".[72] In a letter to my GP in 1981, one of the two American heart specialists I saw made an identical suggestion: "If she persists in her unwarranted concern about her cardiac condition, it would be helpful to obtain some kind of counselling." Not as strongly worded as White or Alvarez but, nevertheless, essentially the same piece of advice, that the emotions, not the heart should be addressed. If tranquilizers, phenobarbitals or mild sedatives, failed to eradicate symptoms, White urged invasive surgery, suprarenal sympathectomy. This surgery involved removal or denervation of the sympathetic nerves connected to the adrenal or suprarenal glands above the kidneys. In 1934, Crile described such surgery, as White proposed, which was being used then as a treatment for NCA and hyperthyroidism and pointed out that it was not without grave risks, even death, principally because the suprarenal glands "cannot be subjected to traction or pressure: and arteries are often invisible"[73] and could be severed in the process. A patient's blood pressure was known frequently to double during such traumatic manipulation, thus posing the threat of cardiac arrest or stroke. This is a heavy price to pay for medical ignorance. Today, doctors still search for hyperthyroidism as a cause of rapid heart beat in the MVP syndrome rather than valvular disease itself. In fact, hyperthyroidism, not IE, was vigorously sought in my case.

Drastic invasive measures like those advocated by White and others reflect the traditional preoccupation of the medical profession with eradicating rather than preventing and call to mind Alvarez's exaggerated claim that women like surgery. Suprarenal sympathectomy has, in effect, the same purpose as frontal lobotomy, to remove parts of the body that are believed responsible for stimulating emotions such as anger or fear. Cutting out some part of the body may perhaps represent a subconscious, instinctive response to deformity or ugliness, Alvarez's poor botched souls, whether it be of the mind or body. It's that self-righteous mixture of morality and medicine of which Lewis was guilty and harks back to the Biblical admonition, "If the eye is an occasion of sin to thee, pluck it out and cast it from thee." If the nerves are responsible for harmful behaviour, especially stimulation of the libido, as Da Costa and Lewis imagined, then this "occasion of sin" should, likewise, be plucked out. In fact, my internist once remarked to me that he would like to take out my spleen to see why it was enlarged.

The Public Good

Until the publication of Barlow's observations in 1963, cardiac neurosis kept the mistaken belief that systolic clicks and murmurs originated from somewhere outside the heart in the forefront of medical thinking. Handling of the patient was thus geared toward avoiding iatrogenically induced cardiac neurosis, and physicians very early on thus adopted the habit of keeping the knowledge of clicks and heart murmurs from the patient. The advice of Gifford Jones in 1983 was the same as that of Franklin Johnston in 1938. Such cases of cardiac neurosis, they said, were "difficult to treat" and the majority of patients were "nervous" and unable to handle the stress of knowing.[74]

Doctors believed that it was not only for the supposed good of the patients that information about their murmurs be withheld from them but also for the good of the public. Cardiac neurotics were, in the eyes of the admirers of Lewis, dangerous, self-serving people. In applying the lessons learned in the war, doctors such as William Evans, who rejected mitral incompetence as irrelevant, issued stern warnings that cardiac neurotics in the civilian population could be as underhanded as their soldier counterparts whom Lewis had said beleaguered the pension office with fake claims. They were not above using the "flimsy evidence" of heart trouble for personal gain and "a systolic murmur in the mitral area," he said, "may loom prominently in older adults involved in a claim for compensation in respect of an accident, when the significance of the murmur will be debated in relation to the injury incurred."[75] Grant had noted a great prevalence of murmurs in ex soldiers, and, even though he rarely found malingering among pensioners, he believed these people exaggerated their symptoms in order to increase their pension benefits.[76]

The assessment of these soldiers depended truly upon the examiner's views. Levine credited these sufferers with more morality. He pointed out that many men retained their symptoms and that "this could not be explained entirely on the desire of these veterans to receive pensions, for some who did not need or accept pensions continued to be handicapped."[77]

Da Costa's imposters, Lewis' malingering soldiers, Evans and Grant's demoralized civilians. It was the war legacy then that shaped the current thinking on MVP: anyone with an apical systolic murmur or a murmur of MVP who complains of symptoms related to the cardiovascular system is, by the same process of reasoning, an imposter. MVP had become a social disease. The beliefs of these giants have fired the current hysteria of the medical profession over malpractice suits. Doctors believe patients on the whole have no genuine complaint but are selfishly and maliciously seeking personal profit.

Da Costa, Lewis, Grant, Wood, White — these are the "giants" cardiologist, Charles F. Wooley from Ohio State University, reveres in his 1976 editorial, "Where are the Diseases of Yesterday?"[78] It is astonishing that, as late as 1972, Paul White and colleagues were still writing about NCA as if the studies of Barlow had never been done. While Barlow was making a connection between MVP and Irritable Heart, Effort Syndrome or NCA, in order to establish a one hundred year old history of MVP as a disease with distinctive pathological and auscultatory features, Wooley was confirming the link in order to establish a history of MVP as a cardiac neurosis. Wooley's editorial was intended to call "attention to the giants on whose shoulders we now stand, to fan the still-warm coals of the earlier studies and to recall Lewis' challenge to bring attitudes of deferred judgement and critical inquiry to our current investigations."[79] Though the fact that MVP has been proven without doubt to be a disease of the valves, Wooley seems to be saying it should be looked at as a cardiac neurosis, the way Effort Syndrome was, and doctors should, therefore, follow the advice of the giants, especially that of Lewis, suspend judgement about the seriousness of MVP and be more critical of the direction research is taking into this condition. There are overtones of Aubrey Leatham's reference to the explosion of information on MVP as "a fiasco".[80] Too much fuss has been created over a "harmless" condition. And, with too much fuss, it follows that anxiety, even cardiac neurosis, is likely to be iatrogenically produced in the patient. This appears to be Wooley's main concern since, nowhere in his paper does he discuss, unlike other writers, the risks of IE to MVP and the need for ABP.

It is, in fact, astounding that, in the face of so much valuable research, that there are physicians in large cities, such as Toronto, who are still promoting the now overturned verdict that MVP is a cardiac neurosis and not a disease with serious complications and risks, and even referring to this condition as NCA. Medical theories, diagnoses, are cyclical. The pendulum has come full swing. Failing to find a satisfactory explanation for MVP and its symptoms, doctors fall back upon convenient labels and unprovable hypotheses of the past. Nothing more effectively relieves the doctor of responsibility than to convince the patient that the head and not the heart is causing all the trouble. Certainly, those doctors who wish to perpetuate the myth of the hysterical, neurotic, hypochrondriacal female would welcome a revival of the great debate over the significance of extra systolic sounds.

Proof that this theory of MVP as a neurotic disorder has never died in clinical practice exists in the medical report, dated June, 1984, of a Toronto doctor to my lawyer at the time of my investigations. This doctor, whom my lawyer asked to prepare a report on MVP, refused to act as an expert witness on my behalf, to say that I had, in fact, suffered further valvular damage because of a lack of treatment, even though my medical records verified my claim. Nor would she speak on behalf of Margo who had her valve replaced. The opinion of this doctor had truly been fired in the crucible of her successors, the giants, Da Costa, Lewis, White, MacKenzie, Evans, Alvarez. My lawyer had sent her copies of my article on MVP, my notes on my condition and my selections from the medical literature. Like Rhodes, Dr. EW's reaction to my knowledge of MVP was the universal one of the medical profession, indignation, scorn and anger that I had invaded the private world of medicine.

In Dr EW's report, I was a cardiac neurotic in no uncertain terms, one of Alvarez's "poor, botched" souls with "constitutional weakness", rather than a valvular abnormality. It was my desire for knowledge of my condition and my attempt at litigation that made me a cardiac neurotic. I did not, Dr. EW said, "understand what mitral valve prolapse was all about". What was MVP all about in Dr. EW's view? What didn't I understand about my condition? I didn't understand, she said, that mitral valve prolapse was *not* a heart disease. Didn't I know, she asked, that MVP was really Neurocirculatory Asthenia and, therefore, it follows, Irritable Heart, Effort Syndrome and even the "escape mechanism" of James MacKenzie? To substantiate her opinion, she referred to a Dr. Gorlin whom she regarded as having discovered the astounding connection in 1962 between MVP and NCA, the year Barlow overturned the 100 year old verdict of innocence.

Dr. EW's history was as shaky as her medicine. If Gorlin was as important as Dr. EW claimed, it was not his medical research or his publications that made him so. Jeresaty, Barlow, even Wooley, whom Dr. EW touts to support her revelation to me, do not mention Gorlin, and none of the historical reviews I have read refer to this doctor. Furthermore, Gorlin wrote a paper on the hyperkinetic heart [81], the term Rhodes once used to describe my heart after my illness. Curiously, although Gorlin found systolic murmurs in all his patients and clicks in half, he described these sounds as "ejection" in quality which, as I've discussed, is something altogether different from MVP and is one of the pitfalls doctors fall into when trying to identify a prolapse murmur. However, Gorlin may well have, as doctors do today, mistaken the sounds of mitral valve prolapse for ejection sounds.

If Gorlin is truly talking about MVP, which he appears to be doing, his opinion is that it is **not** an innocent condition, a normal "anatomic entity" as Dr. EW called MVP. Gorlin described patients, 15 of 24, who had low cardiac output with exercise (lying down and pedalling) and, in six of his patients, there was left ventricular hypertrophy with diastolic overloading or dilatation of the heart which would result eventually in acute heart failure as it did in two of his patients. This was exactly the test I had with almost identical results. These are indisputable signs of the failure of the myocardium to meet the oxygen demands of the body during strenuous exercise. Though Gorlin mentions that stress could provoke an exaggerated cardiovascular response, he does not refer to NCA, and he does not say that the hyperkinetic heart invariably has a favorable prognosis.

Dr. EW's efforts were directed then toward proving that I didn't understand that MVP is a cardiac neurosis and this, she said, in no uncertain terms, was her diagnosis of my cardiac condition. She referred to me as "a woman obsessed with her cardiac murmur", one whom no doctor would be able to convince that "cardiac function is normal", an opinion that reflects Alvarez's beliefs. She arrived at this conclusion without benefit of physical examination. Dr. EW never saw me. She had no x-rays or tests whatsoever, not even the inadequate TMSC records of my hospitalization. To explain the unusual clinical findings during my illness, such as cardiac enlargement, she resorted to a hypothesis that makes James MacKenzie seem clever by comparison. Premenstrual fluid retention had caused my cardiac enlargement. I was just another helpless woman at the mercy of her biology.

To substantiate her claim that I was neurotic because I had knowledge of my MVP, she insisted that I had refused to have the multigated acquisition scan or the wall motion study with exercise. It would, she said, "conclusively prove that she has no impairment of her cardiac function and, therefore, could no longer accuse her physicians" or "she is afraid that her cardiac neurosis will be revealed." It is true that, at the time, I had not yet had this test. My delays, however, were sound. I could not afford to have this test at Mayo, the first place to suggest it, and, until that visit, I had never heard of this kind of test. I'm still not convinced it is necessary to inject the patient with radioactive substances, no matter how infinitesimal the quantities, to demonstrate left ventricular failure with exercise. Some credibility should be given to the patient's report of symptoms of SOB with exercise, in particular if the patient had been active in sports as I was prior to a significant febrile illness. When the test was suggested to me, I was opposed to such an injection, especially after the failure of the spleen scan to show enlargement of that organ. As far as my malpractice action was concerned, I knew that, if such a test showed signs of heart failure with exercise, I would still have to prove that such heart failure was caused by IE in relation to an abscess or dental manipulations without antibiotic coverage. No one had diagnosed IE. I would have to prove to the medical establishment that I had indeed had this infection. In truly horrifying Alvarez judgement, Dr EW advised my lawyer and all lawyers and doctors not to touch me "with a ten foot pole."

The wall motion study did, in fact, show decompensation of both ventricles at the peak level of exercise. And once Doppler echocardiography was employed, tricuspid regurgitation was verified. When I expressed surprise at this finding, my internist blithely remarked, "Well, you've always had that. I told you that a long time ago. It's a totally insignificant finding." He had not told me this, though he had told me nodules were observed on my tricuspid valve. This suggests he knew this information but did not pass it on to me likely for fear of creating a cardiac cripple.

I believe there is a direct causal relationship between my two leaking valves, cardiac enlargement and all the other manifestations during my past illness. In other words, 50 percent of my valvular function is impaired. It was because I was given such inadequate answers that I contacted Dr. John Barlow of South Africa. Dr. EW, of course, said that the number of doctors I had seen was evidence of cardiac neurosis. Doctor shopping, Alvarez had once said, was a certain sign of cardiac neurosis in a woman. I related my entire history to Dr. Barlow and asked his advice. In a letter to me, in March of 1986, he stated, "On the data available to me, you have had infective endocarditis which in turn caused progression of your mitral regurgitation." He arranged to meet me in Detroit in September of that year where he examined me with Dr. Jeff Lakier, his former colleague from South Africa. After this examination, he did not alter his original opinion and, in the course of our long conversation, he referred to my infective endocarditis.

John Barlow is the world's foremost authority on MVP, and his name was once used to designate the syndrome. In 1987, he published a book, *Perspectives on the Mitral Valve*, which was launched at a recent world Cardiology Congress in Washington. Unfortunately, very few lay people will ever lay eyes on this book. His statement about my situation is based on many years of observation of MVP and its association with the disease of IE which appears to be more prevalent in South Africa than in the west. The following excerpt from an article which appeared in the March 1984 issue of *Modern Concepts of Cardiovascular Disease* which Dr. Barlow kindly sent to me sums up his opinion:

> Excepting patients with Marfan's Syndrome, progression to severe mitral regurgitation is uncommon and the majority of patients have little or no increase in the degree of incompetence. An occasional patient presenting at surgery or necropsy with floppy valves, with or without ruptured chordae tendineae, may have a history of a late systolic murmur or click having been heard many years previously. In the absence of infective endocarditis, we have seldom observed such progress.[82]

Since Dr. EW believed in White's NCA theory of the 1930s, she likely also believed White's biased conclusions that cardiac neurosis was found in more women than men. What Dr. EW doesn't know, however, is the fact that other studies have emerged, even in 1984, the year she made her report, which indicate that MVP is found more or less equally in males, 7 percent and females, 8 percent.[83] This should not be surprising to physicians since the disease entity with all its symptoms was first recorded in men. Clearly a severely biased view of women as neurotic, victims of their biology, has lead to a preponderance of peacetime studies of female populations and, inevitably then, to the distortion of the facts.

When specialists, like the one employed by my lawyer, still refer to MVP as NCA and say it is not a disease in 1984 and, when writers like Aubrey Leathem, who regard the whole matter of MVP as rarely causing symptoms "other than iatrogenic anxiety"[84] call the fuss over MVP a "fiasco", we have proof that little has changed in one hundred years in the medical mind. But once again, the medical profession should turn, not to Da Costa or Lewis or White but perhaps even to Libman and certainly to Barlow who cautions that "it is not appropriate for this **important** entity to be regarded as "a fiasco", as described by Leatham and Brigden, to range from a "harbinger of death" to a "variant of normal" as discussed recently by Oakley, or for some aspects to remain "an enigma", which seems to be the current status."[85]

20

Pandora's Box

From the practical clinical point of view therefore MVP seems to be a curiosity, of no greater relevance than an accessory nipple, except perhaps that men over 45 years old with a definite mitral murmur need to be given advice about prophylaxis of infective endocarditis. Unfortunately, 'labelling' someone as having MVP is likely to be harmful in itself and has been documented to cause serious disability. People who believe their heart is abnormal are more likely to adopt an invalid role and to complain of symptoms than if they were unaware of any abnormality. The diagnosis becomes the disease.[1]

Lt. Col. J.H. Johnson "Mitral Valve Prolapse: — The Facts." (1989)
Journal of Royal Army Medical Corps 135. 76-78.

The prolapsing mitral valve presents another conundrum for our consideration. From near total obscurity it suddenly appeared on the scene and now dominates the field of mitral regurgitation like the Colossus.[2]

D.B. Carmichael. "Reflections on Medical Heroes and Mitral
Prolapse." (September, 1987) *The Canadian Journal of Cardiology*
3 (6): 261-262

Once the "diseases of yesterday" were identified with MVP, scientific investigation moved swiftly from the medical into the psychiatric domain. Medical doctors, as well as psychiatrists and psychologists, who cannot accept that the symptoms of MVP are caused by the underlying valvular disease, are engaged in repetitive studies on the psychological nature of these symptoms. No longer able to refute that the auscultatory sounds of MSCs and LSMs are caused by disease, they are out to convince the medical establishment and the public that the cardiac related problems, at least, are not caused solely by the deformed valves but by psychoneurotic or emotional factors. As the debate between the adherents of the psychiatric and disease theories rages, the literature on "cardiac neurosis" and MVP has grown relentlessly over a short period of time and threatens erosion of the solid foundation that took 100 years to establish.

Endogenous Anxiety and MVP

Like their predecessors, the goliaths, Da Costa, Lewis, White and Wood, the modern proponents of the psychoneurosis theory are intent on redefining and relabelling what they conceive as a complex combination of psychiatric and seemingly cardiovascular symptoms. The battleground has shifted dramatically. No longer is there any conflict over the source of the extra systolic sounds, whether they come from inside the heart or from outside, and the question of the significance of mitral incompetence has simply dissipated. For those pursuing the psychoneurotic theory it is not a question, and rarely is the degree of mitral regurgitation (MR) a factor in studies on anxiety and MVP. For these investigators, MVP is once again a nebulous disorder that is still evolving and, therefore, they regard the reliability of well established approaches to ongoing care as questionable. The climate for MVP patients has once again become unstable and dangerous.

The hottest label for MVP now is "endogenous anxiety", and the psychiatric journals contain scores of papers on this topic. According to psychiatrist, David Sheehan, co-author of a study produced jointly by the Department of Psychosomatic Medicine at The Harvard Medical School and The Massachusetts General Hospital, endogenous anxiety is the correct name for all the other "aliases" from Da Costa to the present.[3] Although Sheehan does not specifically include MVP in a list of conditions firmly linked with endogenous anxiety, he does name Irritable Heart, Soldier's heart and NCA, and, by proven association, MVP must, therefore, be included.

The word, endogenous, implies that the anxiety arises internally from within the body, specifically from within the brain and autonomic nervous system (ANS) and that it is triggered by an inappropriate and excessive stimulus, possibly chronic, rather than from an external, threatening source such as a bear, a murderer, a rapist, for example, or a war as in the case of Da Costa's and Lewis' soldiers with whom the great debate all began. The cause has been removed, yet the symptomatology persists. Sheehan defined endogenous anxiety as a "chronic relapsing condition characterized by sudden, unexplained panic attacks and a feeling of helpless terror or impending disaster accompanied by a flight response and autonomic manifestions of anxiety."[4] This anxiety, he said, is in nature phobic, (fear of a particular place, person, thing or situation), hysterical (an acute, irrational response) or hypochondriacal (fear of bodily harm, illness or death, hence cardiac neurosis).[5]

The ANS controls the involuntary muscles, glands and viscera. Viscera, a plural word, refers to the organs housed in the four body cavities, cranium, thorax, abdomen and pelvis, but especially to those of the abdomen. In particular, the ANS governs the pituitary gland which produces the adrenocorticotropic hormone, ACTH, or Hans Selye's stress hormone, often called the anxiety hormone, the discovery and investigation of which created such a sensation in the fifties and sixties. This stress hormone stimulates or controls the chemical activity of the cortex of the adrenal or suprarenal glands, via the splanchnic nerves, and, therefore, the production of adrenalin and noradrenalin or, more correctly, epinephrine and norepinephrine, the substances responsible for all the physical manifestations of fear, such as increases in the heart rate and blood pressure, sweating, dry mouth, increased respiration, chest pain and trembling, the inevitable homeostatic changes in the body in preparation for attack or flight. It was the splanchnic nerves which Paul White had suggested disconnecting way back in the thirties in order to attempt a cure of cardiac neurosis.

War is not really a fair setting for studying the causes of cardiovascular symptoms because soldiers are exposed to unusual, prolonged fear-provoking stimuli and it is, therefore, impossible to determine whether fear or disease is provoking the symptoms, and, yet, attitudes gained from the wars and the study of soldiers have greatly influenced the approach toward MVP today. If the soldiers, who had systolic murmurs that were regarded as unimportant, had not experienced "sudden panic attack" and a "feeling of helpless terror", at the same time as they had cardiac symptoms, it is not likely that these associations would have been made in MVP patients today, and described, as Sheehan has done, as manifestations of endogenous anxiety.

Where is the line to be drawn between emotional and physical disease? The confusion of the cardiovascular symptoms of MVP, chest pain, disturbances in the heart beat and rhythm, tachycardia, extra beats, SOB and fatigue, with a long list of strictly psychological symptoms has rendered that line dangerously fine in the modern era. Included in Sheehan et al's list of psychoneurotic symptoms were not only those highly specific for cardiovascular disease but all those psychoneurotic symptoms in the soldiers described by Da Costa, Lewis, Alvarez, White and others, such as nervousness or shakiness, spells of terror or panic, lump in the throat, fear of being alone, difficulty falling asleep, feeling blue and loss of sexual interest or pleasure.

Certain new diseases were attached to this list, such as hypoglycemia or low blood sugar, the symptoms of which are nervousness, hunger, profuse sweating, alternate pallor and flushing of the face, dizziness and hyperventilation.[6] It is noteworthy that dizziness and hyperventilation have been associated in the medical literature with MVP.[7] The list of psychoneurotic disorders keeps expanding. A doctor who believes in the endogenous anxiety theory would have no hesitation in attributing my two episodes of presyncope, associated with tachycardia, numbness and coldness in the extremities, to hyperventilation provoked by hypochondriacal fear of my heart because of the heavy physical labour I was engaged in.

Agoraphobia, Panic Attack and MVP

Recently the media has devoted much attention to a psychoneurotic or emotional disorder called agoraphobia which manifests as a panic attack. Agora is the Greek word for open market place and, conbined with the word, phobia, means a fear of public places such as shopping malls, buses, theatres and streets for example. Have these heavily populated places, one might ask, become the civilian battleground? A sudden panic attack, accompanied by breathing difficulties, dizziness and sweating sends the agoraphobic individual into flight from crowded, threatening places back to the safety of home and mother. This is the typical picture of the recluse.

Currently, doctors are intensively researching the connection between agoraphobia and MVP. As is usual, women are chosen before men as the guinea pigs in these studies. Kantor et al[8] studied a group of females with MVP at The Long Island Jewish Hillside Medical Centre in New York and claimed that a significant number of these women had agoraphobia. According to these authors, the more nervous MVP patients, who have palpitations, are the best candidates for developing agoraphobia while the more stable, asymptomatic patients merely remain neurotic or anxious. In other words, the patients are not symptomatic because their prolapse is more severe but because their neurosis is more intense.

The opinion of Gifford-Jones, Johnson, quoted at the beginning of this chapter, and others, that doctors should not tell their patients of a MVP, unless, one might infer from Johnson's statement, the patient is a man, is spreading. Prevention of the cardiac symptoms in this unimportant condition lies, therefore, in avoiding the creation of a crippling cardiac neurosis. Kantor and co-workers advised that the mere knowledge that there is a MVP "may be a primary source of anxiety" which initiates the symptoms and the fear of them which, in turn, "further aggravates the symptoms by establishing a feedback loop".[9] The result these researchers envisioned is disastrous. In their view, the palpitations of MVP can lead to a fullblown agoraphobia that imprisons the patient in his or her house. Patients with such a condition are costly to society, Sheehan argued, from the point of view of "long-term unemployment, disability benefits, financial support and chronic health care costs."[10] This is the old argument that Lewis, Evans and others used in their campaign to separate the imposters, both soldier and civilian, from those with genuine cardiac disease, in order to maintain a healthy socio-economic structure.

The literature on panic attack and MVP is accumulating at an alarming rate, and the number of MVP patients said to have this emotional disorder keeps increasing. In 1979, Pariser and co-workers [11] reported panic attacks in about a third, or 6 of 17 patients with MVP. They concluded that panic attacks occurred particularly in women who had cardiovascular problems such as MVP and possibly emotional illness and they urged that physicians look for these diagnoses in such patients. More recently in 1987, Gorman and others from the Psychiatric Department at Columbia University in New York [12] claimed that an assessment of the psychosomatic literature revealed MVP was present in 30 to 50 percent of individuals with panic disorder (PD)or agoraphobia with panic disorder (AgP). Medical opinions are not usually widely accepted within the profession until they are enshrined in textbooks which are then used in the teaching of medicine. Doctors, like Shapiro and McFerran from The University of California,[13] are now suggesting that MVP be included under the heading of Neuroses in the medical reviews of this syndrome and in the standard psychiatric textbooks such as *The Diagnostic and Statistical Manual of Mental Disorders*. Wood's textbook, which placed Soldier's Heart or Effort Syndrome among the psychoneurotic illnesses, was no doubt the model for such proposals.

Biochemical Imbalance — Lactate and MVP

Sheehan and co-workers wrote that "to the best of our knowledge, no substantial evidence has been advanced for the "neuroses having an organic etiology".[14] It must be remembered that the neuroses referred to included those disorders with the well recognized auscultatory feature of a mitral systolic murmur whose seriousness had been undermined for almost a century until their indisputable equation with MVP and valvular disease. The revival of the anxiety neurosis theory of Da Costa, Lewis, White, Wood and others aims to separate the seemingly cardiovascular symptoms from the known underlying valvular disease and prove that, not the valvular lesion, but some biochemical disorder, initiated by anxiety, is the causative factor. To that extent, they are examining the nature of that biochemical aberration. Where once researchers hypothesized that clicks and LSMs had an organic origin, they are now theorizing that the neuroses, themselves, are organic in origin. In effect, this is a revival of the ghost of Gallavardin and his extra-cardiac theory, that the cause of the symptoms is outside the heart. The idea of a biochemical imbalance, like many of the medical opinions hailed as new discoveries, has its roots in a long past. Among the many published reports are those of Paul White and his colleagues. In 1946, for example, Cohen and White conducted studies which they claimed demonstrated chemical imbalances in people suffering from NCA.[15] When these individuals performed strenuous exercise such as walking and running on a treadmill, a test still used today for heart patients and one which I was given even during my illness, or stepping up and down on a 20 inch step, with and without a pack, à la Lewis, blood tests showed excess lactate, a derivative of lactic acid, familiarly recognized as the cause of muscle soreness when sedentary people engage in exercise. Lactate, called a substrate, is acted upon by certain enzymes in order to create oxygen for the myocardium. Along with free fatty acids, pyruvate, ketones and amino acids, the myocardium uses carbohydrates, chiefly glucose, and lactate in the production of oxygen, necessary for chemical and mechanical activity. Rapid rises of lactate to excess levels in the blood indicate interference in the normal conversion of glucose into oxygen. In the myocardial metabolic process, the glucose is converted to pyruvate and, then, to lactate instead of the lactate being converted to pyruvate to be metabolized in the normal way. It has been understood for many years that excess blood lactate is lactate that cannot be utilized by the myocardium and is, therefore, evidence of myocardial ischemia (hypoxia or oxygen starvation), which, if continued, results in myocardial infarction or actual necrosis (death) of heart muscle tissue. In fact, White and Cohen interpreted the excess lactate as a sign the hearts of NCA patients known as MVP today were not, in fact, utilizing oxygen in adequate amounts the way a normal heart would during exercise. Nevertheless, they concluded these individuals did not have disease but were out of shape because they avoided exercise for fear of their hearts.

Naturally the desire to compare men and women preoccupied the early researchers. In the forties, Cohen and White held that women made less use of oxygen during work than men while patients with NCA used the least.[16] Their opinions, based on their measurement of lactate in the blood of such patients and the prevalence of this biochemical abnormality in women provided the exponents of the cardiac neurosis theory with an explanation for the symptoms of NCA and, later, MVP.

In the sixties, some experimenters, like Pitts and McClure, pushed Cohen and White's idea even further by attempting to verify pharmacologically the link between excess blood lactate and what they regarded as anxiety-produced symptoms of a cardiovascular nature. They injected the salt of lactic acid, sodium lactate, into two groups of patients, one with and one without a diagnosis of anxiety neurosis, according to psychiatric records, and certain cardiac symptoms such as chest pain, palpitations, SOB, dizziness and fatigue, the symptoms of MVP. Those with a history of such complaints experienced anxiety along with a recurrence of their symptoms, and the authors concluded that anxiety neurosis could actually interfere with the metabolic activities of the heart and thus cause symptoms. However, as the study pointed out, it has been shown that the rise in blood lactate "per unit of work output per unit of time"[17] in patients with supposedly anxiety neurosis is equivalent to that in patients with coronary artery disease (CAD) and mitral stenosis (MS).

Researchers of the 1980s have repeated these sodium lactate infusion tests of the past, and, likely, in the 1990s, there will be the same or similar repetitious experiments. Unlike most studies on MVP, particularly those on the risk of IE, these biochemical experimentations have surprisingly already been reviewed in the public media by prominent journalists, such as Jane Brody.[18] The conclusions from these studies are identical to those of the past in that they claim high levels of blood lactate are found in anxious patients, especially those with panic attacks or agoraphobia, and the well-known symptoms of chest pain, palpitations, SOB, dizziness and fatigue are being attributed to high levels of blood lactate. What is of great importance here is the question of which information is most beneficial to the public. Is it more important for the public to know that MVP patients are anxious and have panic attacks, as is being reported in daily newspapers,[19] or that there are some very common life-threatening dangers to people with underlying valvular disease that can be prevented? It appears that anything to do with emotional disorders gets to the public faster than that which is lifethreatening.

To sum up, measuring levels of blood lactate in MVP patients and correlating this with anxiety studies to demonstrate anxiety-induced exercise intolerance may be unreliable. Lab textbooks, such as Lynch's, state, "Blood lactate assays are made in the investigation of lactate acidosis in diabetic and cardiac disease or after widespread tissue hypoxia (lack of adequate oxygen supply) and, in combination with pyruvate determinations, in the diagnosis of severe deficiencies of the B group of vitamins. Elevated lactate values have been reported in some neuromuscular disorders and in leukemia. Raised pyruvate levels have been reported in congestive heart failure."[20] Anxiety is the least important reason for elevations of lactate in the blood. A MVP patient who engages in regular physical exercise and consistently experiences SOB may, in reality, have myocardial hypoxia as demonstrated by abnormal lactate-pyruvate metabolism or an insufficient supply of oxygen to the myocardium during exercise.

Coronary Artery Disease (CAD) and Coronary Artery Spasm (CAS) in MVP

The cause of the chest pain in the MVP syndrome has preoccupied researchers. Many have studied the association between chest pain and myocardial lactate abnormalities and have come to different conclusions about the causative factor. In 1975, Natarajan and co-workers[21] found myocardial lactate abnormalities in about 30 percent of MVP patients who had chest pain. Lactate abnormalities were more common with chest pain on exertion. Because five of the patients had chest pain at rest and no lactate abnormality, it could not be concluded that chest pain was caused exclusively by the presence of this chemical substance in excessive quantities in the blood. However, the authors pointed out that this discrepancy between metabolic abnormalities and chest pain exists in patients with angiographically proven myocardial ischemia. Such patients may be those "silent" heart attack victims diagnosed only by myocardial metabolic tests.

Rather than address the question of anxiety, these researchers considered the possibility of CAD because excess lactate is found in individuals who have suffered a heart attack. However, the patients of Natarajan et al had normal coronary arteriograms that showed no obstruction in the arteries of the heart which would herald a myocardial infarction (MI), "though corkscrew appearance of the vessels was frequently noted," which might suggest coronary artery spasm. Traditionally, the blockage of a coronary artery has almost always been implicated in heart attack. Like Cohen and White, however, these researchers believed there must be some degree of myocardial hypoxia or oxygen starvation, such as is found in patients with CAD, even though the patients in the study appeared to have no signs of this disease. The authors proposed that an underlying disease process, involving the myocardium or heart muscle itself, though undetectable, could cause occlusion of the small vessels in the heart, or "abnormalities of cellular metabolism"[22] in the heart could result in myocardial oxygen starvation.

Primary Disease of the Myocardium or Cardiomyopathy and MVP

Natarajan and co-workers raised a very important question which other researchers have taken up. Is the underlying disease of the prolapsed valve and chordae, which is well established, creating a mechanical problem that affects the contraction of the heart and its ability to use oxygen, thus explaining the high levels of blood lactate? Or is a primary disease of the myocardium, which leads to abnormalities in the way the ventricles contract, affecting the function of the valve apparatus? Ultimately, they concluded that the solution to this quandary was to be found in disease, not in anxiety. Their studies pointed to the possibility that an underlying ischemic disease of the myocardium, rather than primary valvular disease, is responsible for the symptoms of chest pain, electrocardiographic abnormalities (ST-T segment depression) and ventricular arrhythmias.

Although the exact relationship between atherosclerotic or CAD, disease of the myocardium (cardiomyopathy) and MVP has not, as yet, been determined, abnormal levels of lactate in the MVP patient may be the harbinger of something far more ominous than anxiety. Studies have documented the click or click and murmur of MVP in patients with established CAD, either immediately following MI or at a later examination. This has lead to the belief that CAD could cause the click and LSM.[23] In one study, 31 percent of patients with angiographically proven signs of CAD and an established history of angina pectoris were found to have MVP with left ventriculography.[24]

Since the cause of the chest pain has concerned researchers, they have attempted to establish a cause other than the generally held view that there is a mechanical factor in the the excessively long chordae and ballooning leaflets that put strain on the papillary muscle, thus causing chest pain. Some researchers have shown a definite relationship between chest pain, which is typically angina-like in some MVP patients, and underlying CAD and, in their opinion, the prolapse results from a collection of abnormalities, including MI, left ventricular dysfunction, ischemic and fibrotic changes in the papillary muscle and myocardium.[25] When the coronary arteriograms are normal, that is they show no narrowing or obstruction from lipid deposition, i.e. atherosclerosis, in MVP patients with chest pain, others believe that coronary artery spasm (CAS) occurs in response to the mechanics of the billowing leaflets in severe cases of MVP and that this causes both the chest pain and MI. In fact, some investigators believe the proof lies in the fact that MI has been documented in patients with known MVP and normal coronary arteries.[26] And recent research in 1987 showed that MVP and MR existed in 8 of 43 patients who were assessed one month after suffering an acute MI.[27] There are researchers, however, who disagree, claiming that MVP is infrequently caused by an acute MI.[28]

The reason this remains a controversial area in MVP studies is that, while CAD, MSCs and LSMs and prolapsed valves have been proven to co-exist, the causative connection has not yet been established. Which is the etiologic factor, the prolapse or the CAD? There are many variables here. Much depends on what standard is taken for identifying the prolapse. Some examiners consider left ventriculography to be definitive while others take echocardiography as the gold standard and, still, many of these studies do not clarify whether the click, considered the hallmark of MVP by most researchers, is invariably present in patients with CAD, prolapsed valves, angina and MI. This is a debate that will likely occupy the medical literature well into the 1990s. But, certainly, this endeavor is more worthwhile than attempting to prove that psychosomatic factors or cardiac neurosis, or even diseased nerves, cause the symptoms since the increases in biochemical substances are not found specifically in MVP.

Myocardial Infarction (MI) and MVP

While the causal relationship between CAD and MVP remains in doubt, there is some very conclusive evidence that MVP causes MI. One such case was published in 1984 in the *South African Medical Journal*.[29] A MVP patient with Marfanoid features was hospitalized for a stroke and was found to have had a painless MI as well. He had no history of chest pain, and his coronary arteriograms were normal, showing no blockage. It was felt he did not have CAS by the testing criteria at that institution, The Tygerberg Hospital, and an endomyocardial biopsy revealed no underlying cardiomyopathy of the sort Natarajan and co-workers had described. The authors of this study concluded that both the cerebral and the coronary embolism resulted directly from the abnormal prolapsed valve. What happened to the patient in this seminal report seems to corroborate the view of some world experts, such as Lawrence Freedman, that valve deformities impede blood flow in the area, thus increasing the potential for coagulation of the blood, and, therefore, the risk of thromboembolism.[30]

This case of MVP with emboli to both heart and brain recalls the case of the tennis player who suffered a painless but fatal MI resulting from IE when an embolus lodged at the division of the left coronary artery in her heart. It is the view, traditionally held, of most physicians and lay people that MI is associated with severe chest pain, but researchers now think completely painless MI is more common than believed. The silent heart attack is believed to represent one third of all MIs. One of the most disturbing reports on silent MI has come out of the longterm Framingham, Massachusetts study of MVP. An update 30 years after the beginning of this study showed that, among the original 5127 patients thought to be free of CAD, there were 708 MIs. 28 percent of the MIs in 469 men and 35 percent in the 239 women were revealed only by routine electrocardiogram examinations. An overall assessment concluded that there were 138 MIs per 1000 of the patients at risk with 42 per 1000 unrecognised and 22 of these per 1000 silent.[31] One possible explanation, in the case of MVP patients, who experience the sudden onset of chest pain, is that they are having a MI or have had a previous silent or painless MI and their current chest pain, while atypical, suggests underlying CAD which has not been clinically detected.

MVP and ANS Defects-Hyperadrenergy

In spite of reports like that from The Tygerberg Hospital in South Africa, the theory that stress or anxiety-activated alterations in body chemistry, rather than the prolapsed valve itself, cause the symptoms of MVP is rapidly gathering momentum. Those engaged in this kind of research presume that the autonomic nervous system (ANS) of MVP patients is in some way defective. Since such studies of the "nerves" of MVP patients have an influence on the treatment recommendations, it becomes important to understand how the ANS works. This nervous system, which controls the involuntary activity of organs of the body, such as the heart and viscera, is divided into two parts. As a general rule, the sympathetic nervous system stimulates and the parasympathetic largely restrains the production of chemical substances. The ANS is controlled by a higher centre in the medulla of the brain which receives impulses or signals and sends out responses. The ANS functions by producing chemicals in the organs it governs. Sympathetic nerves primarily stimulate the production of adrenalin and, as far as heart action is concerned, are responsible for increases in blood pressure, heart rate and the contractility of the heart, therefore improving the pumping action, while parasympathetic nerves largely control the manufacture of acetylcholine which lowers blood pressure and has a marked affect on reducing heart rate. The parasympathetic nerves are sometimes called cholinergic while the sympathetic nerves are called adrenergic. Propranolol, which slows heart action, or blocks the effects of sympathetic nervous stimulation, is, for example, called a nor-adrenergic antagonist. The ANS of MVP patients is said to be deficient in inhibitory mechanisms so that there is chronic stimulation of the adrenergic nerves and thus perpetuation of the hyper-adrenergic state. This is why MVP patients are called "high-strung" or "hyper". In other words, the nerves, themselves, are diseased, and anxiety is, thus, a disease.

Adrenergic hyperactivity or hyperadrenergy means that there is excessive production of particular chemicals, specifically, epinephrine and norepineph- rine, also referred to as the catecholamines, both of which are produced by the medulla of the adrenal or suprarenal glands, situated above the kidneys and at the termination of nerve endings, and both of which ultimately affect the function of other organs in the body as well as the heart. Epinephrine is, in common parlance, the adrenalin which we associate with anger, fear or anxiety. Epinephrine and norepinephrine function in certain ways in the body. Epinephrine does two things: it constricts and dilates blood vessels and relaxes or dilates the bronchioles, which would improve breathing in patients with CHF. Norepinephrine has only an inhibitory effect, constricting almost all the blood vessels in the body thus making the heart work harder and so causing a rise in blood pressure and an increase in heart rate. It is this excessive production of adrenalin-like substances that causes the chest pain, palpitations etc. according to some medical researchers.

Just as they have done in the case of excess lactate, researchers have attempted to calculate the amount of norepinephrine and epinephrine in the circulation of MVP patients with a view to establishing that, not regurgitation or the prolapsed valve, but anxiety-produced adrenalin is causing the symptoms. A group of researchers from Ohio State University College of Medicine,[32] including Harisios Boudoulas, who has done much research on MVP and hyperadrenergy, and Charles Wooley, who has cited the connection between MVP and the earlier disorders on the basis of anxiety-like symptoms, have measured 24 hour urinary excretions of epinephrine and norepinephrine and plasma catecholamines in symptomatic MVP patients during treadmill and handgrip exercises. They found these levels to be abnormally high, especially in patients who experienced frequent premature beats or extrasystoles. In their conclusion, Wooley, Boudoulas and their colleagues advocated further study of anxiety to unravel the mystery of how "stress-mediated or stress-activated biochemical mechanisms",[33] which cause a hyperadrenergic state, relate to the many symptoms of MVP.

Heart Failure and MVP

These studies raise some intriguing questions. Why do the symptoms of MVP and the laboratory findings of chemical aberrations with exercise testing closely resemble those found in patients with heart failure? Is the increased production of the catecholamines an indication of high anxiety levels or proof that the heart of a MVP must work harder than a normal heart to carry out the same physical functions? In other words, do these hearts show signs of failure in varying degrees, according to the strenuousness of the exercise?

Since high levels of epinephrine and norepinephrine in the blood and urine are found in heart failure patients as well, they are no more unique to anxiety than elevations of lactate in the blood. It is known that exercise causes marked increases of these chemicals in the blood of heart failure patients, and it is well established that the over-production of catecholamines via the ANS in such patients is a reserve or compensating mechanism to increase the output of blood from the heart during exercise when it must work harder. Epinephrine and norepinephrine cause increases in heart rate and blood pressure and, thus, ultimately, dilatation of the heart to accommodate the increased blood volume. Often dilatation is accompanied by hypertrophy of the heart muscle since overwork thickens it as it does any muscle in the body. The hyperadrenergic state is perpetuated in order to maintain or prolong life. In fact, injections of epinephrine were once used to stimulate the heart after a myocardial infarction when part of the heart muscle had been deprived of oxygen and was, in fact, dead or necrotic. Is it possible that the increased production of these chemical substances works in MVP patients in the same way it does in heart failure patients? Are they thus a means of improving a cardiac output that becomes inadequate, according to the strenuousness of the exercise, because of a faulty valve mechanism and mitral regurgitation that prevents maximum oxygen supply to the muscles? This would especially be true in patients with moderate to severe regurgitation which would not permit satisfactory cardiac output during exercise. And, if the strenuous exercise were to be continued, would cardiac arrest intervene in MVP patients whereas it would not in those without?

My rest and exercise wall motion test, called Gated Equilibrium Pool Scintigraphy, which was done in 1984, revealed several abnormalities which the examiners interpreted as uncertain, such as prominent left atrium indicating possible enlargement, decreased contractility of the right ventricle, borderline increases in pulmonary blood volume and abnormal left ventricular end systolic volume. This exercise test pointed to an inadequate cardiac output or what the examiners referred to as "a degree of decompensation of both ventricles at the peak level of exercise". It is now known that I have tricuspid regurgitation which, if not associated with the structural abnormalities of disease, either prolapse or a healed or active IE, "is invariably caused by pulmonary hypertension or right ventricular dilatation and failure."[34] In retrospect, as the test suggested, there was, in all probability, some pulmonary congestion which would account for my SOB during the testing and with any strenuous exercise and my inability to go the last lap of the test. It is likely that, at that time, there would also have been high levels of norepinephrine and epinephrine in my blood and urine. But, clearly, they would not have been associated with anxiety.

Boudoulas, Wooley and co-workers rejected the idea of heart failure in their MVP patients, concluding that their patients had good left ventricular function (LVF) and no evidence, on examination, of severe regurgitation or cardiac enlargement. Their testing included phonocardiographic observations and the measurement of systolic time intervals, echocardiograms, treadmill exercise and isometric hand grip exercises. It did not include the kind of test I had which more accurately evaluates LVF. As I've pointed out elsewhere in this book, patients, thought to have minimal regurgitation and excellent cardiac function have shown, with left ventriculography, moderate to severe regurgitation of blood into the left atrium. Where does good left ventricular function leave off and heart failure begin? Margo was said to have good left ventricular function when she was dying, and Doug played hockey right up to the time of his admission and a diagnosis of IE and left ventricular failure for which he required mitral valve replacement. As long as a patient is functioning satisfactorily, despite compromised activity, with or without medication, doctors will not reveal that cardiac function is in any way impaired. I have known people who clearly have heart failure who are totally unaware of this fact. If they are young, they attribute their shortness of breath to being out of shape, as Lewis would have believed, and, if they are past forty, to getting old.

In a popular book for the public about heart disease, Alistair Hunt, a British doctor, says " . . . let us clear up a popular misconception about heart failure. Laymen usually think that this term means the heart has stopped and that life is at an end. This can be the cause of some misery until they understand how doctors use the term differently. Their meaning is nearly always only that the heart is beginning to show signs of strain and finding difficulty in meeting all the demands on the circulation."[35] Such a statement explains why many doctors disguise heart failure with explanations to the effect that the patient is either out of shape, getting old or neurotic. No one wants to have a diagnosis of heart failure. Knowing becomes important when there is a danger to the patient and when the anxiety of not knowing affects the patient adversely.

The group from Ohio State University has published a number of reports on the relationship between anxiety and autonomic nervous system dysfunction in the MVP syndrome, and it has concluded in its 1984 report in *Psychopathology*[36] that "an independent, biochemically-mediated anxiety state existing in an individual with MVP" may explain the symptom complex. This report acknowledged the group's indebtedness to Da Costa, Lewis, Wood and others. The contention that women have more symptoms than men and that anxiety plays a role in causing the well-known symptoms associated with the heart is a revival of those earlier beliefs. Boudoulas, like many doctors I have encountered, has suggested that MVP patients may be "hyper" or "high-strung", and Klein has referred to the "prototypical patient" as "a woman with migraine and Raynaud's phenomenon who's either short and thin or long and lanky."[37] Raynaud's phenomenon is a condition in which exposure to cold turns the extremities white, then cyanotic or blue, then red, over a period of a few minutes, and is caused by the constrictive effects of norepinephrine on the blood vessels. Alvarez said Raynaud's phenomenon was found in individuals with NCA and nervous disorders,[38] and, it will be recalled, that he believed migraine was always associated with neurosis. It would not be surprising if that famous picture of the male with Da Costa's syndrome hanging in the Royal Postgraduate Medical School were to be replaced with that of a short and thin or tall and lanky woman with MVP and a depressed countenance.

That anxiety should produce exactly the same symptoms in every individual with the same underlying disease seems, however, too coincidental. Anxiety has a predilection for different parts of the body in different individuals depending upon their early childhood conditioning. The classic example is the over-anxious, insecure individual with irritable colon and diarrhoea or constipation whose toilet-training has been begun too early and carried out in an atmosphere of anxiety. And, if researchers were to select more men, or at least an equal number of men, with MVP, for their studies, perhaps the misconception that women outnumber the men would gradually be exposed. After all MVP was once thought to be a male disorder simply because men were studied in great numbers. When the number of women, as in the Ohio group's studies, is three to nine times the number of men, there is a kind of optical illusion that makes more women than men appear to have MVP and more women than men to have complaints. MVP in the medical mind begins then to be associated almost exclusively with women. The individuals in this 1984 report of Boudoulas, Wooley and others were not differentiated as to the severity of the prolapse and the corresponding severity of the mitral regurgitation. Arrhythmias, fatigue and dyspnea are more common in MVP patients with more severe regurgitation. Could the fact that these symptoms were found more frequently in the women suggest that these women had more severe mitral and/or tricuspid regurgitation?

Some very elaborate tests that no doubt require a lot of time and money have been undertaken to study how anxiety, rather than mitral valvular disease, can cause the symptoms of MVP and inadequate cardiac performance. In 1979 Gaffney and co-workers published an article which compared the cardiovascular response in MVP patients with that of a control group without the disorder during and after certain tests that were more stressful than physically demanding. Again, the subjects, 35 in number, were all women. These tests to measure how the heart performs included pharmacological interventions, such as the intravenous infusion of phenylephrine, a drug which acts like adrenalin to increase the heart rate and blood pressure, the diving reflex which involved dunking the face in a bowl of water at 0°C and the use of the lower body negative pressure device (LBNP) in which the legs are sealed in an airtight chamber resembling that used by NASA to test the cardiac fitness of astronauts for their space environment.

The MVP patients, unlike the control group, demonstrated various abnormalities in different degrees according to the type of test. Some of the abnormal cardiovascular responses included ventricular arrhythmias, higher heart rates and heart rates that did not decrease as blood pressure increased or did not return to normal resting values as quickly as in patients without MVP. Though blood pressure remained stable or rose in some patients, cardiac output fell by 20-25 percent and there were decreases in stroke volume which is a measure of the amount of blood pumped out of the left ventricle with each contraction. MVP patients also showed increased venous and arterial vasoconstriction. This means that, although the heart is working harder under the stressful conditions, there is greater resistance to blood flow in the narrowing or constricting of veins and arteries and this affects the total cardiac performance.

The inadequacy of the cardiovascular response in these MVP patients is similar to that found in patients with heart failure. However, Gaffney and co-workers concluded, like the Ohio University group, that there was no left ventricular dysfunction and no hypertension or CHF. And while these researchers remarked that anxiety was not likely to have played a part because the patients were relaxed and even dozed during the testing, with the exception of the diving reflex, they concluded, again like the Ohio group, that the cardiovascular abnormalities could be attributed to a hereditary defect in the autonomic nervous system which they referred to as "an inefficient homeostatic control system". The normal regulatory or restraining mechanisms in the ANS that keep heart rate, blood pressure, stroke volume, cardiac output and venous or arterial vasoconstriction within normal limits did not function adequately.

These authors summed up the problem as one of "defective sensing, inadequate central processing and output or altered end organ responsiveness, with or without structural abnormalities of the nervous system."[39] Such a conclusion reminded me of the "poor botched souls" with constitutional weakness that Alvarez had described. Like the giants of the past, these researchers asked whether MVP patients might not benefit from physical training with graded exercises. In short this is the treatment Da Costa and Lewis recommended 100 years ago for the same symptoms.

MVP and the Small Heart

There may yet be another explanation for the symptoms of MVP which is to be found in the earlier literature. However, modern researchers have ignored this aspect. In 1943, Arthur M. Master, writing for the United States Navy Bulletin, came to essentially the same conclusion as Gaffney et al, but with an entirely different explanation for the abnormal cardiovascular responses.[40] Master examined 30 men who manifested SH, ES or NCA and refused them admittance to the United States Navy. These men, he said, were slenderly built. They suffered all the common symptoms that are associated with the MVP syndrome: tiredness on effort, SOB, palpitations, chest pain, tachycardia, dizziness, syncope, decreases in myocardial oxygen consumption that Cohen and White later described, and electrocardiographic evidence of T-wave inversion on electrocardiogram when changing from the resting to the sitting or standing position, a finding in MVP patients associated with sudden death which I will discuss later.

In Master's view, x-rays provided the most significant evidence of deviations from normal physiology. These men had hearts smaller than those of persons without the syndrome characterized by the distinct set of symptoms. Master indicated that he had reviewed the literature on the subject of the hypoplasia of the heart or the underdeveloped heart. This suggests that a substantial body of knowledge existed at the time on the subject of hearts that are smaller than normal for age, sex and size. Noteworthy were Master's references to Alexander MacLean. In 1940, MacLean demonstrated that his testing with the mercury manometer, used to determine pressure pulses in the arteries, showed that the radial pulse of Effort Syndrome patients disappeared entirely, something which did not occur in normal individuals. The conclusion was that ES or NCA must be organic in nature and that the small heart contributed to the problem.

Master referred to the studies of Graybiel and Paul White who reported in 1935 on the now well established observation that, when NCA individuals with small hearts changed their posture from recumbent to sitting or standing, their T-waves on electrocardiogram became inverted. It is surprising that Paul White made such observations but still insisted the symptoms of these patients were caused from anxiety. Master interpreted this fact as evidence of insufficient circulation and return of venous blood to the heart. Of some significance also is Graybiel and White's comment that, in patients with NCA and small hearts, the electrocardiographic abnormalities that showed circulatory deficiency occurred frequently in relation to certain infections. One can only wonder if such infections were undiagnosed IE since electrocardiographic abnormalities are common in this disease. Dysrhythmias, in particular tachycardia, occur frequently in IE. Electrocardiographic abnormalities of ST segment depression were observed during my febrile illness when I had an abscess in relation to ongoing endodontal work.

Starr and Jonas published a paper in 1940,[41] on individuals with subnormal circulation. Those with "functional heart disease" represented one half of the patients in the study. These people, many of whom were considered to have NCA, would represent the MVP patient today since their symptoms were those commonly associated with MVP, dizziness, especially when they stood up, which modern physicians now recognize as orthostatic hypotension, weakness, fatigue, dyspnea on exertion, lightheadedness and fainting spells as well as coldness of the extremities which may well have been Raynaud's phenomenon that Klein said was present typically in MVP patients. Of most interest was their finding, like Master's, of a heart size that was generally smaller than it would be for age, size and sex. Some hearts were said to be "extremely small", as mine was described. In association with the subnormal circulation and small heart were arrhythmias and a cardiac output said to be 56 percent below the average in some cases. Starr and Jonas referred to these characteristics as a syndrome and sought an explanation which is of particular significance. They said, "It soon occurred to us that this group of symptoms is characteristic of patients convalescent from the severe infectious diseases", among which was "prolonged pyrexia of unknown origin". Their observations only confirmed Graybiel and White's. This was 1940, the pre-antibiotic era, and one cannot help but think of Libman's studies of healed and healing IE and that these infections sounded suspiciously like IE. Once again, I stress the fact that my case is an example of the latter since I was never diagnosed or actually treated with IV antibiotics at any time during my illness and had only a series of short courses of oral antibiotics. While these observers obviously considered the small heart to be of importance physiologically, Lewis did not, even though he had referred to it in his works, a point which Master makes.

Master, following the leads of the past, showed that such patients with smaller than normal hearts, had low cardiac output with exercise and inadequate circulatory responses with insufficient return of blood to the heart. After exercise, the heart rate and blood pressure in Master's patients did not return to normal resting values as quickly as they did in normal patients. Gaffney et al's patients showed the same abnormalities. Master's observations confirmed the presence of a definite organic abnormality which he defined as "a constitutionally small heart which does not eject enough blood per minute to nourish the heart, skeletal muscles and organs of the body adequately in response to effort." Unlike Lewis and others, Master did not believe the exercise tolerance of such men could be improved with physical training because the size of the heart was the chief factor in poor effort response. This is the reason he rejected such men for the strenuous life of the navy.

Much later, Samuel Levine, in his 1958 textbook, took up Master's observations and found that patients with NCA or Soldier's Heart had smaller than average hearts on x-ray.[42] However, modern researchers after him have not investigated the possibility that MVP patients have smaller than normal sized hearts and that this may be the cause in part for their symptoms. Enlargement of such hearts during the course of the patient's history, even though within normal limits, may be a clue to an undiagnosed IE and thus the reason for the development of severe regurgitation after the infectious episode and eventual replacement of the mitral valve. I now have cardiac enlargement, but I am told it is insignificant. Nothing can be proven because my earlier x-rays which showed my "tiny" heart vanished during the traumatic period when I tried to seek help just after my release from hospital the first time. Doctors have always believed that "significant" cardiac enlargement must be present before they will make a diagnosis of chronic heart failure, even though many patients who develop CHF after MI are known to have only slight mitral regurgitation and slight cardiac enlargement. Da Costa, Lewis, MacKenzie and others all considered enlargement and hypertrophy or thickening of the heart muscle to be the hallmarks of a failing myocardium. When my heart enlarged, it was still within what Dr. Austin viewed as normal limits. He only knew it was enlarged because he had consecutive x-rays before him. It stands to reason that the majority of cases of cardiac enlargement in the MVP syndrome would be missed if, in fact, such patients were to have, at the outset, congenitally smaller hearts than normal people. A smaller than normal sized heart could also explain why some researchers define the problem in MVP as one of a valve being too large for the ventricle.

Doctors who accept that a heart can be failing only if the heart muscle is hypertrophied or if the heart is greatly enlarged will naturally not interpret classic signs of heart failure in a normal sized heart as evidence of failure with exercise. Da Costa had dismissed the SOB and peripheral edema associated with the Irritable Heart Syndrome as unimportant and transitory and, today, there are doctors, such as my internist, who hold the same opinion of these findings and, ultimately, therefore, the mitral and tricuspid regurgitation become insignificant. When a MVP patient engages in strenuous or stressful exercise, abnormal increases in epinephrine and norepinephrine production, in blood lactate, in venous and arterial vasoconstriction, in heart rate and blood pressure along with abnormal fall in cardiac output and dilatation of the heart do not prompt researchers, as these reports suggest, to relate such findings that could indicate heart failure to the prolapse per se, to any left ventricular dysfunction, hypertension or to potential heart failure with exercise.

Joseph S. Alpert in his book, *Physiopathology of the Cardiovascular System* says " all patients with symptomatic cardiovascular disease have in one sense or another developed heart failure. That is one of the myriad functions of the cardiovascular system has failed."[43] This would mean that symptomatic

MVP patients have heart failure which only becomes evident with strenuous exercise or other stresses to the body as Master pointed out. Hence the danger of strenuous exercise. It is also possible that the small heart, described by Master, could create the potential for heart failure or sudden death with strenuous activity in an otherwise healthy individual. When I experienced tachycardia and presyncope in association with heavy physical labour, I was told that the disturbances in heartbeat were unrelated to exercise and, in fact, I was told I could continue on with this indiscriminate, Herculean work. No doubt, it was thought I would become a cardiac cripple if I were told the truth. From his letters to my GP, Dr. Austin's purpose was clearly to avoid a cardiac neurosis. Perhaps the test results Wooley, Gaffney and others have reported, despite their own conclusions, are warnings that stressful or strenuous activities are not without risk to the MVP patient and that the advocation of physical training, à la Lewis, is inappropriate and possibly dangerous. Such tests should perhaps lead doctors to explore more carefully the relationship between congenitally small hearts, rather than anxiety, and cardiovascular symptoms.

It is evident that there is great danger to the MVP patient in this unparalleled pursuit of the anxiety neurosis theory. There can be no more potent a sign of such danger than in the recent "fiasco" over a single case that appeared in the medical literature. This case and the attitude to it call to mind the power and influence of Gallavardin which far outweighed the significance of his few autopsied cases. The patient in question was a 28 year old man who complained of palpitations, syncope and chest pain and was hospitalized at least ten times, according to his observers, in the Philadelphia-New Jersey area of the U.S.[44] Doctors recorded that the patient was a chronically ill-looking man with Marfanoid features, a high arched palate,[45] MVP with MSC and LSM [46] and had electrocardiographic abnormalities involving the T wave and ST segment.[47] Many different medications were included in his treatment: quinidine, an analgesic and anti-inflammatory drug, propranolol which slows the heart rate, digoxin, a synthetic digitalis which strengthens the heart muscle, and Warfarin, an anti-coagulant. Causes of hospitalizations were listed as chest pain, decompression sickness and gastrointestinal hemorrhage which was acknowledged as "secondary to aspirin or Coumadin ingestion or both,"[48] since these are anti-coagulants also. His examiners at one of the hospitals noted a cutdown scar on the patient's chest indicating cardiac investigations [49] and his hematocrit and hemoglobin were appreciably decreased.[50] These were the true facts or observations made by examiners.

Certain aspects of the medical history provided by the patient, however, could not be verified. He claimed that, while he was in Germany, he had been twice admitted to the Nymphenberg Hospital for catheterization and told he had a blocked coronary artery, cardiomegaly and a myocardial infarction after which a pacemaker was inserted in his chest. However, doctors in the U.S. discovered that catheterizations were not done at that hospital in Germany [51] and that the dates when he was supposed to be in Germany conflicted with hospitalizations in the U.S. At one institution he represented himself as a student at Yale while at another Princeton.[52] His sister was not at an address he furnished, and he could not remember the name of the doctor who had prescribed nitroglycerine for angina-like pain over a period of four years.[53]

However, the patient's testimony was not altogether untrue. His statement that the German hospital's echocardiogram showed MVP was, indeed, verified in the American hospitals. Obviously investigations had been carried out there, but he was mistaken about dates, something which may be an understandable oversight. The information that his grandmother had Marfan's disease was, in all probability true, since the patient, himself, had Marfanoid features. That the patient stated he was taking anti-coagulants seemed to have been true from the evidence of lowered hematocrit and hemoglobin, an indication of hemorrhage, and from the fact that he had been hospitalized for gastrointestinal bleeding. The scar on the patient's chest was proof of some kind of investigation, whether this was in the U.S. or Germany. While the patient gave an incorrect date for his hospitalization at one of the American hospitals and an incorrect address for that institution, his medical records were ultimately retrieved from the said institution.[54] Doctors from the three institutions reporting on this patient said he signed himself out each time. On one occasion, this was to enter a rowing competition after he had been admitted for chest pain. Despite some provable facts, the inconsistencies in the timing and place of investigations in his story and his behaviour in signing himself out lead his examiners to declare he suffered from "a severe personality disorder".[55] He was called a classic "cardiac cripple" because he had been told of his MVP.[56]

While the patient may well have a personality disorder, neverthless, some important information he gave could be verified. Errors in medical histories are known to take place frequently, incorrect dates of events, incorrect names etc. The patient, it does appear, was able to control his chest pain with nitroglycerine. This may explain why he signed himself out without waiting for further tests, and, certainly, patients become frustrated when they get neither information nor explanation for their symptoms. If he were taking anti-coagulants, Coumadin or Warfarin, a doctor must have given them to him as they are not available without prescription and, though he may have signed himself out, he did not admit himself nor perform surgery on his own chest. And, surely, without reason, no doctor would resort to such invasive measures. One would want to prove beyond a reasonable doubt that this unusual case of MVP was truly one of severe personality disorder and one would want to see many more such cases before using this one as evidence of the MVP-neurosis equation.

Doctors labelled this MVP patient a case of Munchaüsen's syndrome or pathological malingering, which harks back to Lewis and Da Costa's malingering soldiers and Wood's cowards. This name for chronic fictitious illness comes from the German fabulist, Rudolph Raspe, whose book, *Adventures of Baron Munchaüsen*, is a collection of unrealistic, exaggerated tales that defy rationality and truth. Munchaüsen's Syndrome, which is also called Hospital Hobo's syndrome, is described in *The Merck Manual of Diagnosis and Therapy* which every doctor has in his office. This means that every physician is expected to be familiar with this bizarre psychological condition. The Manual gives a very complete description and warns that such patients are able to produce "the clinical picture of myocardial infarction, hematemesis (vomiting of blood), hemoptysis (spitting of blood from the larynx, trachea, bronchia or lungs as in tuberculosis), acute abdominal conditions, or a pyrexia of unknown origin . . . symptoms of cerebral tumor or disseminated sclerosis with uncanny skill". These patients, the Manual warns, are not averse to conducting surgery on themselves. "A patient's abdominal wall may be a criss-cross of scars and a digit or a limb may have been amputated." One begins to wonder if his cutdown scar on his chest was viewed as self-inflicted. They may also infect themselves. "Pyrexias are often due to self-inflicted abscesses, and the culture, usually Escherichia coli, clearly indicates the source of the infecting organism."[57]

Of most significance in this masochistic list is fever which the Manual says is usually from a self-inflicted abscess infected with the patient's own feces. With the popularization of the MVP-neurosis equation, will doctors be looking for the Munchaüsen bogeyman, as Evans once called mitral regurgitation, in every symptomatic MVP patient? And will doctors consider a fever of unknown origin, in the absence of other symptoms of IE, to be self-induced? Doctors already have great difficulty in identifying IE and, if they are conditioned to look for Munchaüsen's syndrome, they might, tragically, be even more likely to misdiagnose IE.

The dangers of generalizing about this rare instance of a psychosis, if, indeed, that is what it is, in the MVP syndrome are overwhelming. Authors who describe this case, warn that such a patient is "a medical economic factor".[58] This was the same opinion expressed by Lewis, Evans, White, Wood and others. The cost factor is an argument many psychiatrists, psychologists and medical doctors are currently using to persuade their colleagues that it is inadvisable to tell patients they have a heart disease called MVP since such knowledge will make them cardiac cripples and they will then become a burden to society.

There are only three references to this "Munchaüsen case" in association with MVP in the medical literature, all brief letters addressed to the editors of the journals. Robert Jeresaty, in his book on MVP, referred to it in his discussion on psychiatric manifestations in the MVP syndrome,[59] and one is reminded of the suggestions that MVP be included in the sections on cardiac neurosis in the psychiatric textbooks. Had the patient been a woman, it is quite possible that hysteria would have consumed the medical world, and there would truly have been a "fiasco", to quote Aubrey Leatham. There is, indeed, evidence that the search for this bogeyman may become routine in MVP patients. In the section on psychiatric manifestations in his book, Jeresaty cited the results of the administration of *The Minnesota Multiphasic Personality Test* (MMPI) to fourteen patients with MVP. Of the six patients with symptoms, "five had abnormal scores for hysteria and hypochrondriasis," he pointed out, and "four had abnormal scores for depression, psychopathic deviation and schizophrenia, and three abnormal scores for psychasthenia."[60]

I am reminded of the diagnosis of "labile mentality" and "pathological anxiety" that was accorded me during my febrile illness. Jeresaty concluded that investigation of the psychiatric symptoms of MVP is warranted and that patients in mental institutions should be routinely tested for MVP.

It is not difficult to imagine in our Orwellian world in which the masses are controlled by a few powerful groups, that all MVP patients may be required to take the MMPI test some time in the future. What is most frightening is that this test is old, dragged out of the ark like the laurels of the giants, Lewis and Da Costa. Constructed in the early 1940s, the MMPI was used for the measurement of psychoneuroses in medical practice, the same reason for which Alvarez had written *The Neuroses*, so that doctors might distinguish genuine from fake illness and thus quickly pass the patient on to the appropriate specialist, specifically the psychiatrist. The 550 MMPI questions [61] relating to gastrointestinal, cardio-respiratory and genitourinary habits, family and marital background, education, occupation, sexual, political, social and religious attitudes, phobias, delusions, hallucinations, depressed and manic states were designed to elicit proof of psychosomatic illness. It is easy to see how the list of endogenous anxiety symptoms was formed. It was this evidence, proof of psychosomatic illness, that Dr. Adami, a former psychiatrist, was after when he questioned me, during my third hospitalization to find out the cause of low-grade fever, clubbing and spleen enlargement. His series of questions followed the format of the MMPI test.

The attitude of the MMPI's creators, McKinley and Hathaway, manifested the intellectual and social snobbery of the elite, and it is disturbing that such a test should still be used. Like Alvarez, the creators of the test favoured the word, "moron", for many of their troubled patients.[62] For instance, McKinley and Hathaway give highly selective information about a woman they diagnosed as neurasthenic, hypochondriacal and hysterical. She had the same cardiovascular symptoms found in the condition known today as MVP: chest pain, dizziness and fainting spells. It was said that "her general knowledge seemed considerably restricted to religious topics. Her intelligence quotient was 110. It is difficult to understand how she became the high school valedictorian unless the scholastic competition was very poor in her class."[63] How, it might be asked, can such a biased opinion throw any light on the cause of the chest pain, dizziness and fainting spells? Because this woman's cervical ribs were very long, they were removed in the all too familiar resort to surgery, to cutting out the offending part of the body, in imitation of the Biblical commandment. Symptoms, however, continued as before.

That such a narrow perspective clouded their judgement was manifest in another case of multiple sclerosis which these doctors misinterpreted as hysteria, though once the woman's diagnosis was made definitively, her MMPI tests all showed normal scores. Drastic results ensued for this patient who suffered partial blindness while she waited for proper treatment. Doctors made an identical error in judgement just recently in the eighties in the case of a farmer from Bradford, Ontario who died from viral encephalitis which was likewise mistaken for hysteria and correct treatment delayed for 24 hours.[64]

How competent are doctors, who have no specialty in psychiatry, in interpreting what is anxiety and what is disease? The Psychiatric Department of the University of Toronto in association with Toronto General Hospital published a report in 1980 based on the examination of the medical records of all patients with MVP, between the years 1972 and 1977, who underwent left ventricular angiography. The physicians examined the records to determine, in their own words, by "statistical means, whether in fact, patients, with MVPS as a primary diagnosis, are perceived by their physicians as psychologically more disturbed than either patients with other cardiovascular conditions in whom MVP is found coincidentally or patients with cardiovascular conditions with no MVP."[65]

During the patient's hospitalization for the test procedure, the treating physicians who recorded the presence of psychological disturbances were not necessarily psychiatrists. The majority appeared to be interns who have little experience with patients, residents who have somewhat more and internists who have the most experience though their training is still not specifically in the area of psychiatric illness. The patient was considered to have a psychological disorder if one or more examiners observed signs of anxiety or depression dating from admission up to 24 hours before the invasive procedures.

Even though the authors regarded their evidence as "statistical", they admitted imperfections existed in their study. The patients, they said, had symptoms which their doctors regarded as sufficiently alarming to justify invasive tests, such as ventricular angiography and, therefore, these patients could not be regarded as typical of all MVP patients. And, unlike patients with more clearly defined cardiac disease, MVP patients, the authors recognized, are "less aware of their disorder".[66] As I have pointed out, many doctors do not believe in telling their MVP patients of their heart condition, and what this statement suggests is that an informed patient is a less anxious patient. An uninformed patient will naturally ask more questions than an informed patient, and thus will, inevitably, appear more anxious. It was repeated frequently, in the medical records during my hospitalizations that I was "unusual" or "anxious" because I asked a lot of questions. Surely, too, such invasive procedures and the hospital setting by its very nature would naturally produce some level of anxiety in most people, and, as the authors pointed out, the symptoms of these patients were important enough to justify these invasive measures. When serious disease is present, these researchers said, physicians were not as apt to note psychological disturbance. It might be added that psychological disturbance in a very ill person would be taken for granted. Other studies, these authors confessed, show that depression is more often overlooked in patients who are hospitalized for long periods of time since familiarity with such patients disinclines doctors to note neurotic behaviour while "residents tend to select for psychiatric referral younger patients with less serious medical illnesses."[67]

Considering doctors' attitudes to MVP, it is not surprising that complications such as IE, the development of SOB, slight cardiac enlargement, peripheral edema and even left ventricular dysfunction would not be regarded as seriously in a MVP patient as in a patient with RHD and mitral stenosis. The "beauty", or in this case, the "depression", the anxiety, is in the eyes of the beholder. Despite these variables that related to the accuracy of their study, these authors concluded that endogenous anxiety or depression existed in 57.8 percent of the group with MVP as principal diagnosis compared to 22.8 percent in the group with coincidental MVP and 18 percent in the control cardiac group without MVP.[68] Such impressive results could influence the treatment of MVP patients, and, yet, the study was, as its authors suggested not without its imperfections.

In Canada, MVP research began to take the same disturbing direction as in the United States once the syndrome was equated with what had formerly been regarded as a set of neurotic symptoms. The treatment of MVP has quickly fallen into the hands of psychiatrists or medical doctors who choose to treat a disease as a psychiatric disorder. The suggestion runs through the medical literature that doctors should return to the old treatments because the symptoms of psychoneurotic origin could be cured with graded physical training à la Lewis. The MVP patient must be forced to accept that exercise is not going to hurt and will not bring on the symptoms because the underlying disease does not affect the function of the heart.

A study involving MVP patients, undertaken at The McMaster University Medical School in Hamilton, Ontario in the eighties, showed a return to Lewis' ideas. Dr. Arthur Cott, psychologist, Associate Professor of Medicine at that institution and Director of the Behavioural Medicine Unit of St. Joseph's Hospital in Hamilton, headed this project. He and his colleagues studied two groups of patients with "chest pain or pressure, tightness and palpitations", one with, in their words, the "benign condition of MVP" and one without heart problems.[69] Typical of contemporary opinion, there was no acknowledgement in the prospectus announcing this study that these symptoms were, in any way, related to genuine disease of the mitral valve. They were attributed to emotional attitudes, pain and a lack of physical fitness and fear of a heart attack with strenuous exercise. The aim of this study was to increase the patient's level of physical functioning through psychological conditioning and, as if doctors were dealing with Effort Syndrome, exercises, in the Lewis tradition, formed the backbone of this project. The organizers of the study designed their program to reduce a patient's "unnecessary disability" [70] and increase his or her productivity. The study did not, of course, address the far more important issue of deterioration of the prolapse nor how to prevent this by informing patients of the risks in the syndrome and the appropriate protection available.

This study demonstrates that the long link with the past remains unbroken, and the role of the medical professional is the same as it was in Lewis, Evans or Wood's time: defender of society by forcing the patient to throw off his or her cardiac neurosis and rely less upon the use of medical facilities. As in the past, doctors believe that exercise, not knowledge, prevents cardiac crippling which this St. Joseph's project was specifically designed to avoid. Once again the blame is suddenly shifted to the patient. The patient's attitude, not the heart, is diseased, and the cure lies only in the doctor's ability to exorcise the "medical economic factor" of the Munchaüsen bogeyman.

The Panic Attack Clinic — and the Use of Antidepressants

Studies of the neuroses and MVP have enormous influence on the medical establishment. On November 16, 1983, it was announced in a local Toronto newspaper that a panic clinic would be established at Toronto General Hospital.[71] This clinic was designed to treat patients with agoraphobia which, as I have already pointed out, some researchers are claiming is found in fifty percent of MVP patients and is the basis of symptoms. Given the present climate surrounding MVP, it is likely that many MVP patients, whom doctors feel have developed psychological disorders, specifically cardiac neurosis, over their symptoms, particularly those who have been told of a MVP, will be sent to this clinic. Considering the psychiatric diagnosis, the label "pathological anxiety" and a "labile mentality", that was made in my case, despite abscessed tooth, chest pain, tachycardia, sweats etc., would I have been sent to such a facility, if such a clinic had existed? Perhaps, in the future, we will see doctors, who are convinced their MVP patients have hypochondriacal fears, packing them off to panic clinics instead of addressing the underlying disease.

While the panic clinics themselves may appear to be harmless, and even beneficial, they could become a factor in overlooking real disease such as IE which may be regarded as a neurotic or psychotic disorder. Doctors are using tranquilizers to treat agoraphobia at The Toronto Panic Attack Clinic.[72] Treatment regimens have their origin in the United States where most research has been done on agoraphobia, endogenous anxiety and MVP. This treatment consists of tranquilizers and antidepressants. According to the American experts on these psychiatric manifestations in the MVP syndrome, Drs. David Sheehan and Donald Klein, whose work I have already referred to, the most effective way of treating panic attack is with the tricyclic antidepressants such as imipramine and the monoamine oxidase (MAO) inhibitors such as phenelzine. The implication is that these drugs are being used in significant amounts since, as the authors have indicated, the drugs can take a long time to work, up to "six weeks of treatment with steadily increasing doses before the drug's effectiveness is apparent."[73] Klein and colleagues have written an article on the use of imipramine with MVP patients who suffer panic attack. They reported that they had success in diminishing both the autonomic malfunctioning which they believe causes the panic attacks and the panic attacks themselves which they say are caused by the knowledge of the presence of MVP.[74]

The treatment of MVP patients for panic disorder is not limited to Canada and the United States. Grunhaus et al from Hadasah University Hospital in Israel reported they found MVP in 39 percent of psychiatric patients with RSPA, Recurrent Spontaneous Panic Attacks, and that clomipramine, another tricyclic antidepressant like imipramine, reduced both the panic attacks and cardiac symptoms in 20 patients.[75]

However, the treatment of symptoms of genuine disease of the cardio-vascular system with drugs specifically used to treat neurotic or psychotic disorders is frightening and for MVP patients even dangerous. Phenelzine, for instance, is normally used in the treatment of patients described as "atypical, neurotic or reactive" according to the CPS.[76] Doctors described myself and many of the other women who wrote to me in exactly this way. Patients treated with these drugs are said to have anxiety or depressive disorders that manifest as phobic or hypochondriacal, and, currently, much effort is being made to link MVP with these two emotional disorders.

There are some serious risks attached to the use of these antidepressants. The MAO inhibitors, such as phenelzine, trade name Nardil, have side effects that are well established problems in the MVP syndrome. These drugs were originally manufactured to treat psychotic depression but it was observed that a side effect was hypotension and they were then subsequently used in the treatment of hypertension.[77] Hypotension is a common symptom of MVP and, of course, could precipitate syncope. The other side effects of phenelzine, according to the CPS, are dizziness, drowsiness, weakness and fatigue and the drug may potentiate hypoglycemia as well as being contraindicated in patients with CHF.[78] All of the above problems have occured in MVP patients. As I've pointed out a MVP patient can develop CHF and in its early stages doctors will not recognize or accept it for what it is. For instance, propranolol or Inderal can cause cardiac wheezing in patients with early heart failure. While my internist has suggested I discontinue it, he gives me as reason that I have suddenly late in life developed asthma.

The other antidepressants currently being used in panic clinics to treat panic attacks, agoraphobia and endogenous anxiety, such as clomipramine (Anafranil) and imipramine, are not MAO inhibitors, and impramine, in particular, should not be used in conjunction with such MAO drugs as phenelzine, according to the CPS. Both clomipramine and imipramine have been used to treat psychotic conditions, including manic depressive states and psychosis. These drugs, like phenelzine, have similar risks. The CPS warns that they should be "administered with extreme caution" in patients with a history of cardiovascular disease and both have potential dangers for patients with kidney damage.[79] If the MVP patient has CHF or chronic glomerulo-nephritis, (GN) these drugs could be dangerous. However, as I have pointed out, the signs of CHF, SOB, edema and fatigue are not accepted as such in MVP patients, especially in young people, no more than they were in Da Costa's or Lewis' time. And if a patient has had an unrecognized IE, he or she may have a symptomless GN which could deteriorate with the administration of these drugs.

These antidepressant drugs can also cause serious arrhythmias, known to occur in the MVP syndrome, which predispose the patient to death. Like the MAO inhibitors, clomipramine and imipramine can precipitate orthostatic hypotension with manifestations of dizziness, lightheadedness or syncope, typical symptoms of the MVP syndrome. Of most significance to the MVP patient is that these drugs can cause myocardial infarction and stroke, and unexpected deaths have occured in non-MVP patients using these antidepressants. The ECG changes which clomipramine can produce, such as flattening or inverted T waves have been associated with sudden death in MVP patients.[80]

Abnormal Platelet Activity, Thromboembolism (stroke) and MVP

Many reports have been written on the cerebral complications in the MVP syndrome. In fact almost as much attention is being given to this topic as to IE. Researchers agree that cerebral ischemic (Gk. ischaimos=to stop blood) complications are a most serious feature that urgently requires investigation. Those, such as Grunhaus and co-workers, who are experimenting with the antidepressant drugs are aware of the association between cerebral ischemic complications in young patients and MVP and advise that more work needs to be done in that area.[81] One third of all cerebral infarctions (strokes) in young adults under the age of 45 occur in patients with MVP.[82]

The history linking MVP and stroke goes back a number of years, as does most any other recognized problem associated with this disease. It was Barlow, the physician whose name was once given to the syndrome, and Bosman in 1966 who made the first observation of an incompleted stroke in a MVP patient who was left with only temporary weakness in her arm.[83] Barlow and Bosman did not comment upon the association between MVP and this episode of cerebral ischemia.

The first report of a definite connection between MVP and cerebral ischemia was made in 1974 by a Canadian doctor, J. M. Barnett, Professor and Chairman of the Neurology Department of The University of Western Ontario. In his introduction to his report on Transient Ischemic Attack (TIA), Barnett said "the extent of the stroke problem is staggering. It is the third cause of death in most developed nations, ranking behind heart disease and malignancy . . . by 1980, one out of five persons will die of stroke."[84]

Barnett was speaking of stroke in general and, though he only mentioned MVP briefly, his comments became an ironic prelude to the storm of research that would take place in the seventies and eighties on MVP and cerebral ischemic complications. Barnett admitted that, in the past, he had excluded MVP and orthostatic hypotension as unrelated to TIAs and stroke. However, in his 1974 paper, he readdressed the issue. He defined a Transient Ischemic Attack (TIA) as "an event of swift onset over a few seconds producing a focal neurological deficit lasting commonly a few minutes and not more than 24 hours."[85] When the blood supply is cut off to a specific area of the brain for only a short period of time, there are no lasting effects. Barnett lists three factors associated with TIAs, orthostatic hypotension, tachyrhythmia and cardiac decompensation (which it was suggested I had with my wall motion exercise test in 1984). All of of these problems occur in the MVP syndrome. In fact, tachyrhythmia or rapid heart beat of varying seriousness is one of the most common complaints, as I have already pointed out. The patients with MVP who had TIAs in Barnett's study had cardiac arrhythmias including paroxysmal atrial fibrillation. Barnett indicated that the relationship between cardiac arrhythmias in the MVP syndrome and cerebral and retinal embolism cannot be denied.[86] Another mechanism said to produce TIAs is emboli from the mitral valve, and it was Barnett who first put forward this theory. This is not difficult to accept when we remember the explanations Lawrence Freedman offered on how NBTVs are formed because of damaged endothelium of the mitral valve and the mechanics of billowing valves.

Barnett and his colleagues from the University of Western Ontario have studied the relationship between cerebral complications and MVP and have produced a series of reports in 1975[87], 1976[88], 1977[89], 1980[90], 1982[91]. In his 1980 study, it was found that 40 percent of 60 young patients under the age of 45 with a history of incomplete stroke and TIA had MVP as compared to a 6.8 percent incidence in the control group which did not have MVP and was matched on the basis of age and sex. When six of Barnett's patients with other known causes of cerebral embolic attacks, such as birth control pills, were extracted, the incidence of TIAs and incompleted or minimal stroke was still 30 percent.[92] This factor alone pointed to the dangers of oral contraceptives or any medication such as MAOs or tricyclic antidepressants that can cause stroke.

Other researchers agree with Barnett and colleagues on the seriousness of cerebral ischemic complications in the MVP syndrome. Sandok and Giuliani, in 1982 put the risk of stroke in young people with MVP at four times that of the normal population and this, they said, is a "conservative estimate."[93]

The picture is a confusing one, and there are many seeming inconsistencies regarding the identification of MVP patients at most risk of these complications. Frequently, arrhythmias are found in association with cerebral ischemic attack in MVP patients. Yet, stroke has been found in 50 to 75 percent of patients with only **minimal** prolapse and unimportant signs on Holter monitor, which records the heart's rhythm and rate, and many people who have stroke do not know they have prolapse.[94] Others have the usual symptoms of chest pain and palpitations.

One of the most common arrhythmias associated with stroke in MVP patients is atrial fibrillation which is both a rapid and irregular heart beat. It has been found in 60 percent of MVP patients with cerebral ischemic complications, and the authors of the report, Nishimura et al, warn that patients with this symptom could be at very high risk of TIAs or completed stroke.[95]

A group from Boston University School of Medicine analyzed a series of studies covering the years 1977 to 1985 involving 114 MVP patients. The complications ranged from mild to severe with 32 percent suffering from only transient TIA, 66 percent experiencing completed stroke and 32 percent of the patients retaining permanent neurologic damage after their first attack. 20 percent of these patients had recurrent ischemic attacks either months or years apart. It is believed that the solitary event or one that recurs only after a long period of time usually results in more severe brain damage, and the risk is greater if more than one valve is damaged by the myxomatous process or by IE.[96]

What all this suggests is that MVP patients, especially those with particular kinds of arrhythmias, which are usually associated with moderate to severe regurgitation, are at very high risk of a cerebral ischemic attack whether that be a transient or a completed stroke with resulting brain damage of varying degrees. An arrhythmia slows down the movement of the blood out of the heart and thus encourages the formation of clots especially in the crevice between the ballooning valve leaflet and the atrial wall. The prolapse is responsible for the cardiac arrhythmia which then in turn favours the formation of thrombi.

A 1981 study presented some grim facts about MVP and the whole question of the relationship between hyper platelet activity and thrombogenesis or how thrombi or clots are formed. In this study there were 29 patients with MVP. Nine of them had a history of thromboembolism, cerebral, retinal or deep venous in nature. Eight had temporary loss of vision i.e. retinal emboli and twelve had neither thromboembolism nor visual attacks. Three groups manifested varying degrees, 100, 75 and 58 percent, of hypercoagulability on blood testing or a higher than normal tendency to form clots. Overall, 76 percent of the 29 patients with MVP had evidence of platelet coagulant abnormalities.[97]

Platelet hypercoagulability means that the platelets, which are responsible for stopping excess bleeding but are also implicated in the formation of bacterial vegetations in IE, clump together or aggregate faster in people with MVP than in people without this heart disease. Such a blood abnormality increases the potential for thrombotic or embolic formation. A thrombus (pl. thrombi) is a blood clot which remains in the place where it was formed while an embolus (pl. emboli) is a blood clot which travels via the blood stream to another site in the body. The prefix "em" suggests that the clot emmigrates or moves away to another site. Travelling clots or emboli can lodge anywhere in the body, in addition to the brain or heart. They may lodge in the central retinal artery or its branches, arterioles, of the eye causing visual disturbances, blindness, which may be permanent or transient, or they may lodge in other organs of the body such as the kidney, lungs, liver or bowel. The smaller the artery or its branches, the more silent the infarction. The risk of embolism is appreciably greater if the regurgitation is more severe and if the patient has more than one leaky valve.

The list of researchers from medical centres all over North America and the rest of the world who are involved in the study of MVP and thromboembolism is a long one. They are studying the neurologic complications which include TIA, complete stroke, partial or total blindness called amaurosis or, if fleeting, amaurosis fugax, from the Latin word for fleeing, retinal vascular disease and even migraine. Researchers uniformly agree that neurologic disturbances present an important problem and that the incidence is high in the MVP syndrome. I list only a few of these people involved in these studies who have produced significant papers worth reading: Waldoff et al, 1975,[98] Kimball and Hedges, 1976,[99] Saffro and Talano, 1979,[100] Caltrider et al, 1980,[101] Hart and Easton, 1982 [102], Jones et al, 1982,[103] Scharf et al, 1982,[104] Kouvaras and Bacoulas, 1985,[105] Kelley et al., 1988.[106] It is of interest that three of these classic articles appeared in the same issue of the medical journal called *Stroke*. What this shows is that MVP is, indeed, a Pandora's Box of ills, and it may be found, in the future, that a great many diseases that physicians think are separate entities may be associated with prolapse of the valves.

Recently, researchers have identified a relationship between MVP and migraine headaches. Five percent of the general population,[107] according to Adams and Griffith in *Harrison's Principles of Internal Medicine*, suffer from migraine and most sufferers appear to be women. A 1978 study by Litman and Friedman of the Akron General Medical Centre in Ohio found that 10 percent of women are subject to migraine headaches. Over one quarter of these women, about 28 percent, have MVP. There is a higher incidence of stroke in these people. Individuals with migraine complicated by visual and neuro-logical disturbances such as various degrees of transient blindness and paralysis are those at greatest risk of stroke. Litman and Friedman believe that these complications are caused by "repetitive emboli from the mitral valve",[108] an opinion that is in accord with the report on the Tygerberg patient who suffered both a cerebral and coronary embolism, and migrainous infarction has been documented.[109] Litman and Friedman recommend that all individuals with migraine should be screened for MVP and, if this condition is present, these patients should be protected against stroke as well as IE. One of the ways of preventing migraine and stroke, these authors, say, is by avoiding birth control pills. Other researchers have suggested the use of antiplatelet or anticoagulant drugs, including aspirin one gram per day in patients with MVP and TIA and, if TIA persists despite the use of aspirin, then anticoagulation with warfarin is indicated. It was also recommended in the same study that MVP patients be screened for protein S deficiency which can be occasioned by oral contraceptives, pregnancy and the nephrotic syndrome which, as I have discussed, results from IE. Deficiencies of both protein S and C are associated with recurrent arterial and venous thrombosis.[110] Obviously smoking should also be eliminated since it shows a link with stroke. And the antidepressant drugs and the MAO inhibitors are, likewise, not wise choices of therapy. The appeals of writers like Litman and Friedman suggest, as usual, that there are many people with MVP that have not yet been identified.

Strong evidence that birth control pills are dangerous to MVP patients exists in a very interesting case in the Canadian medi-legal literature. In 1971, Pauline Buchan, a young woman of 23, suffered a paralyzing stroke while using Ortho Novum birth control pills. She sued the drug company on the basis of inadequate packaging information which did not convey the risks to women. Her story has only recently emerged when, in 1984, the court awarded her over $800,000 in damages. [111] I followed Buchan's trial and suspected, even before her MVP was revealed in the press, that she had this heart disease on the basis of what I had read in the medical literature about the propensity for stroke in the MVP syndrome.

In the wake of the Buchan case, it would seem reasonable that the drug company would have updated its insert in the birth control package. However, in the year following the settlement of this case, the Ortho contraceptive information, though much more detailed, still did not spell out MVP among the risk groups. And at the time of this writing, in 1989, the insert still does not list MVP specifically in the general references to underlying cardiac disease.

Who is responsible for the information provided in the pill package? The major influence behind this literature intended for public information is the medical profession itself, rather than the drug company. It is the doctors who advise drug researchers. At the time of Buchan's trial, a medical committee had been set up to advise the government on the nature of the information that should accompany the pill. Doctor Kinch, testifying at the Ortho trial as head of this committee, said the doctors believed that the American inserts, at the time Mrs. Buchan was using the pill in 1971, were "too detailed" and "too terrifying" to be given to Canadian women, but, as Barbara Seaman pointed out, there was a financial factor since, after the introduction of stern warnings on the U.S. package inserts, sales of oral contraceptives dropped from 10 million to 6 million. [112] A decline in the use of the pill, of course, means a decline in the number of visits to the doctor.

Doctors were also quoted as saying, in a report from the Canadian Medical Association, "we do not want anyone upsetting our patients with scary stories about the pill. [113] Women are, in the medical stereotype, little girls whom daddy must protect from knowledge that might make them anxious. This and similar statements made at the trial reflect the chronic condescension and paternalism of the medical profession, especially towards women, and, no doubt, the typical protective instinct of doctors. The less information the public has, the less dangerous it is. With such influence and with doctors' views regarding the dangers of telling patients they have MVP, it is not difficult to understand why the package information for contraceptives still does not specifically mention MVP as a condition that increases the risk of embolism. And, indeed, the pill manufacturers would be likely to support the doctors' opinions since the less information about risks the better from a financial point of view. Since it is the medical profession which determines what information goes into the pill package, doctors are also at fault for inadequate warnings, and it might be pointed out that the drug company was likely sued because rarely can a doctor be successfully sued in Canada.

While it is true that, at the time Pauline Buchan had her stroke, there was little knowledge of the connection between MVP and cerebral complications expressed in the medical literature, this relationship was more than well established at the time of her trial in 1984. However MVP never became an issue. Her personal physician stated, in his testimony, that he would prescribe the pill today "given similar circumstances".[114] One must ask if he meant by this statement that he would prescribe oral contraceptives for women with MVP. There are millions of women throughout the world who have MVP who are likely using oral contraceptives and, therefore, this aspect of MVP should be further investigated, and MVP should be specifically mentioned in the birth control inserts.

The comments made at Pauline Buchan's trial about "upsetting" women imply once again that doctors view women as emotionally unstable, unable to handle in a rational manner negative truths about the risks to their health, that, in fact, they will become neurotics. It is the old tradition going back to Alvarez and much further which established that the female has, by virtue of her biology, a propensity for hysteria, a belief that has likely lead to an excessive number of hysterectomies in women to prevent them from becoming emotional cripples.

It is not difficult to find cases reported in the media about the deaths of young people that are particularly tinged with a diagnosis of anxiety neurosis. Subsequent to Pauline Buchan's sensational trial, two young Canadian women died from complications evidently linked to oral contraceptives. On April 30, 1982, Carol Rosenberg, a university student, died from a pulmonary embolism. This young woman reported symptoms of shortness of breath, rapid heart beat, exhaustion and fainting.[115] It can be seen at a glance that these symptoms, attributed to the contraceptives Carol was taking, are identical to those of a cardiovascular nature found in MVP. Three days before her death, four doctors who examined this young woman failed to diagnose a pulmonary embolism. Her x-rays had shown abnormalities, dilated pulmonary arteries and a raised diaphragm. As in Margo's case, one doctor diagnosed viral infection or "flu" and attributed Carol's symptoms to neurosis or anxiety over her examinations.[116]

A month before Carol's death, another young woman, Catherine Fitzpatrick, from Ottawa, died from the same cause. Once again, the symptoms, including chest pain, were related not to the pill but seemingly to endogenous anxiety in that Catherine was treated for "back spasms" and told not to worry.[117] The overriding question here is whether or not these two women had MVP but, apart from that very real possibility, which only a thorough and accurate pathological report could verify, what should be stressed in these two tragic deaths, is that doctors must stop regarding symptoms, associated with the cardiovascular system, as indicative of anxiety or neurosis, especially in women, as was obviously a factor here.

The spectre of psychoneurosis, manifesting as hypochondria, panic attacks or endogenous anxiety, unfortunately plays a very significant part in the doctor-patient relationship. It determines what kind of prevention and treatment of complications, if any, are instituted. Underlying disease is not likely to be addressed if the symptoms are regarded as psychoneurotic in origin. Whenever there are symptoms related to the cardiovascular system, neurosis rears its ugly head so to speak, especially in young people. Unless a patient has heart disease that can no longer be disguised with diagnoses of unfitness, or in the past soldier's heart, weightgain from lack of exercise, or some other popular diagnostic scapegoat, such as late developing asthma, that the public accepts, a doctor is not likely to tell the patient of heart failure. A very sad story was told to me recently of a young woman, aged 42, who suddenly, within one year, developed, what the doctor diagnosed as a cardiomyopathy. The patient was not told she was extremely ill, in fact, dying, even though her husband reported that he had to prop her up in bed at night because she was drowning in her own fluid, as he put it. For many months, the doctor told them she was simply gaining weight from eating too much and not exercising though the husband protested vigorously that she ate very little. She, of course, could not exercise because of her extreme SOB. The woman was eventually told that she required a heart transplant but now refuses to accept this. Margo was not told she was dying until the moment she was wheeled to the operating room. If the patient has symptoms, especially those of MVP, but is not told they are related to an underlying heart disease, that patient will have anxiety which arises from not knowing and, therefore, from a lack of control. As someone so wisely said to me, if the chest pain, tachyrhythmias, cold, blue hands, SOB, dizziness, fatigue, fainting were indeed caused by anxiety why do all anxious people, even those without prolapse, not have these same symptoms of a cardiovascular nature.

Hypochondria or neurosis was a feature in the medical histories of two very well known performing artists, Glenn Gould and Maria Callas, and raises some pertinent questions about their unexpected, premature deaths. Their egocentricities were regarded generally as evidence of obsession with their health, neurosis or hypochondria. One may recall Callas' notoriously frequent cancellations and public tantrums and Glenn Gould's predilection for wearing gloves when he played and scarves and overcoats in hot weather, according to a friend of mine who was his schoolmate.

However both these famous people had evidence of organic disease and of general ill health. Even more interesting is the possibility that they had MVP. In the case of Callas, there is the familial factor of "heart trouble". A sister was known to have some sort of recognized cardiac disease.[118] Although there was some suggestion that Callas committed suicide, the final medical decision appears to have been a coronary embolism or heart attack.[119] Certain physical features of MVP were present in the singer, a high arched palate, deformities of the thoracic cage, such as an unusually long rib cage, long arms relative to her height and long, thin fingers or arachnodactyl[120] as well as extreme myopia.[121] These skeletal abnormalities are characteristic of MVP [122] and, when combined with myopia and a high arched palate, increase the chances of MVP to 60 percent.[123] The singer was also known to have chronic low blood pressure.[124] A fall in blood pressure in the standing position or orthostatic hypotension is a characteristic of MVP. Photographs of Callas reveal other physical characteristics found with MVP or one of the associated connective tissue diseases. For instance, she appears to have had a high, rounded rib cage, which, like the high arched palate may also have contributed to her great gifts. Both pectus carinatum or the pigeon breast and its opposite, the indented sternum, pectus excavatum, as well as prominent ears which Callas had, are found in MVP and associated diseases such as Turner's Syndrome[125], a disease characterized by infertility caused by a chromosomal defect that adversely affects the reproductive system. The latter may explain Callas' infertility. According to Meneghini she had early menopause at the age of 34.[126] MVP, itself, is associated with infertility. Of 71 women who were having gynecologic treatment and a cardiac exam at a fertility clinic in New Orleans, 96 percent had MVP.[127] Long after the famous weight loss which transformed the singer into the typical asthenic looking individual with prolapse, Callas's photographs showed ankle edema which could point to early heart failure from either mitral and/or tricuspid regurgitation which would also predispose her to embolism.

But did Callas have yet another complication known to occur in MVP? She was frequently unwell during her singing career with fatigue and febrile illnesses related to the upper respiratory tract. One of these bouts, when she was more ill than at other times, lasted two months in May and June of 1949, and was characterized by fatigue, exhaustion, extreme weight loss and gauntness of facial features, a temperature spiking to 100° F each afternoon, cough, and what she, herself, described in her letters as "strange unremitting headache" and skin blemishes. This illness was diagnosed as "flu" or viral infection and oral antibiotics were given for several months.[128] Such symptoms could have been those of IE which would leave the singer with further damage to a pre-existing slight valvular lesion such as MVP. Callas' physicians considered her "crazy"[129], and her frequent complaints of this nature were often taken for hypochondria. At the time of her sudden death, she complained of similar symptoms, a malaise with very low blood pressure,[130] which could suggest a recurrence of an unhealed IE and possibly the embolic complications that lead to her death in much the same way the athlete, described in my introduction, died from a coronary occlusion caused by IE, manifesting solely in this way or did she die from a coronary embolism issuing from the mitral valve as in the case at the Tygerberg Hospital described in the South African medical literature.

The Canadian pianist, Glenn Gould, died from a cerebral embolism or stroke, yet there are some facts surrounding his death which raise questions. It is curious that he was said to have primary hypertension or high blood pressure as a family inheritance[131] when, in fact, his mother died in advanced age and his father, at the time of this writing, is still living. Essential hypertension, unrelated to anything else, generally does not become a problem until the age of sixty or even older. Gould died just after he turned fifty. Can his unexpected, premature death be explained solely on the basis of a primary hypertension? Barnett and colleagues have said that while MVP should be considered as the underlying cause in stroke in patients under 45, this condition should be diligently sought in older patients who die suddenly of stroke.[132]

Gould, like Callas, after her weight loss, was asthenic looking. He had the long arms and spidery fingers of a Marfan's individual and was tall, gangly or lanky, as Klein had described the typical MVP person. Such physical characteristics may acount for why he preferred such a low chair to play the piano. Furthermore, he may have had Raynaud's phenomenon since he had cold hands and some circulatory problem which made him soak his hands for lengthy periods of time prior to performance. Patients with Raynaud's phenomenon are known to do this in order to restore colour and warmth to their fingers. This action, like the wearing of gloves to play the piano, or in hot weather, was regarded as hypochondriacal or eccentric but may have, in fact, been the indication of a genuine disease.

While Gould's biographers have maintained that he inherited primary hypertension and that this caused his death by stroke, there are renal authorities who have shown that there must be a specific etiology for essential hypertension and that this cause is the kidney. There may be functional or structural abnormalities or a glomerulonephritis. Medical evidence does not exist for relating hypertension to "excessive sodium ingestion, emotional stress or obesity"[133] or even diet. However, hypertension is associated with hyperadrenergic abnormalities or excessive sympathetic nervous system stimulation as well as Raynaud's phenomenon, secondary to pulmonary hypertension, both of which are found in MVP patients.

Gould was being treated with several drugs that affect the nervous system, including Valium, the anxiolytic Librax, an anticholinergic drug that acts on the parasympathetic nervous system, and Stelazine[134] which is used in the treatment of psychosis and, since it can cause tachycardia, should be given only with certain precautions to patients with heart disease. Obviously there was some attempt to address a problem of a nervous or psychiatric nature.

The health facts leading up to his death also suggest an underlying cardiac disease such as MVP and possibly the complication of IE. Gould, like Callas and, many people with MVP, suffered from several episodes of "flu" like illnesses with fever and upper respiratory symptoms. In the summer of 1958, on one of his extended tours, he suffered from a particularly prolonged febrile illness which was diagnosed as a flu or virus with concentration in the upper respiratory tract and the bronchioles and was characterized by night sweats with high temperatures to 101°F that spiked in the evening. Gould recorded a general unwell feeling or malaise at that time. During this illness, there was also associated kidney involvement with symptoms of back pain. Gould was prescribed bed rest on a non-protein diet in an effort to heal the kidneys according to his biographer, Otto Friedrich.[135] Was this in fact a strep infection or a strep viridans IE superimposed on an existing cardiac disease with prolapsed valves which went unrecognized as IE can?

Throughout his life he appears to have been treated for symptoms in association with the heart or kidneys though some people might say that the involvement of these two organs was secondary to the hypertension. Hypertension occurs in both cardiac and renal disease[136] and, in glomerulonephritis, which is always associated with IE, hypertension occurs in 90 percent of patients.[137] Gould took both anti-hypertensive medications and diuretics, hydrochlorothiazide which are used to remove fluid from the body in cases of heart failure and kidney impairment, and was troubled with symptoms that could be both cardiac and renal in origin.[138]

In fact, Gould was treated with a vast array of drugs for disease in addition to drugs for anxiety or neurosis, even psychosis,[139] information about which can be found in the CPS, and the impression is that he could not find help for his mysterious symptoms and so consulted several physicians. However, the drugs he was taking imply a diagnosis was made each time, unless such drugs were given as anxiolytic measures, just as I was given propranolol, digoxin and diuretics. All of these drugs Gould was taking are prescription items and, therefore, had to be given on the basis of a physician's decision. In addition to the anti-hypertensive and diuretic drugs, Gould took Zyloprim or allopurinol[140] which is used in the treatment of gout which he was said to have though it usually manifests in an acute way. However, it was said that he had only mild arthritic pain in his fingers. According to textbooks on internal medicine, colchicine is "the only treatment for acute gout of a specific diagnostic value."[141] This means that, if a doctor wants to be sure a patient has gout, he would begin a trial of colchicine. But Gould did not appear to have taken this drug, even though gout was not a definitive diagnosis in his case.

Given Gould's history of febrile illnesses and the involvement of the kidneys, it is not unlikely that he had a nephritis. When the glomerular function is impaired, uric acid solutes cannot be filtered out of the blood at the same rate as in a healthy person.[142] Therefore, gout is also found in glomerulonephritis which is initiated by a streptococcal infection and maintained by immunological stimulation.

The possibility arises then of a combination of underlying cardiac and renal disease, IE and GN, or a classic case of Libman's bacteria free stage of endocarditis with continued immunological damage. Arthritic pain or myalgias, as already discussed, are often an indicator of either rheumatic fever (RF) or IE in the right setting. An indication that Gould did, in fact, have some kind of underlying cardiac disease, likely the common MVP, is in the fact that he took Inderal or propranolol which, as I have shown, is a drug frequently prescribed for MVP patients for "palpitations" or other more serious arrhythmias. If a doctor considers the palpitations to be of an anxiolytic nature, as Austin did in my case, then the underlying cardiac disease will not likely be addressed. Gould was also taking tetracycline, a bacteriostatic drug that can mask a serious infection, as it could have done in Margo's case, since it keeps the bacteria under control but does not destroy it. The same could be said for chloromycetin, an antibacterial drug, which the CPS warns should not be used to treat influenza (flu), colds, infections of the throat, in other words, trivial, self-limiting viral infections. The use of these antibacterial and bacteriostatic drugs, as well as Resteclin, an anti-fungal drug which is no longer used, suggest that Gould must have had some ongoing bacterial infection unless one has to assume viral infection for which he would have been incorrectly treated since such antimicrobials do not attack viruses. A combination of all these drugs could confuse the picture and certainly disguise a serious endocardial infection or, give rise to mutant strains, not easily detected in the laboratory, of more common bacteria.

Towards the end of his life, at the time of his death, he suffered, as Callas had, from a flu-like illness, similar to the lengthy one of 1958.[143] Was this a recurring IE and GN? He recorded many signs that could indicate IE in his notebooks, for example shaking chills, night sweats and nocturia, which could be associated with heart failure or chronic renal disease, or, possibly, with diuretics if he were in fact taking them at this time, though it is unlikely that, if properly advised, he would take these drugs before going to bed. As well, he recorded high temperatures, myalgias, irregular heart beat, tachycardia, which he described as a hammering in his chest, pain and tightness in his chest, both complaints of MVP patients, irregular pulse, abdominal pain, gastrointestinal disturbances and chronic sore throat. Curiously, he recorded spasms, twitches and stiffness, all of which could be indicative of neurological complications of IE. He was said to be gaunt-looking, which may suggest weight loss, a non-specific symptom of IE, though he also reported weight gain, which could be fluid retention in association with heart or kidney failure. Observers noted that he had the appearance of a sick and rapidly aging man, though his illness was interpreted as a virus and his massive cerebral embolism as an isolated event.

As I have shown IE is an embolic disease and, in prolonged cases, cerebral complications are frequent. One must ask whether Gould's death was in any way the result of a fatal cerebral embolism in association with an undiagnosed IE and underlying, unknown MVP? Or even a late occuring cerebral embolism from a previous IE. Brain embolism is essentially a manifestation of heart disease and does not usually occur in its absence[144] and is, as in the case of MVP patients, usually caused by a serious arrhythmia, whether that is atrial fibrillation or some other chronic dysrhythmia. These are questions which cannot be answered without a thorough pathologist's report and they are likely never to be answered since public access to certain of his papers has been "restricted", and the papers in question, including his own notes of his symptoms at the time of his death, are those dealing with his health.[145]

Arrhythmias and Sudden Death

The whole question of sudden death in the young and middle aged requires investigation to determine whether MVP is responsible. Are there, in fact, warning signs which identify the patient at risk long before the fatal event but which may be overlooked if the patient's complaints are viewed as neurotic. In the U.S., sudden death is the cause in two-thirds of 600,000 deaths occurring annually from heart disease. The usual precipitating factor is a cardiac arrhythmia, specifically ventricular tachycardia.[146] In Canada, deaths from cardiovascular disease have averaged around 80,000 annually from 1981 to 1986, when the number was 79,259. This figure represents approximately 44 percent of the total number of deaths annually (184,224 in 1986) in Canada, an astonishingly high number. There were 47,461 deaths from ischaemic heart disease in that year in Canada, of which 27,072 were from MI. As well, in 1986 there were 2,602 deaths from dysrhythmias and 1,822 unspecified cardiac arrests.[147] MVP is the most common underlying cardiac disorder and, therefore, it is not unreasonable to ask how many of the sudden deaths, deaths from MI and deaths from dysrhythmias in both countries were related to an unrecognized MVP?

It has been suggested throughout the medical literature that, in cases of sudden death, where there is no history of actual cardiac disease, indicated by a murmur and/or cardiac enlargement, that MVP should be routinely searched for at autopsy. It is important to stress again that cardiac enlargement, which remains within normal limits, may not be recognized in a MVP patient if the heart, to begin with, is smaller than normal for size, age and sex, and no ongoing documentation over a period of years exists to prove that the heart has actually increased in size.

MVP patients commonly suffer from cardiac arrhythmias and, more rarely, from ventricular tachycardia which is a precipitating factor in sudden death. Such arrhythmias have been documented on echocardiogram (EKG) and have served as premonitory signs of fatal events. For example, MVP patients are known to have EKG abnormalities that might herald sudden death, such as inverted T waves and prolonged Q-T interval[148] as well as abnormally low levels of blood potassium which can precipitate cardiac arrest.[149]

It is appropriate to understand briefly here how the electrocardiogram records the electrical activity of the heart. In the posterior wall of the right atrium, at the point where the superior vena cava enters the heart, there is a mass of fibers called the sino-atrial node or SA node. This bundle of fibers connects with the ANS and is the normal pacemaker of the heart that begins the cardiac cycle and sets the heart rate. The electrical stimulus from the SA node positively charges the cells of the atria causing them to contract. The electrical impulse spreads in a manner similar to the wave formation created when a pebble is thrown into water in that each successive wave provokes the next. The cellular change from negative to positive is called depolarization and is represented graphically on the EKG as a P wave. The impulse from the atria spreads to another node, the AV or atrial-ventricular node. A pause follows, before its stimulation, in which the blood moves from the atria to the ventricles through the mitral and tricuspid valves. The ventricles become depolarized or positively charged and this electrical activity forces them to contract and thus pump the blood into the aorta and the pulmonary artery. Ventricular contraction, on the EKG, is called the QRS complex. There follows a flat segment in the electrocardiographic picture which is called the ST segment and, if that is depressed, as it was during my illness, it may represent ventricular strain. The ST segment is followed by the T wave which represents the repolarization or negative charging of the ventricles so that they can again be stimulated by the series of events beginning with the SA node's stimulus. This complete cardiac cycle of P wave, QRS complex and T wave with the measured pauses, such as the ST segment, is repeated endlessly throughout the life of the human being. This is only a brief and general description of how the electrical activity of the heart operates.[150]

Sudden death of MVP patients has been reported in the medical literature, in particular when this disease is found in other members of the patient's family.[151] An arrhythmia is generally the cause. In 1976, Koch and Hancock's follow-up studies of the natural progression of MVP over a ten year period showed there was a 12.5 percent incidence of sudden death, 5 of 40 patients.[152] These patients were 9, 30, 32, 50 and 64, and three of them had multiple premature ventricular beats. By 1987, it was established, from an analysis of the literature dealing with arrhythmias in MVP patients, that many potentially dangerous arrhythmias occur frequently in these patients, such as atrial premature complexes or contractions which have been recorded in 35-90 percent of patients, atrial tachycardia in 3-32 percent, ventricular premature complexes or contractions in 58-89 percent of MVP patients in study groups and, in adults, there is a 43 to 56 percent incidence of complex ventricular arrhythmias and ventricular tachycardia in 5 to 21 percent of patients.[153]

There is, as with every aspect of MVP, considerable controversy over the seriousness of cardiac arrythmia in the MVP syndrome and its actual link with sudden death. Kligfield et al from the cardiology division at The New York Hospital-Cornell Medical Center have conducted valuable research in the area of cardiac arrhythmia and MVP. These researchers are of the opinion that the most definitive proof that an arrhythmia is responsible for sudden death in the MVP syndrome comes from the fact that "the only abnormality in survivors of cardiac arrest and in patients referred for management of refractory, symptomatic complex ventricular arrhythmias" is MVP.[154] If this is, in fact, the case, it may be of tremendous significance in view of the statistics in Canada, for example, that showed 1,822 deaths from cardiac arrest in 1986.

According to Kligfield and co-workers,[155] MVP patients with lethal arrhythmias usually have what is called a "depressed ejection fraction" at rest. The ejection fraction is a mathematical computation which indicates how well the heart works as a pump, how much blood is put out during a cardiac cycle. A depressed ejection fraction points to an insufficient volume of blood being ejected from the heart into the aorta and the rest of the body during a complete cardiac cycle. The end result is that blood that should be pumped out remains in the ventricles and, therefore, the heart dilates and eventually the muscle thickens or hypertrophies from a prolonged effort to meet the oxygen demands of the body. And, if blood remains in the ventricle, there is a tendency for coagulation and thus the formation of thrombi. Patients who have died have had LVEF of 45 percent and a RVEF of 29 percent, and Kliegfield et al say that death occurs in such patients with depressed ejection fraction as the result of a sudden arrhythmic episode or from acute failure of the ventricle to pump out enough blood. Normal ejection fraction is said to be around 50 percent.

In fact, it is well known that "heart failure from any cause", hence from severe mitral and/or tricuspid regurgitation with dilatation of the heart, "may initiate atrial fibrillation".[156]

Some researchers have attempted to determine statistically the exact nature of this risk of arrhythmia to MVP patients, but the results remain somewhat uncertain. Unmanageable and dangerous ventricular arrhythmias are said to be about four to twenty times more common among MVP patients than among those without according to the calculations of Kligfield and group.[157] Other recent studies in *The New England Journal of Medicine* in 1985 of Nishimura, McGoon and co-workers[158] suggest an annual mortality rate of 40 per 10,000 among patients with few or no symptoms of their MVP, and when the large MVP population is taken into consideration, this becomes a significant figure. This figure is twice that for sudden death in the general adult population. It also suggests that there must be a higher rate among those with more pronounced symptoms.

The general physician should thus be on the alert for MVP patients who could be at risk of sudden death, but the situation is not likely to change until MVP itself is regarded as important and the symptoms are no longer attributed automatically to neurosis, specifically arrhythmias that are passed off as a few insignificant palpitations or a nuisance as Austin called my episodes of paroxysmal atrial tachycardia with heart beat in the 200-250 range. In 1984, Cheitlin and Byrd[159] provided a definitive portrait of the MVP patient at greatest risk of sudden death:

> The young or middle-aged woman with a late systolic or pansystolic murmur, with or without a nonejection click (usually symptomatic), with an abnormal ECG (most often with ST-T wave changes and occasionally with prolonged QT interval), and with multiple arrhythmias on ambulatory ECG and marked mitral valve prolapse, usually of both leaflets, on the echocardiogram.

Cheitlin and Byrd's description proves that patients at risk of sudden death can be identified and that even those with mild regurgitation, as evidenced by a LSM, are at risk. While propranolol is likely the drug of choice to minimize the more common arrhythmias, other strategies must be adopted to prevent the more serious dysrrhythmias. Prevention of a LSM or a PSM is, of course, the ideal measure. This means further investigation of the pathogenesis of prolapsed or billowing valves and, in my view, intensive research into the relationship between MVP and IE.

Researchers have isolated unquestionably a subset of patients within the MVP syndrome who are at greatest risk of sudden death and attempted to evaluate that risk. Logically, they are those with mitral regurgitation (MR), and the risk appears dependent upon the severity of the regurgitation. According to Kligfield and his group at the Cornell Medical Centre in New York, many of whom were involved in the long term Framingham study of MVP, the risk of sudden death could be as much as "50 to 100 fold greater in patients with MVP who have MR."[160] These are very frightening odds.

More dangerous arrhythmias have been found more frequently in patients with MVP and MR. All this effort on the part of researchers points clearly to the fact that MVP should not be considered as a cardiac neurosis, that there is justifiable grounds for serious investigation. On the subject of the importance of sudden death in the MVP syndrome, Barlow, whose studies provided the turning point in MVP research, said in his book, *Perspectives on the Mitral Valve*:

> In 1970, we subjected 12 patients with the primary BML (Billowing Mitral Leaflet) Syndrome to submaximal effort test and detected multifocal ventricular extrasystoles in three. We therefore emphasized the importance of exercise in precipitating premature ventricular contractions and warned of a risk of sudden death, should multifocal ventricular ectopy develop. At that time, sudden death was not a recognized complication of the BML syndrome ... however, numerous studies on BML and MVP, as well as our own increased experience, revealed that the BML syndrome was highly prevalent.[161]

Our age is obsessed with fitness and preaches that exercise is the magic route to health, but for those individuals with unsuspected arrhythmias and MVP, exercise may be dangerous. As stated elsewhere in this book, exercise may make you fit but it will not make you healthy. I have no doubt now that the advice which Dr. Austin once gave me, at the time of my episodes of arrhythmia during a daily staggering work load of restoring my house, was neither professionally sound nor safe. The ancient Romans believed in the truism, in media res, or a moderate course in everything. The MVP patient may do well to heed this advice.

MVP and Pregnancy

Although MVP is unanimously acclaimed the most important disease of this century, the public knows less about it than about many other disorders. Its risks, its connections with other well established conditions offer the medical profession extensive territory for worthwhile investigation, but an obsession with psychoneurotic studies will only impede the progress towards understanding this common disease. There are very few reports, for example, on MVP and pregnancy. That from Rayburn and Fontana of the Ohio State University in Columbus, in 1981 appears to have been the first in the obstetric literature.[162] They described a 25 year old patient who experienced CHF, premature labour and preeclampsia (toxemia associated with headache), proteinuria and increased blood pressure. Although the authors pointed out that this patient's CHF was completely reversible with no significant effect on the fetus or the mother, the long term effects on both are simply not known. The authors suggest that possibly the patient had an underlying cardiomyopathy, a frequently advanced theory to explain the nature of the tissue abnormalities and the symptoms in the MVP syndrome, in particular chest pain. They also suggest that the therapy used to treat the premature labour can precipitate heart failure when an underlying disease is unknown. However, it is also possible that the degree of regurgitation in this patient may have been more severe than was suspected. If she, in fact, had hemodynamically significant regurgitation, failure would be more likely during pregnancy when there is an increase in blood volume which, according to these researchers, accounts for the changes in the click and murmur. The murmur, for example, becomes louder and longer. It is, therefore, not inconceivable that a heart, compromised by valvular damage, would be unable to handle such an increase in blood volume.

A significant number, 10 or 24 percent, of deliveries in this study were cesarean sections because of "failure of the labour to progress, breech presentation, repeat cesarean section, or suspected fetal distress."[163] While the authors reassure that complications appear to be well tolerated and not appreciably greater than in patients with no cardiac disorder, more statistical evidence is required before any unassailable conclusions on pregnancy in the MVP patient are formed. Identifying the underlying MVP is imperative if drugs are to be chosen safely for dealing with such complications in pregnancy as premature labour or toxemia.

CHF is not the only complication reported in pregnancy in MVP patients. In 1988, a case was reported for the first time in the journal, *Obstetrics and Gynecology*,[164] of TIA in association with pregnancy and MVP. According to the writers, stroke is rarely seen during pregnancy and has been recorded only once in 26,099 live births in Rochester, Minnesota during more than a twenty year period from 1955 to 1979. At 26 weeks gestation, the woman suffered diabetes and at 37.5 weeks, a loss of consciousness lasting four minutes with no recollection of the episode. The thromboembolism was related to the underlying MVP, and the woman experienced transient weakness in her left hand at the time that labour commenced. The patient's delivery was, as in the other study, by cesarean section. There was no complication in the delivery, and the patient's mild paralysis subsided almost immediately. She was treated with aspirin, 325 mg twice a day for three months, to prevent a recurrence of TIA. During a second pregnancy she received the same treatment up to two weeks before delivery by cesarean section. The woman then made the choice of using contraceptives. Such cases underline the fact that investigation is required in this area. Both these reports recommend the use of ABP during delivery in MVP patients with mitral regurgitation.

MVP and Sleep Disturbances

MVP should be diligently sought in any incompletely understood condition, especially if there are symptoms or physical characteristics associated with the cardiovascular system. Recent studies have shown that such apparently innocent symptoms as drowsiness, narcolepsy (attacks of deep sleep of short duration) and sleep apnea occur frequently in MVP patients. Sleep apnea is defined as a transient, involuntary suspension of respiration due to a decrease of carbon dioxide tension in the blood. The Clinical Research Center at Ohio State University College of Medicine reported on 120 patients with primary sleep disorders.[165] The results were astounding. Half of 35 patients, or 49 percent, with narcolepsy and 58 percent of the 24 patients with excessive drowsiness had MVP. Of the remaining 61 patients with sleep apnea, 20 percent had MVP. Sleep apnea, the study said, "leads to lowered partial pressure of oxygen in the blood, which might trigger ventricular premature beats if it got low enough." In fact, dangerous ventricular dysrhythmias were found in 26 percent of their MVP patients with sleep apnea on 24 hour ECG Holter Monitor, though the authors cautioned that the dysrhythmias could not be proven to be associated exclusively with the sleep apnea. Nevertheless, these figures are very significant when we recall that, in most cases of sudden death, the cause is ventricular tachycardia, and sleep apnea may well be implicated in sudden death from dysrhythmias. Dr. Nancy Snyderman of the American College of Surgeons recommended the avoidance of such things as alcohol and other depressants but said that such antidepressants as imipramine had been used with success in sleep apnea patients.[166] If MVP patients are prone to sleep apnea, this could be one more reason why a doctor might prescribe imipramine or another antidepressant which would only add to the complications in the syndrome. It is interesting to recall how frequently the patients of Da Costa, Lewis and others reported rapid heart beat at night or other disturbances in sleep patterns or an inability to lie on the left side without provoking rapid heart beat, a symptom which many MVP patients have personally reported to me and which I myself have experienced.

Sleep apnea, unassociated with MVP, is being studied in infants. Dr. Bohlman from the University of Maryland Medical Schools advises that children and infants should be checked for sleep apnea and, in particular, those infants who die from Sudden Infant Death Syndrome (SIDS).[167] If none of the usual complications exist in these children, that is breathing difficulties from enlarged tonsils, small and receding jaws, abnormal muscle control of the tongue and pharynx or a central abnormality governing the muscles of respiration,[168] is it possible that they could have an unsuspected cardiac abnormality, specifically MVP, which doctors find difficult to diagnose in infants? According to the Merck Manual, 10-15 percent of autopsies in SIDS cases do, in fact, reveal an unsuspected cardiovascular or CNS abnormality, the latter disorder known to be at the basis of excessive adrenalin or catecholamine production in MVP patients. But, more surprisingly, in that group, there is also "evidence of overwhelming infection".[169] Is it too tenuous to suggest that such an infection could be unsuspected IE imposed on an equally unsuspected prolapsed valve? After all, as Kaplan points out, in children under the age of two, the pathologist, not the clinician, usually diagnoses an IE.[170]

The Pathogenesis of MVP

The cause of the tissue aberrations which produce valves that billow, bulge, balloon or prolapse still remains a mystery and is a matter of some controversy. As a group of researchers from Israel expressed the problem: naming a disease is not understanding it nor explaining its pathophysiologic mechanisms.[171] The research into the pathogenesis of MVP is scanty. Running through the medical literature is the suggestion that MVP is, like mitral stenosis, an acquired disease rather than a congenital disorder.

Some researchers have attempted to explain the prolapsed valves in terms of a genetic problem involving embryonic mesenchymal tissue that is a pool of undifferentiated cells. From that source, connective tissue of many different kinds develops, forming the supportive part of bones, cartilage, breasts, and the various adipose, elastic, fibrous connective and lymphatic tissues. Connective tissue contains the supportive protein component of collagen. One group of researchers, Rosenberg et al, from The University of Michigan, has proposed that, in the early stages of pregnancy, there is abnormal development of the mesenchymal cells which are responsible for the formation of the heart, smooth muscles, blood vessels and blood. Rosenberg et al say the disturbances in the growth pattern occur in the sixth week of fetal life when the mitral valve "undergoes embryological differentiation"[172] and assumes its ultimate form. At that time, the stage is set for adult breast development which is also dependent upon mesenchymal cells. According to these authors, poorly developed breasts, or hypomastia, are related to prolapsed mitral valves and are often a clue to the presence of this cardiac defect.

As I've pointed out, an abnormally small heart may correlate with underdeveloped breasts and smaller chest dimensions in men and women and, likewise, may offer a clue to MVP. In the older literature, subnormal heart size was frequently noted in patients with Soldier's Heart, Irritable Heart and NCA, the precursors of MVP, and with orthostatic hypotension which is a common symptom of MVP. Starr and Jonas back in 1940[173] found, like the moderns, Gaffney, Wooley and others, that such patients with what they called "functional" heart problems and small hearts, "most frequently in the lower half of the normal range" or "definitely subnormal" had low cardiac output and insufficient return of blood to the heart.

Although Rosenberg et al do not comment upon heart size in the MVP syndrome, it seems logical that a mesenchymal cell abnormality could prevent the heart, as well as the breasts, from attaining its full, normal size, especially if it is crowded by an indented sternum. These writers pointed out that the thoracic cage and vertebral column, like the mitral valve and breasts, also begin their differentiation in the sixth week of fetal life, and the defect of sternal indentation or pectus excavatum is established at this point in time. The smaller chest dimensions and skeletal deformities found in MVP may in some way curtail the growth of the heart.

According to Rosenberg and his group, "mesenchymal dysplasia may be the unifying concept that explains many of the associated conditions seen with mitral valve prolapse."[174] In MVP and many of the connective tissue diseases, the acid mucopolysaccharides in the spongiosa portion of the mitral valve increase, crowding out the sturdier fibrosa component composed primarily of dense collagen, thus undermining the structural supports of the mitral valve. Some of these diseases linked with MVP are Marfan's Syndrome, Turner's Syndrome, myocarditis, Ehlers-Danlos Syndrome, lupus erythematosus, muscular dystrophy, osteogenesis imperfecta, Wolff-Parkinson-White Syndrome, pseudoxanthoma elasticum and Noonan's Syndrome, to name a few, an explanation of which is impossible in this text.[175] Those people who have these diseases should also be investigated for MVP.

Some other researchers, however, would disagree with Rosenberg and co-workers. They are of the opinion that the abnormalities which occur in the sixth week of fetal development may be caused, not by something within the maternal environment but by something introduced from outside. In 1976, O'Rourke and Crawford drew attention to laboratory studies which showed that the ingestion of a certain kind of foodstuff, lathyrus peas, produced myxomatous degeneration of the valve leaflets and skeletal aberrations in laboratory rats. Such peas contain a foreign chemical or toxin, beta amino-proprionitrile. The authors postulated that prolapse could be "the result of fetal exposure to toxic agents during the early part of pregnancy."[176]

Earlier, in Chapter Three, I discussed the question of whether IE itself produced the myxomatous degeneration that causes the valves to become heavy, thickened and floppy after repeated mild episodes until the prolapse or billowing is severe enough to permit regurgitation of blood backwards into the atrium during systole. If the introduction of a foreign chemical can, in fact, produce myxomatous degeneration of valvular tissue, one wonders if bacterial endotoxin, which is composed of certain substances including polysaccharide derived from the cell wall and released with decomposition of the microorganism, could do the same thing. It is a question then of whether, during the crucial early weeks of pregnancy when the fetal heart and valves are forming, the mother suffers a transient bacteremia or a mild IE of the sort Libman described, in relation to dental work, for example. MVP, most likely the "silent" variety, may or may not be present. A bacterial infection at this time could alter the collagen content of the valve by increasing the acid mucopolysaccharides through deposition or accumulation of the bacterial endotoxin antigenic complex in the developing valves. A second question would concern whether or not these products of bacterial decomposition, the endotoxins, can cross the placental barrier. Since there is already acid-mucopolysaccharide in the valvular composition, polysaccharide endotoxin may not be perceived by the barrier censors as foreign. The presence of either the bacteria or the endotoxins in the blood stream would stimulate platelet aggregation and thus the adherence of these polysaccharide end products to the developing mitral valve to commence the myxomatous process. Alternatively, one might ask if the developing fetus is in some way affected by immunological changes in the mother in response to a transient bacteremia or a mild IE.

Although researchers have discussed the possibility of injurious mechanisms producing the changes in the collagen content of prolapsed valves, they have not, apart from the studies on toxins of lathyrus peas, considered that this injurious factor may be a disease mechanism, a bacterial endotoxin. Some researchers believe that the valvular injury is acquired, rather than genetic, and is mechanical in nature. This view of the pathogenesis of prolapsed valves is called "the response to injury hypothesis".[177] It is thought that minimal structural alterations in the valvular parts, which are not explained, exist at birth, create stress during systole and lead to damage of the healthy collagen core of the mitral valve. The explanation for these slight structural changes in the chordae tendineae and leaflets is said to be, however, a genetic one and, therefore, the injury hypothesis may co-exist with the theory that an abnormal development of the mesenchymal cells is responsible for the valvular abnormalities. It is not inconceivable that an undersized heart, its growth having been restricted at a critical time by thoracic developmental abnormalities, may also play a part in the mechanical injury theory.

In the words of Joseph Perloff and John S. Child of the Cardiology Department at UCLA Center for the Health Sciences[178], the "response to injury hypothesis" poses a challenge to the idea of an isolated mesenchymal dysplasia.

> The primacy of a developmental defect of mitral connective tissue is challenged in favor of the "response to injury hypothesis". In a study of the types and characteristics of the collagens in normal and myxomatous human mitral valves, it was concluded that in the latter, the fibroblasts produced additional collagen (especially type III) similar in composition to tissues undergoing repair. Repair implies injury, and injury results in weakening of the central collagen core allowing leaflet expansion, chordal elongation, and annular dilatation. The "response to injury hypothesis" proposes that minor "normal" congenital variations in the architecture of the chordae tendineae and leaflets leave parts of the cusps relatively poorly supported . . . Disproportionate systolic stress on these relatively vulnerable, less well-supported segments of the tensor apparatus sets the stage for minor injury, repair, and recurrence of injury culminating in progressive collagen disruption, weakening, stretching, and expansion of the leaflets, chordae tendineae, and annulus recognized clinically as mitral valve prolapse.

This damage from wear and tear is seen to be perpetuated by the slight alterations in the valvular apparatus itself, followed by natural healing. With time, the valvular function would become significantly impaired. This is in line with the theory, already discussed, of the loss of supportive collagenous connective tissue because of the natural process of aging according to Ariela Pomerance.

However, the same changes take place when tissues are undergoing healing from injury caused by an inflammatory disease as from an injury caused by mechanical trauma as described by Perloff and Child. There are increases in the white, fibrous connective tissue, which is a kind of collagen, as part of the repairing or scarring process. The multiplication of fibroblasts to form the collagen fibers leads to thickening or fibrosis of the tissues. This is what is called scar tissue. This kind of connective tissue is different from that which forms the healthy collagen core that gives support to the valve itself. With repeated inflammatory episodes the reparative connective tissue thickens, becomes more dense and contracts and thus interferes with the function of the organ, specifically the valve leaflets, chordae and annulus. Pathologists have found fibrosis or scarring in prolapsed valves in association with healed vegetations from IE and this can be seen as the lumps and bumps that determine the degree of prolapse measured ultrasonically with the echocardiogram. This fibrosis exists side by side with the excessive mucopolysaccharides and may account, for instance, for the thickened, shortened chordae that are found alongside those that are stretched, long and thin from excessive acid muco-polysaccharide. Either disturbance in structure could lead to ruptured chordae. As explained earlier in this book, the mitral valve is composed of two kinds of tissues, the fibrosa, a collagenous or connective tissue, which lends support and shape to the valve, and the spongiosa, composed of acid mucopolysac-charides which proliferate in prolapsed valves. Instead of proposing that the spongiosa has increased, as many researchers believe, and that this involves a mesenchymal cell abnormality, Perloff and Child believe there is overgrowth, in response to the wear and tear of mechanical stress during systole, of the white, fibrous connective tissue of the healing process so that the normal healthy collagen core is eventually threatened. However, since increases in both fibrosis and acid mucopolysaccharides have been found in the presence of IE and prolapsed valves, one could ask if this injury that causes transformations in the normal healthy collagen content of the valve might not be IE, as was believed in the pre-antibiotic era.

It is these and many other questions about MVP that must be resolved. Rather than waste precious time and effort as well as financial resources on proving MVP is a neurotic disorder, it might be more useful to explore the old belief of the connection between pericarditis and the click-murmur syndrome that was so popular in the first half of this century! Efforts to disentangle the neurologic-biochemical-biological triangle of MVP are valuable but, when psychology is stressed at the expense of pathology, or, when the true "cries of the heart for help", as Obrastzow, in 1905,[179] so eloquently called the auscultatory sounds of cardiac disease, are mistaken for cardiac neurosis, the patient suffers. There is little benefit in undertaking studies primarily concerned with relating endogenous anxiety to MVP without analysing the etiologic role of stress in disease and without investigating the relationship of the biochemical abnormalities to the histological aberrations found in MVP.

Fortunately, there are medical scientists who are studying the myriad aspects of MVP and those who are boldly challenging the charge of endogenous anxiety or cardiac neurosis. There are those who are studying autonomic dysfunction and hyperadrenergy who reject the idea that anxiety is the cause. In 1981, Santos et al.,[180] like the older researchers, explained the symptoms of giddiness, lightheadedness, dizziness, syncope, as the "pathophysiologic mechanism" of orthostatic hypotension, that is a fall in blood pressure with postural change from the sitting to the standing position. In other words, the orthostatic hypotension itself, which may relate as Master said to the small heart, not stress, causes the symptoms and, clearly, in the view of Santos et al, there is underlying disease. These authors advise that orthostatic hypotension can be corrected with the use of beta-blockers such as propranolol or Inderal.

There are others who agree with Santos et al and who endeavor to correct the one hundred year old misconception even more emphatically. Coghlan and co-workers from The University of Alabama School of Medicine studied 600 symptomatic MVP patients and boldly declared that they were "far from neurotic", even though, like Wooley, Boudoulas, Gaffney and others, they attributed symptoms to hyperadrenergic activity.[181]

Like most other disease concepts, orthostatic hypotension is not new. Researchers had begun studying it years ago in the late thirties when it was said to occur in patients with Effort Syndrome or Soldier's Heart, Irritable Heart and NCA. In 1940, MacLean and Allen published a paper on Orthostatic Hypotension and Orthostatic Tachycardia, also known to accompany MVP, and determined that the problem was one of insufficient return of venous blood to the heart in the standing position[182] and, it follows, during exercise. This, once again, was the view of Master and others who attributed the problem to a smaller than normal heart.

In an interview reported in *The Journal of the American Medical Association*, Dr. Boudoulas declared that "in future we may be able to say that anxiety itself is due to a biochemical disorder."[183] However, there is a very significant difference between anxiety neurosis and stress. The stress of being without a job, of a financial crisis, of the loss of loved ones is very real and can lead to organic disease, which even Alvarez recognized, while neurosis always suggests a fictional element, that there is no cause for the anxiety, that it is fear of unknown, imaginary illness and that the symptoms are, therefore, psychosomatic.

A 1983 Australian study[184] reported that 103 MVP patients, who were given tests for neuroticism, the Eysenck Personality and the General Health Questionnaire, were found to have scores that were not different from those of the control group with other cardiac diseases or from those of patients in primary care centres. Of most importance was the observation that, in 50 patients with agoraphobia, **no prolapse** was found. Furthermore, the authors Hickey, Andrews and Wilcken, bravely criticized the diagnostic criteria of several prominent researchers, Pariser, Ventakesh and Kantor who claimed that the symptoms of MVP are related to chronic endogenous anxiety. Hickey et al found "a disturbing lack of detail" and inadequate evidence that MVP actually existed in all the patients in these studies. "The questionable accuracy of diagnosis of cases previously reported (i.e.MVP and chronic anxiety), and the present findings, based as they are on large, carefully diagnosed samples of patients, clearly refute the notion that there is an association between mitral valve prolapse and neurosis."[185] Such studies are of great benefit to millions of patients with MVP while screaming headlines in the press, "Panic — Sudden Waves of fear linked to a physical disorder" from which "more than a million Americans, most of them women" suffer[186], are not and would only cause further panic, while strengthening the doctor's view that women, in particular, are neurotic. Although Jane Brody, its author, does not specifically mention MVP, one of the doctors whom she interviews, Dr. Donald Klein, to whom I have already referred, has intensively studied agoraphobia in the MVP patient, and much research, as I have pointed out, concerns the relationship between panic disorder and MVP.

In a recent 1986 paper, "Prevalence of Anxiety Disorders in Patients with MVP", authors, Mazza et al, reviewed the efforts of researchers to link the cause of symptoms with the anxiety disorders.[187] This group logically claimed that, if the symptoms are caused by an impaired autonomic nervous system, then the treatment should be pharmacological rather than psychotherapeutic. These authors also criticized the evidence linking MVP and any of the anxiety disorders because such evidence was "in direct conflict with psychodynamic formulations of anxiety and phobic symptoms and this raises the question of the appropriateness of treatment based on these formulations."

What this means to me is that the researchers whom Mazza et al refer to are overlooking the psychological and emotional conditioning necessary for the formation of an anxiety neurosis. Mazza et al's patients with MVP and a control group without the condition were given tests for anxiety and depression according to a rating scale established by a psychiatrist and were also interviewed by a psychiatrist who lacked knowledge of the presence or absence of MVP. The data from these tests showed there was no appreciable difference between the MVP patients and the control group with respect to signs of panic or phobic disorder or anxiety neurosis. Mazza et al concluded that the argument to establish MVP as the primary etiology in the pathogenesis of anxiety neurosis is highly questionable. Before applying such titles as Hyperventilation Syndrome or Endogenous Anxiety Syndrome, doctors should reflect on the warnings of these researchers.

With the emphasis on the anxiety disorders, it is not surprising that there are some doctors who have gone so far as to question the value of using ABP to prevent IE in MVP patients, even though it has taken almost twenty years since the introduction of antibiotics to accept this proven preventative strategy. Some influential researchers, who have adopted to go against mainstream opinion on ABP and MVP, have said that "no prophylaxis and penicillin prophylaxis would result in a similar number of deaths."[188] But the conclusions of these writers are not based on the study of actual cases of MVP and IE but on predictions derived from their calculated estimates of the efficacy of certain regimens such as intramuscular (IM) injections of penicillin combined with oral administration from which they conclude prophylaxis would result in seven times more deaths than if there were no prophylaxis. They included deaths from reactions to the penicillin itself. But IM injections, which the AHA recommends only if the patient cannot take oral medication, may well be more risky since they may cause hemorrhage. A regimen of oral penicillin alone was not included. Conclusions such as this are, ultimately, predicated upon the opinion that IE is extremely rare in general and in the MVP syndrome in particular, though extensive research proves otherwise. The very first line of Lawrence Freedman's important book, *Infective Endocarditis and Other Intravascular Infections* states, "The most important example of intravascular infection is infective endocarditis (IE), a **common** (my italics) and serious disorder in man."[189] This was the opinion of Emanuel Libman, Horder, Glynn, Osler and others of the first fifty years of this century.

To bolster their argument, the opponents of this protection for MVP patients attempt to convince the medical establishment that "the prevalence of MVP and estimates of the risk of infective endocarditis are inflated" and they even ask whether, in fact, MVP and IE are related at all.[190] However, since the true etiologic relationship between IE and MVP, that is whether repeated episodes of IE, either treated with oral antibiotics or healing spontaneously, actually cause the floppy, ballooning valves, has not yet been established, discarding antibiotic protection could be a regressive and dangerous route. Patients with histories similar to mine should be studied. Some of the researchers who question the use of ABP in the MVP syndrome like to make the statement that the efficacy of ABP to prevent IE remains unproven, yet extensive animal research and repeated observations that individuals do improve with **early** treatment demonstrate that this protection does work. Such writers tend to see the whole issue as one of economics, the cost-benefit ratio. Oral prophylaxis is very expensive and IV ABP, such as Margo had to take because her prosthetic valve made her a very high risk patient, are not "cost-effective" at all they say. Costly to whom one asks? Whether it is private or socialized medicine, the patient pays the same as anyone else. And certainly the cost is greater to that individual who suffers further valvular damage and CHF or death as a result of IE! Such writers make these statements while candidly admitting that their "decision analyses" . . ."are obviously susceptible to challenge because they themselves are based upon assumptions that are at best **crude** estimates."[191] Such efforts on the part of researchers can only inspire fear in the MVP patient. The same can be said for the relationship between stroke, heart attack and MVP. This complication also requires further study. All practitioners, not just researchers writing for the medical journals, should be making observations about their patients with MVP. To give up now would jeopardize the knowledge that has accumulated so slowly about MVP. For-tunately, so far, the majority of research would disagree with the conclusions of these writers. However, what may be shaping up is another costly and protracted debate, like that of the past over mitral incompetence and, specifically, over the cardiovascular features of the syndrome now known as MVP, with little or no benefit for the MVP patient but, rather, significant danger. The cost benefit argument is used all too frequently. At my recent hospitalization in September of 1989 for a febrile illness, when I suggested that more than six sets of blood tests might have to be done in an effort to grow the microorganism from my blood, the internist argued that six sets had cost $180, and the hospital had to take the cost-benefit argument into consideration before doing more blood tests. This attitude was extremely offensive, particularly in view of my medical history of which he was aware. I pointed out, in Lawrence Freedman's book, with which he was not familiar, the recommendations of the standard 6-8 blood samples and Freedman's advice that up to twenty might have to be done if a positive culture cannot be easily obtained.[192] Is the patient's life not worth $180.00? I began to wonder if this was a little bit of propaganda to make Canadians think that the reason health care is imperfect is because there is not enough money in a socialized medical system and that we ought to lobby our government to permit privatization of medicine which the Canadian doctors want because it would give them the financial benefits of their American brothers.

It has taken 100 years to put science at the service of humanity in the matter of MVP but it may be only a brief period before the non-disease-neurotic architects erode that 100 year old foundation upon which the MVP patient's health and safety rests. Let us prevent doctors from throwing Barlow's gold back under the white reef into the deepest part of the ocean.

21

The Pied Pipers

I'm able,
By means of a secret charm to draw
All creatures living beneath the sun,
That creep or swim or fly or run,
After me so as you never saw!
And I chiefly use my charm
On creatures that do people harm,
The mole and toad and newt and viper;
And people call me the Pied Piper.

Robert Browning: *The Pied Piper of Hamelin*

Doctors may regard this book as an act of neurosis, evidence of hypochondria and an obsession with my health, perhaps even proof of Munchaüsen's Syndrome. How dare I, a puny female, cast myself in the role of a David, directing my slingshot against the Goliaths of medicine? Like the doctors who banished detailed information from the oral contraceptive package, they will say I have no business writing a "scary" book about a benign condition. They will say that this book is the work of their "intellectual subordinate", in the words of Dr. Geoff Issac, and the daughter of a laborer, who could not possibly, "get past the eighth grade in school"[1], in the words of Dr. Walter Alvarez. This book might even give rise to their fears of dangerous, subversive activity of the kind Lewis once suggested might lead to a revolt of the lower classes through feigned illness in order to withdraw from the labour force on a disability pension.

However, this book has not been written to drum up fear; it has been written to inform and to reveal. It is meant to bring to the attention of the public knowledge about MVP and to emphasize the yawning chasm between the information patients receive and the information that *exists* and to encourage people everywhere to read the medical literature with a view toward assisting in the prevention of deterioration in their health. MVP is a serious disease which commands public attention. An informed public can exhort uninformed professionals to adopt the preventative strategies available to them. MVP **must** become a household word just as heart attack, stroke and AIDS have become. If this book appears to be a "scary" book, the only truly frightening aspect is that doctors and dentists are failing in their duty to protect their MVP patients.

Proof that very little progress has been made among physicians since my first encounter with IE in 1979-80, is forcefully demonstrated in the confusion I encountered at my second hospitalization in September of 1989 for an acute fever of unknown origin. This illness began with shaking chills and, several hours later, I had a temperature of 40°C accompanied by severe aching, frontal headache and lower abdominal pain. My GP immediately pronounced my symptoms indicative of a virus, or a flu, and it was only with considerable persuasion that I obtained consent to have blood tests done to rule out IE. I needn't point out how commonly IE is mistaken for flu. Upon presentation at hospital emergency, I then had to convince the internist of the wisdom of such blood tests.

I had seen this internist once back in 1976 after I had experienced the two episodes of paroxysmal atrial tachycardia. It was he who had sent me on to Dr. Austin who diagnosed MVP and, yet, neglected to provide me with the necessary ABP for dental and surgical procedures. If I had been treated appropriately in the past and if I had in my possession copies of my medical records, especially those echocardiograms and x-rays that had strangely disappeared, there would have been no necessity, at the time of this second illness, to give a summary of thirteen years of medical history in ten minutes. This created stress, confusion and, needless to say, the waste of precious time. Nor are doctors willing, given the present inequitable relationship, to accept a precis of the medical history from the patient. This internist was, like my GP, on the verge of dismissing my fever as viral in origin. A "virus" is a catch-all term frequently used for most maladies associated with fever, especially those the doctor cannot easily diagnose. Apart from the well-known viral illnesses, such as rubela, influenza, measles, mumps, chicken pox, for which most people have been vaccinated, the doctor will tell the patient that there are several hundred viruses, many of a mysterious nature, which he cannot possibly identify. However, the majority of these viruses only rarely produce acute disease and the most common ones found in Canada and the U.S. are usually readily identified.[2] And, in my own case, there have been only two occasions when I have suffered from acute fever of 40°C, or 105°F, the one I have related and the one of 1989.

Once persuaded of the logic in testing my blood for bacteria, the internist had to be convinced that more than three blood samples might be necessary to grow the microorganisms. Once again, I stress that it was only my hard-won knowledge gained as a result of my previous episode of IE and my subsequent reading that made it possible for me to insist that my blood be tested for bacteria. And this time I arrived at the hospital with a fever and **two** murmurs! However, the internist was unable to hear my tricuspid murmur though I and my husband can hear this distinct blowing sound with our stethoscope at the lower right sternal border, and tricuspid regurgitation has been shown on echocardiogram. My white blood cell count was 18,000 and is usually not elevated in viral infections. On the basis of the medical history I gave him, this internist started IV antibiotics, 2 million units of pen G every 4 hrs. and 80 mgm. of gentamycin every 6 hrs. While my blood was drawn before the antimicrobial treatment, the echocardiogram was done towards the end of almost ten days of treatment. If there had been vegetations, the antibiotics would have greatly reduced their size. However because my blood had not grown anything by that time and because my internist did not see any vegetations on the echocardiogram, he made the decision, without the assistance of any other specialist, to release me rather than complete the full course of 4-6 weeks. Even at the time of my discharge, he repeated his belief that the illness had been a virus. Later tests would show that my blood was negative for viral antibodies. Two days after my release, when a cardiologist looked at my echocardiogram, he said he saw vegetations on the tricuspid valve and signs of "something other than thickening" on my mitral valve. Nothing was done, however, and two days later he amended his interpretation to healed vegetations.

If what this cardiologist saw was, in fact, healed vegetations, they are indisputable evidence that I had suffered from IE in 1979-80. Alternatively, these may have been recent vegetations healed by the antibiotics. The echocardiogram, as I have pointed out, cannot accurately distinguish between healed and unhealed vegetations, old or new vegetations. The tricuspid regurgitation becomes a symptom of IE, if active vegetations were, in fact, present, or possibly a sign of new activity in old vegetations suppressed but never cured. In any case, the IE, if not cured, could then become chronic or subacute with a duration of months to years acording to the older writers, especially Libman, exactly as it had done in the past. Those individuals with the highest risk of IE, according to Lawrence Freedman, are patients with prosthetic valves or a previous IE, as already pointed out.

In spite of all that I had learned, I felt very timid in requesting blood tests for IE although such a step, in the case of a patient with murmur and fever, should, as one researcher has said, be a "reflex reaction". The reason, of course, was the feeling of impotence in challenging the medical establishment. However, with public support, which I hope this book will encourage, patients will not feel so alone nor frightened of contradicting a doctor. Involvement in one's own health care is a positive step towards therapy.

This experience raises, once again, the issue of prevention of IE in the first place. If this fever indicated an IE, a possible cause exists in the periodontal bleeding occasioned by brushing or flossing a crowned tooth. Like any prosthetic device, crowned teeth generate problems. They are particularly susceptible to plaque adherence and thus inflammation and bleeding of the gums. This problem existed for a period of two months prior to seeing my dentist at the end of August, 1989, two weeks before the onset of fever. However, as related in this book, the reason for the crown goes back to the time when the majority of my teeth were drilled and filled during my teens when I was a totally uninformed patient. The cycle is endless. Restored teeth generate problems and frequently have to be crowned to save them. The lesson: healthy, natural teeth are the best prevention against IE.

Since IE is most frequently caused by interventions related to teeth or to septic conditions in the mouth, the prevention of IE cannot really be addressed without examining the attitudes of both dentists and the public toward teeth. It has been proven scientifically that sugar working with bacteria in the mouth causes dental decay, specifically streptococcus mutans found in plaque, as already discussed. The caries, in turn, can cause IE either immediately or at a later date. It is known that, among civilizations with low sugar consumption, there is less dental decay. It would be valuable to know if there were also less IE. Although there is justice in blaming the patient for bad diet, governments have also failed to convince the public through education programmes of the scientific evidence in this regard. One might conceive of government regulation that requires sugar and all sticky, sugary and starchy foods, which are also known to cause decay, to carry a warning, as in the case of cigarettes and alcohol, of the risks to one's health. The streptococcus mutans found in plaque assists in the production of excessive amounts of dextran "which serves as a determinant for its ability to adhere to damaged heart valves and cause bacterial endocarditis" and has been implicated in 14% of the cases of streptococcal endocarditis.[3] But, as in most matters of health, rather than attack the cause or educate the public to change detrimental eating patterns, expedient antidotes are used, such as fluorides which may later prove to have serious side effects.

Dentists should discourage people from eating sugary substances, but many do not. Recently, several dentists I spoke to, insisted that sugar was not linked to caries. Prevention of dental decay is simply not profitable for the dentist. Dentistry is a business, and it's the bottomline that counts. If tooth structure is severely weakened from restorations for dental caries, work will eventually be provided for all specialties of dentistry, in particular endodontics and periodontics. In an American survey, for example, as high as 89 percent of 451 dentists said that they performed endodontal work in some or all of their patients rather than pass them on to specialists. Profit was one of the common motives.[4]

A continued controversy exists between general dentists and periodontists, which dramatically emphasizes that the profit motive is prominent. Dr. Paul Keyes, who has worked with the National Institute of Dental Research in the U.S. for 27 years, has developed a simple, non-surgical method for treating periodontal disease. According to Keyes, his mixture of hydrogen peroxide, baking soda and salt, kills the "bacteria" in the dental plaque which is responsible for periodontal disease. This is actually an old home remedy that is used in conjunction with deep cleaning to remove calcified bacteria from the teeth and roots. Patients can apply the mixture at home. Periodontists, however, are angry and are challenging Keyes because they are being done out of work. General dentists want to use Keyes' method to replace income lost from less drilling and filling because of preventative fluoride measures and, thus, they are not referring their patients on to the periodontists for surgery.[5]

Oral hardware, crowns, bridges, dentures, quick and easy to insert, like prosthetic valves, allows the dentist to work much faster, reduces his decision making and, therefore, his risk, and, ultimately, is more profitable. Business management courses, part of the dentist's training, emphasize dollars instead of professional ethics. "When he's told over and over again by the one conducting the course," one American dentist lamented, "that if he 'sells' more bridges, inlays, crowns, dentures etc., every month his annual income will be increased by "x" number of dollars — then the dollar sign becomes paramount."[6] What is most disturbing about this "complaint" is that the dentist assumes no responsibility for his own avarice; it was instilled in him by his teacher.

Alvarez charged that bad teeth in a woman meant "lack of good sense or of good discipline or a great fear of pain,"[7] another stereotypical response to the female patient. Attitudes are shaped by the individuals or groups who possess the knowledge. If the public believes that natural teeth are a frill or luxury, dentists and doctors, not the patient, are to blame. Comments like this in the media, "But look, let's be realistic, do people die from toothaches?"[8] reflect the public's lack of knowledge about the relationship between the teeth and the heart.

The absence of government subsidized dental care and the resulting high prices dentists charge make dental care a luxury, an idea perpetuated by public ignorance and the belief that the teeth have nothing to do with serious health care. A lack of knowledge compounded by poverty automatically breeds a sense of defeat regarding the care of one's teeth. "I truly believe," one woman wrote to the journal, *Dental Economics*, "the major reason for not having one's mouth fixed is simply the lack of funds. Dentistry is a luxury, not a necessity. It is a fact that man can live without teeth . . . it creates true hardships on some to go to the dentist for simple fillings."[9]

Dr. D. W. Lewis of the Faculty of Dentistry, at the University of Toronto, Ontario, speaking at a health conference summed up public feeling that can only have been fostered by the government's and the dental profession's indifference to a very important aspect of health. "Dental disease relative to the main issues of society today is not important. The status dental health has in our society is largely culturally defined . . . we have been conditioned to expect our beauties and principal entertainers to have white, shiny, straight teeth."[10] The majority of people, Lewis maintains, believe that losing teeth is inevitable when, in fact, natural teeth can be kept into old age.

Some statistics from Ontario, for example, reveal that only 48 percent of all persons visit a dentist at least once a year and, even then, treatment is incomplete. Other facts are equally distressing. 54 percent of the total number of decayed teeth of seven year old children go unfilled. This figure is as high as 73 percent in eastern Ontario. And, while one in five chidren, aged thirteen, require orthodontic care because of severe malocclusion, only one in twenty-five receive it.[11] In the U.S., 90-95 percent of Americans have dental caries which, in 90 percent of cases, is preventable through restriction of sweets, proper brushing and flossing.[12] Prevention then begins with diet.

In Northern Ireland, both dental and medical care are subsidized by the government, and public education is a priority. The results are astonishing. An effort has been made to assist parents in caring for the teeth of their children with heart problems. Each year, these children go to one of three cardiac clinics for a combined cardiac and dental examination and, where it is appropriate, antibiotic coverage is explained and employed. This correlation of dental and medical care, involving the parents, resulted in a significant reduction in the number of children requiring dental extractions, from 208 in 1972 to 98 in 1975-76.[13] Not only do such measures ultimately save lives but they protect the child against the future need for dentures which, even doctors and dentists admit, severely "degrade the quality of life."[14]

But most dentists in the U.S. and Canada object to any kind of government subsidized dental care. Dr. A. J. Harris, former President of the Ontario Dental Association objects because he believes people will abuse such a system. Harris paints a picture of "five million people" suddenly knocking on the dentist's door, all of them thinking "it's all free now. Just make an appointment and whatever damage has been done to your mouth, regardless of who's to blame, will be repaired at no cost to you."[15] Patient abuse of benefits is an old argument which has its origin in Lewis and Evans' fears that malingering soldiers or depraved civilians would cheat pension boards or compensation funds. There is a certain punitive tone to Harris' words. Dentists should not have to "repair" teeth ravaged by patient neglect or some other past dentist's mistakes. That he sees the patient as largely to blame is clear from the following statement: "Part of the problem with that 50 percent (those who do not receive regular dental care) is that these people are not aware of what preventative dental care will achieve and how simple it is to maintain proper personal oral hygiene."[16] To increase public awareness there must be more widespread education programs, which are the responsibility of the government, and encouragement of the individual to inform him or herself.

However, the dental, like the medical profession, is largely responsible for keeping the public in ignorance. The protective instinct motivates dentists to oppose public education because knowledge results in demands for "more", and dentists, like doctors, see the educated person as dangerous. Dr. Kenneth Pownal, former Registrar of the Royal College of Dental Surgeons in Toronto, the governing body of the profession, says "the public attitude has shifted from fatalism to skepticism, to high expectancy of success. High expectation leads to deeper disappointment; deeper disappointment leads to the lawyer's office; in many cases the lawyer issues a writ and a malpractice suit is underway."[17] It is clear that the bogeyman is the malpractice suit. Public education enables people to recognize incompetence among dentists as well as doctors. Knowledge erodes the power of special groups. Informed people demand, not more, but better dental care.

The ideals of self-reliance and self-determination have emerged as a challenge to the anonymous forces that move individuals about like pawns on a chessboard. People want to believe that they have control over their lives, their destinies and their health. The emphasis on exercise, whether jogging or pumping iron, diet, vitamin subsidies, herbal remedies, the spiritual therapies of a variety of cultures, yoga or shiatsu for example, or any of the alternatives to institutionalized medicine promise restoration of equilibrium to the body and the soul. But, whether the curative is vitamins, expensive jogging shoes, live cell treatment at a luxurious European spa or just plain, old traditional medicine, health care is big business. The industry puts out its feelers, picks up the demand, infinitely multiplying it with hard-core selling, and speedily manufactures the supply, frequently transforming even the harmless, esoteric interest, with perhaps more psychological than physical benefit, into a major industry with all its inherent vices. What looks like freedom is actually control.

Doctors and dentists have likewise exploited this innate desire for control over one's life and acceptance of responsibility for one's health. Blaming the patient for disease has thus naturally become a kind of common therapy. But this may be just another means of maintaining power over the patient. The doctor's edict that changing one's lifestyle can cure may foster the illusion that patients are in control or have parity with the doctor or dentist. In a familiar anecdote of the patient who dies either from smoking or eating too much food high in cholesterol, Gifford-Jones once remarked in one of his newspaper columns, "Look, God didn't kill your husband! Nor has he died because of fate or what this hospital has done. His death didn't just happen. Your husband killed himself." This piece, which begins with, "What would God do if He were a surgeon?",[18] is a subconscious appeal to the patient to trust the doctor unquestioningly, as if he were God, whether the doctor is blaming or treating, and, in fact, the two might mean the same thing subliminally.

If the patient can be convinced an illness is self-caused, rather than acquired through the negligence of the doctor or hospital, or if the patient can be convinced he or she is responsible for complete recovery, the bogeyman, malpractice, is scared off. In this effort to shift the management of disease to the patient, something as implausible as laughter can assume the status of a curative.

To attribute cardiovascular symptoms associated with MVP to endogenous anxiety is an indication of the shift of responsibility from the doctor or dentist to the patient. Blaming the patient is the therapy, and it is to be understood that removal of the anxiety would remove the symptoms. And, accordingly, when complications appeared, both doctor and dentist, in Margo 's and my cases, gave us diagnoses of hysteria, labile mentality, pathological anxiety or cardiac neurosis. Margo's dentist claimed that he had informed her of the risk of IE and the need for ABP for all procedures, though no such advice was recorded in his records, and that, in her carelessness, she disregarded this information. Her neglect resulted in near death. My periodontal abscess was blamed on my inability to tolerate crowns not on malocclusion, a cracked root or inadequate endodontal treatment. When my complications accumulated, including the enlargement of my heart, my general dentist repeated, "I told you at the beginning that crowns don't work for everybody," and "an enlarged heart means nothing. There are athletes who have enlarged hearts."

Popular health writers like Jane Brody have fallen into the doctors' trap. "Self-blame", Brody claims, assists the individual in coping more efficiently with disasters including illness. Appealing to the patient's desire for control, she said, "helplessness is the most destructive of all feelings after being a victim."[19] Thus the patient must assume a good measure of responsibiity. When my medical records vanished mysteriously while my health deteriorated, no amount of self-blame would ever have had any effect on relieving my feelings of impotence, let alone curing my illness. An individual cannot recover through self-blame but by having the power to redress a wrong or change the system that permits the wrong.

A chasm exists between scientific knowledge and practice. Until every physician breaches this gap, disease will never be conquered no matter how much responsibility the patient assumes for illness. Why, for instance, should two Chiefs of Cardiology in two major hospitals in the same city hold diametrically opposite views about the use of ABP with MVP patients? Since the medical colleges set the standards these individuals are to follow, we have the right to ask whether they are fulfilling their obligation. Should the standard be that of Richibuctoo, Thunder Bay or even Toronto or should it be that of the major medical centres of the world? The responsibility of the Colleges is to assure that every doctor is giving his patient the best advice and care that medical science has to offer. Yet, the College of Physicians and Surgeons of Ontario (CPSO), for example, did not issue a bulletin, equivalent to the 1979 Dispatch of the Royal College of Dental Surgeons of Ontario, regarding ABP and MVP.

The CPSO, like most governing bodies of the medical profession anywhere in the world, does make attempts to regulate members. For instance, in the early eighties, it tried to ascertain how many doctors, particularly among the elderly, were up to date. Over a period of three years a peer assessment committee reviewed a sample of doctors' files, and, in 1983, found that 13 percent of doctors over fifty "practiced medicine in a fashion that caused serious concern" or "kept grossly deficient records" and 49 percent of doctors over 70 were practicing medicine that was disturbingly out of date.[20]

However, most such attempts to regulate the profession and to establish an accounting system are vigorously opposed. The General Secretary of the Ontario Medical Association (OMA), Dr. Edward Moran, at the time of that report, considered such close monitoring to be age discrimination, an attempt to put these older doctors "out to pasture when they're in full possession of their faculties".[21] Though old doctors can maim or kill, just as old motorists can, they are not, in Moran's view, in the same category and do not require skill testing and refreshment courses.

Random attempts of the governing body to review doctors' work in general have met with stiff opposition here in Canada and likely elsewhere. In 1982, for example, a group called the Association of Independent Physicians (AIP) responded to such policing by launching a legal suit against the College to prevent unauthorized visits from the Peer Assessment Committee. In its defense, the AIP used the Canadian Charter of Rights, Section eight, dealing with "unreasonable search and seizure" to prove the College could not legally force a doctor to hand over a patient's medical records for examination of treatment methods or billing checks.[22] The action of this group was not surprising. Their resistance to any kind of control has lead to their opting out of the government medical care system on the basis of the right to set their own fees for their services.

Doctors had been dragged unwillingly into the government medical plan at its inception. Their resistance to control by their governing College or the government is longstanding and is an indication of their old desire for the U.S. style of free enterprise health care. Canadian dentists already have this, and there is little chance of subsidized dental care in Canada at the present time because of the political power of that profession and the limited understanding of the public about the importance of good dental care.

Healthcare in the U.S. is big business, and technology has largely been responsible. The alliance with industry has propelled the move away from prevention and proven treatment procedures toward replacement of diseased organs as if they were the assembly-line parts of an automobile. Modern medicine has become heroic through technology; it is salvation medicine. By contrast, prevention of disease or treatment of disease, as in the case of IE with 4-6 weeks of IV antibiotics, looks unexciting without the stardom that prosthetic valves fashioned by a glittering technology offer. Traditional early signs of disease may, in fact, be disregarded, or at least the patient may not be told of them. Kidney disease, for example, illustrates an interesting point. Protein in the urine has always been regarded as a sign of CHF or GN. In 1970, a medical surgical nursing textbook showed normal urine chemistry values for measurement of protein over 24 hours as "zero".[23] The values in the eighties, according to the *Lippincott Manual of Nursing Practice* (1982)[24] and Wallach's *Interpretation of Diagnostic Tests* (1983)[25] are now 100 mg. per 24 hours. In the seventies, many studies of IE and GN reported that patients were dismissed after antimicrobial treatment for IE with a final diagnosis of "no protein in the urine" which would imply that this was one of the final goals of treatment.[26] Richard Saul Wurman, in *Medical Access*, a very valuable book published in 1985, which explains test procedures for the public, states, "A functioning kidney does not allow protein molecules to pass through so there should be no protein in the urine."[27] According to Harrison's *Principles of Internal Medicine*, "Slight to moderate proteinuria is the rule in patients with heart failure."[28] I, therefore, cannot understand why my internist regards 115 mg. of protein over a 24 hour period as an insignificant finding.

Do these variations point merely to differing opinions, as in the case of MVP and ABP? Or are they an indication of the approach doctors commonly take toward telling patients of disease? Or do they represent a change in the concept of disease itself provoked by the technological boom? As I've pointed out, 50 percent of kidney function can be lost before symptoms appear. Thus, if a patient had laboratory evidence of GN resulting from IE, yet had only non-disabling symptoms, doctors would not likely reveal this abnormality, no more than they would reveal CHF to a breathless MVP patient, if, indeed, testing for such abnormalities, had ever been done prior to the appearance of marked symptoms. After all, there is no cure known to medical science for an immunologically related GN. When the kidneys cease to function, salvation medicine, dialysis and kidney transplant, would come to the rescue. Will the time come, one asks, when doctors accept a certain level of blood in the urine as normal? Such a statement may seem exaggerated, but doctors, in Margo's case, initially overlooked this classic sign of GN in association with IE. Has medical science reached a stasis or has it, in fact, regressed?

The headlong rush toward technological hardware to replace body parts has had a disastrous effect on treatment methods for valvular disease. Although ideally the best treatment is prevention of naturally occurring deterioration or of IE that damages the valves, there are thousands of individuals whose valves are not protected against infection and who, inevitably, because of severe regurgitation, must have surgical intervention.

Prosthetic valves are likely regarded as the greatest invention since penicillin. Once open-heart surgery techniques were in use by 1955 with cardio-pulmonary by-pass, the development of the prosthetic valve was not far behind it. According to historical reviews, following- the introduction of prosthetic valves in 1961, techniques for repairing or reconstructing valves damaged by disease declined for the next twenty years in the U.S., and likely in Canada if, in fact, they had ever been done on a major scale, and reports describing this kind of surgery virtually disappeared from the American medical literature during the period from 1955 to 1985.[29] Currently, doctors in the U.S. and Canada rely almost exclusively on valve replacement with mechanical or bioprosthetic devices, made either from porcine or calf tissues, rather than repair of the patient's own natural tissues.

However, valvular replacement is being widely criticized. For example, in Canada, The Alberta College of Physicians and Surgeons, in a 1983 report, complained that there are too many valvular replacements in that province and that doctors "in the process of obtaining specialist qualifications" are doing valvular surgery. In fact Alberta has the highest surgery rate in Canada. This fact suggests how easy it is to replace valves, and the report boldly states that money is the incentive.[30] Replacing a valve is faster than repairing it, or even treating for IE, and, therefore, more profitable.

Technology has lead to the loss of manual skills. This is particularly apparent in the decline in the physician's auscultatory skills with the advent of the echocardiogram as a diagnostic tool for MVP. The echocardiogram, though inferior to the stethoscope, has become the preferred method of identifying MVP for many doctors. Likewise, the younger surgeons today unfortunately do not want to learn the tedious, time-consuming skills of valvular reconstruction using the patient's natural tissues. Unexpected decisions must be made during the surgical procedure. This puts stress on the surgeon and increases the risk of failure which could affect the surgeon both psychologically and financially. At an annual meeting of The Samson Thoracic Surgical Society held in Banff, Alberta, in 1976, a group of surgeons from California summed up the reasons why mitral valve replacement has become the standard treatment for mitral regurgitation. "Valve replacement," they said, "often involves a decision made preoperatively on the basis of cardiac catheterization and angiographic data and requires less intraoperative judgement," and prosthetic valve replacement is easier to accomplish.[31] Industrial technology has made prosthetic valves so readily available that valve replacement has become, in the words of these researchers, "the primary treatment for mitral valve disease", superseding the "techniques and skills" of surgeons once "gifted in the art of reconstruction."[32]

At the Sixty-third Annual Meeting of The American Association for Thoracic Surgery in Atlanta, Georgia in 1983, the guest speaker, Parisian cardiovascular surgeon, Alain Carpentier, who pioneered work in reconstructive valvular techniques, provided a humorous but frightening anecdote of the attitudes, which are prevalent in the U.S. as well as Canada, and even among the most high profile cardiovascular surgeons, toward treatment options for diseased valves:

> I was invited to the Texas Heart Institute to give a lecture on valve reconstruction. After the lecture, Denton Cooley invited me to watch him operate upon a patient with mitral valve insufficiency. He opened the atrium in 2 seconds, took out the valve in another 2 seconds, and then, with the valve in his hand, said: "Let's see what we can do to repair this valve, now." For mere ordinary surgeons such as myself, valve analysis requires more time and should be carried out step by step.[33]

This anecdote is reminiscent of a scene in Tennessee Williams' play, *A Streetcar Named Desire*. Stanley Kowalski, the testy, young man nagged by his wife, Stella, and his sister-in-law, Blanche, to clean up his mess from gorging on his supper shoves everything on to the floor with one swipe of his large arm and says, "That's how I'll clear the table."[34]

Denton Cooley co-invented a prosthetic valve which became known as the Cooley-Cutter prosthesis. Though it was popular with surgeons and gave its creator a brief moment in the sun, it is now no longer commercially available, and the commonly used mechanical mitral valves now on the market are the Starr-Edwards ball valve, the St-Jude Medical bileaflet and the Medtronic-Hall valves.[35]

Valvular repair was revived in the 1970s but was confined mostly to Europe: in Britain, Shore et al., in Spain, Duran et al., and, in France, Alain Carpentier et al.,[36] the major pioneer in the renaissance of mitral valve reconstruction. The famous Clinique Lériche at the Hôpital Broussais in Paris, a 732 bed hospital, on the left bank of the Seine, is devoted entirely to cardiovascular disease. Valve surgery comprises 46 percent of the average 2000 cardiovascular operations a year.[37] Carpentier and his group of cardiovascular surgeons have described their techniques for replacing the stretched mitral or tricuspid valve ring with a prosthetic device, the Carpentier ring, cutting out excess tissue from floppy leaflets, shortening of elongated chordae and repair of chordae that are fused, shortened or thickened. [38] All of these pathological features have been found in MVP. The techniques of the Parisian group have been adopted by cardiovascular surgeons in other countries.

Cardiovascular surgeons returned to valvular reconstruction because, as Bonchek summed up in 1982, "All prosthetic valves have inherent disadvantages."[39] Whether the valve is mechanical or a tissue bioprosthesis, there is a very high risk of IE, and thromboembolism occurs in two to five percent of patients per year. Anti-coagulants are necessary during the remainder of the patient's life, even with tissue valves, but these drugs cause hemorrhage in one to three percent of patients per year. Mechanical valve action is unpleasantly audible to the patient, and sudden death from mechanical failure is a serious problem.[40] Tissue valves or bioprostheses last about ten years in about 80 to 85 percent of patients, and it is predicted that the fifteen year durability rate will be considerably worse.[41] The overall survival rate for prosthetic valves, mechanical and tissue, has, in one group of 66 patients, been as low as fifty plus or minus eight percent at the five year mark.[42] Porcine valves may deteriorate in as little as three years according to Bonchek.[43]

On the other hand, reconstruction of the valves, using the patient's natural tissues, encourages earlier operation, when the heart is only minimally damaged. Surgeons feel the reduction in complications and the improved durability in cases of repair outweigh the risks of early operation. Valvular reconstruction is even recommended for patients who are asymptomatic but have evidence of dilatation of the heart or a fall in ejection fraction with exercise.[44] However, valve replacement is usually done when the patient is dying from severe heart failure with symptoms at rest. Such patients are in Class IV of the New York Heart Association Classification (NYHA) for heart failure. It is generally recognized that, within five years of receiving a valve replacement, 20-40 percent of these patients are dead, according to Galloway et al of the New York University Medical Centre. On the other hand, valvular reconstruction can still be carried out with good results when a patient is in Class IV heart failure.[45]

Repair or reconstruction gives the best results in cases of mitral incompetence and degenerative valvular disease, which largely includes patients with prolapsed valves and all the common pathological features in varying degrees of severity associated with that condition. In 1983, Carpentier reported the results of a series of 1421 cases of valve repair between the years 1969 to 1982. The mortality rate during the surgery was 3.6 percent for those with mitral disease and 8.6 percent for patients with both mitral and tricuspid disease. This rate, Carpentier said, declined, in the year following this study, to 1.6 and 3.2 percent respectively suggesting that the techniques continued to improve. The re-operation rate for his series of patients with degenerative valvular disease was very low, at 0.7 percent per patient-year, and the thromboembolic rate was almost negligible at 0.6 percent per patient-year. Repair, Carpentier pointed out could also be performed during IE after a fifteen day course of antibiotic therapy in 60 percent of patients by cutting out the vegetative lesions.[46] In a previous report in 1980, Carpentier had concluded that the survival rate, when deaths at surgery were excluded, was 88 percent at nine years for his entire series of patients.[47]

Various studies show that, with mitral reconstruction, 95 percent of patients are still free of thromboemboli at five to ten years. This compares favorably with the 10-35 percent of patients with mechanical valves who have serious thromboemboli within five to ten years after valve replacement[48] and with the tissue valves that require anticoagulation since up to five percent of patients per year experience thromboemboli. By 1987, the comparative results still showed reconstruction is superior to replacement with mechanical or tissue valves. A Swedish report concluded, from various studies, that about 90 percent of patients in the degenerative disease-mitral regurgitation group are alive 5-8 years after reconstructive surgery and more than 50 percent do not require reoperation even after 15 years. "Mitral valve repair," the report concluded, "is associated with fewer valve related complications than replacement and even without anticoagulant therapy, there are hardly any embolic events."[49]

There are two important centres in the U.S. where reconstruction rather than replacement is the mode of treatment, the New York University Medical Centre and the Los Angeles Heart Institute. Galloway et al.[50] from the New York institution share the same opinions as the European cardiovascular surgeons that, in over 90 percent of cases of valvular disease with mitral insufficiency, as in the case of MVP, valvular reconstruction can be successful, and they have shown, like the Parisian surgeons, that reconstruction is particularly suited to valves damaged by IE. As they pointed out, the risk of IE is greatly reduced when the patient's natural tissues are retained. Most researchers agree that valve reconstruction or repair is superior to replacement and should be the preferred method of treatment even for IE patients with longstanding disease that becomes refractory to medical management. Why then are there 2900 valve replacements in Canada per year?[51]

Despite the decline in popularity of valvular repair in the U.S. once the first prosthetic valve, the Starr-Edwards ball-valve, was introduced, some singular surgeons persisted with the more time-consuming, difficult skills of reconstruction. The chief pioneers, Jerome Kay and his team at The Los Angeles Heart Institute at the University of Southern California have been practicing the art of valvular reconstruction since 1959. The lengthy experience of the Los Angeles group in repairing valves with serious regurgitation coupled with 15 years of experience with prosthetic valves has shown that repair is far superior than replacement with either mechanical or Starr-Edwards and Hancock glutaraldehyde-treated porcine tissue valves. It is noteworthy that they, unlike Carpentier, do not use a prosthetic ring so that all of the natural tissue is preserved. The Los Angeles team strongly urges surgeons everywhere to reconstruct natural valves before considering replacement with a prosthetic device.[52] Carpentier ended his address at the American Association for Thoracic Surgery with the same advice as Kay and his group. His humorous anecdote of the hypothetical surgeon who is attending a similar conference in the year 2050 in the hope of finding the perfect prosthetic device suggests that mitral replacement will never be the ideal therapy.[53]

What is most disturbing is that MVP was the cause of the serious regurgitation in the majority of Kay et al's 216 patients in his 1978 report which compared the merits of repair and replacement.[54] This was the same year that I was told I did not require ABP with dental work. Such an opinion becomes a disturbing aberration when one considers the extent of research that was being carried on in all facets of MVP at that time, even in Canada. MVP is "the single most common cause of moderate or severe regurgitation", Guy and co-workers at Victoria General Hospital in Halifax said, and was the underlying cause for valve replacement in 50 percent of the patients in their 1980 study.[55] This opinion has not changed, and the percentage of patients with MVP as a cause of replacement has even increased. Waller et al found MVP was the cause of severe regurgitation in 62 percent of patients requiring mitral valve replacement.[56] Doctors should, therefore, be asking themselves why such a stable condition is deteriorating so frequently to the point where surgical intervention is necessary. Perhaps it would be wise to heed the warnings of researchers, like Galloway et al, who said that "it is well known that with mitral insufficiency significant, irreversible ventricular injury (manifested by dilatation, hypertrophy, and a fall in ejection fraction) can **insidiously evolve with few or no symptoms.**"[57] There are likely thousands of people with experiences similar to mine: a case of IE associated with dental work, which goes unrecognized either by the patient or the physician involved, perhaps treated inappropriately with inadequate doses of antibiotics that suppress the microorganism for long periods of time but do not kill it so that the patient ends up with mitral and/or tricuspid regurgitation and heart failure a half dozen years or more later. By then the cause, if it were ever sorted out, would be long forgotten.

The direction medicine has taken in the treatment of valvular disease is a natural outcome of the belief that technology, rather than pathology research, can conquer anything, can even "triumph over disease". But at base of the illusion is something even more disheartening. The obsession with technology is, as in any other area of endeavor, motivated by human greed, the desire to accumulate wealth. Richard Brown, author of *Rockefeller Medicine Men: Medicine and Capitalism*, says that the popularity of technological products of "questionable usefulness", and I would include prosthetic valves, is the inevitable outcome of the marriage between business and medicine.

> Once a product or service is developed, the major medical interest groups determine its market. The commodity's producers extol its advantages and push for acceptance and sales. If the drug, instrument or procedure increases the technical effectiveness of physicians, it is likely to be ordered by them.

If it increases the status or incomes of physicians, it is also likely to be used. If its availability in a hospital is likely to attract physicians or otherwise produce income, hospitals will want to buy it. If third party payers will foot the bill it is a certain winner![58]

The message here is clear, that medicine, like any other profit-making institution, will promote a product, or even a technique such as mitral replacement, not purely out of charismatic interest in the wellbeing of patients and only if its profitability can be verified. The fact that doctors invent and patent devices, whether prosthetic valves or artificial hearts, such as the Jarvik 7, no longer used in the U.S. but still used in Canada, confirms the symbiotic relationship between industry and medicine. In a way, the rush to get into the market for medical technological devices and equipment is like the gold rushes of the past where the prospectors, hoping to make their fortune, rushed to stake their claims before anyone else in a promising territory. If other easier, less risky methods are available, how can prevention of valvular disease or micro-surgery to repair damaged valves be popular when both are fraught with difficult decision making, are time-consuming and carry high risks for the doctor in psychological and financial terms no matter how much better they might be for the patient?

It takes knowledge on the part of the public to criticize the medical or dental professions, and this knowledge is not easily come by because it is controlled by the professions themselves. Thus patients would rarely have or even be aware of the informational resources that would enable them to evaluate the justification for the high number of valve replacements. It took lay people a long time to realize that too many hysterectomies and too many by-passes were being done. Patients without knowledge simply have to wait and trust that the profession will promote what is in the best interests of humanity. It is not surprising, therefore, that patients might "expect too much", might expect "miracles" from a profession that shrouds its activities in mystery and keeps its mistakes and weaknesses hidden while proclaiming its accomplishments that invite simplistic awe from a public kept in the dark ages. A patient who has been snatched from the brink of death has considerable difficulty in weighing in an objective manner the relative merits of valve reconstruction or replacement. He or she is just glad to be alive, feels gratitude for having been rescued and usually regards the doctor as a hero. The public must become informed, and therefore critical, as well as supportive, about the progress of medicine as about anything else and refuse to "foot the bill" for these pioneers in science-fiction medicine with their polyurethane and aluminum hearts, teflon valves, plastic veins or silicon breasts which have superseded prevention of disease.

Technology, whether employed in surgical procedures or diagnostic testing, permits the doctor to be even more inaccessible while having even more control over the patient. The doctor can literally hide behind the machine. With, for example, the lengthy, complex wall motion study, the patient is surrounded by intimidating technological equipment and remote, time-conscious technicians who give little explanation, other than that the procedure is harmless, even if the patient is able to formulate questions about the abstruse objectives of such mathematical computations. Of course, the patient's doctor is nowhere in sight and meeting with him would not elucidate the meaning of such terms as end diastolic volume, ejection fraction, pulmonary blood volume ratio etc. because he becomes immediately antagonistic when the patient poses questions, especially those of a sophisticated, technical nature because they represent, frankly speaking, a threat to the doctor who is, by the nature of his risky profession, unwilling to share. And why, one asks, are complex technological devices with injections of radioactive substances, no matter how insignificant they are purported to be, necessary to determine heart failure with exercise? Why isn't the patient's symptoms and poor exercise performance in daily life sufficient evidence? And all the factors that might have influenced the judgement of a pre-antibiotic physician to treat for IE, in the presence of very high fever, murmurs and high white blood cell count, become subordinate to the one piece of evidence, the echocardiographic picture. In the end, the doctor can blame error not on himself, but on the machine. Technology renders the doctor's activities all the more inscrutable, his mystique more impenetrable, his power and prestige more unshakable. Gone are the days of black bags and bedside medicine, but there is a powerful lesson to be learned from the marriage of medicine and technology and that is that the public is old fashioned and out of date in its attitude towards technologized, computerized medicine.

The reaction of Canadian doctors to the new *Canada Health Act* introduced in 1984 illustrates the true nature of the 20thC doctor-patient relationship. It is no longer one of children and daddies or supplicants and gods; it is a business relationship. This document fixed the price the doctor could command for a particular service. The Canadian federal government withheld an equal amount in health care grants to the provinces for every dollar extra-billed to the patient above the government's established fee. In a sense, this ruling penalized the entire health care system for the sins of the doctors. Not only did the doctors want to set prices but they also wished to keep these prices secret from the patient until after the service was performed. The *Canada Health Act* was followed by a statute in 1986 banning extra billing and instituting a system of fines to penalize this illegal practice.

A look at some of the issues of this controversial battle establishes that the modern doctor does not regard his role primarily as altruistic, that of caregiver or public servant, but as businessman in the privileged position of offering an essential service. At an annual meeting of the OMA in Ottawa in June of 1983, Dr. N.R. Fink confirmed in the language of the marketplace the source of the doctors' outrage over this bill. "The law," he declared, "is incompatible with our status as private and independent businessmen, let alone physicians . . . we're entitled to set our prices."[59] However, not notifying the purchaser of the price prior to the purchase is contrary even to the spirit of capitalism. Who buys a car, home, fridge, pair of shoes or automobile tune-up without knowing the price and shopping around for the best buy? The trouble is the patient cannot always wait and he or she does not have enough information to know what is the best buy.

In keeping with their role as businessmen, the doctors hired a public relations agent to sell their indispensable product and promote support for their interests. This publicity agent, the National Citizens' Coalition, NCC, is a right-wing lobby group, headed, at that time, by a millionaire, Colin Brown, who had campaigned against many other measures viewed as socialistic. The OMA urged its members to donate money to the NCC to fight the Canada Health Act. The NCC attempted to convince the public, by a fantastic distortion of facts, that banning extra billing, designed solely to increase the doctor's income, would hurt the patients, that the quality of health care would deteriorate. This is the underlying sales strategy of the marketplace, that the better the product, the higher the price. A full-page appeal in Toronto's conservative business paper, the *Globe and Mail*, called upon the public to pressure local politicians by signing an accompanying petition and donating money, using the form provided, to assist that organization in defeating the *Canada Health Act*. Individuals who fell for this were, in effect, cutting their own throats. While Canada's health care system has flaws, it does fulfill the principle that such care is a right, not a privilege to be enjoyed only by the wealthy.

The subject matter of the NCC's appeal confirmed the "status" of the doctors as businessmen who do not want to be classified socially or financially with postmen, tax department officials, teachers and other civil servants. The language unequivocally separated the doctor-businessman from the worker and the humble patients. It was the typical, insulting "ticker-belly-bum talk-down" language doctors employ with patients, full of children's words, "gee", "yeah", "piffle", "How'd you"[60] and implied in tones, reminiscent of Alvarez and Issac, that the patient is the "intellectual subordinate" whom the doctor can control and ultimately hoodwink with grammatically impaired, folksy speech designed to make him or her feel at home.

This NCC document was hyperbolic, underhanded and full of threats and all for the purpose of getting public support for increased physician income through extra billing. The best doctors, it claimed, would flee the country, leaving only the inferior behind. Recent statistics reveal, however, that there is actually a surplus of doctors in Ontario.[61] This was the same argument that Dr. Austin had used when I asked for an investigation for IE and the removal of my abscessed tooth with IV antibiotic coverage. He would be better appreciated he said in the U.S. where he would have less criticism. The cries of the NCC, "How'd you like to . . . go to special courses to keep yourself updated on everything new that's being discovered and then be told by the government you can't earn any more than the one who's too lazy to take the special course," are, in fact, untrue since specialists earn salaries considerably higher than those of the GP, and the Alberta report on surgery indicated that some doctors performing the work of specialists are unqualified to do so. This fomenting document, entitled, *So How'd You Like Your Open Heart Surgery Done by a Civil Servant?*, ended on an ironic, rather brutal note of subliminal coercion in the advice to citizens to "scream in pain" against the new *Canada Health Act.*[62]

Doctors went to great lengths to elicit public sympathy in this significant conflict. In appropriately vitriolic language, they painted themselves as victims of violence who had been robbed of their rights, and their contest with the government was a "power-play", a noble struggle for "freedom" from "slavery".[63] The federal government had inflicted everything from "fraud"[64] to "rape"[65] upon the doctors. The former President of the doctors' national union, the Canadian Medical Association (CMA), Dr. Everett Coffin, vowed that the CMA would "sanction" any strike as a retaliatory measure.[66] In this prolonged struggle against, in the words of Dr. Earl Myers, then President of the OMA, "an excessive and oppressive use of government power" that resorts to "an act of violence"[67], doctors viewed themselves as powerless peasants storming the Bastille in a courageous revolution against injustice. That the system they attacked was designed to assure that rich and poor alike have equal access to the same medical services only underlined the inappropriateness of the doctors' imagery.

Women have been the targets of medical injustice for so long that it is not surprising that, in this campaign to protect their incomes, doctors used women in a particularly despicable fashion. It is frequently said that a picture is worth a thousand words. The OMA's repeat photographs in the daily papers at that time showed an elderly doctor examining a pregnant woman.[68] The accompanying words represented the doctor's denunciation of government intervention in Canada's health care. Our system is more "well-balanced" than the American free enterprise system it claimed. The response of the patient could only be guilt if she did not support the doctors in their demands for more money since our system and the doctors are "superior". The statement, "It's not uncommon to hear of Americans taking out crippling bank loans to pay for lengthy illness or surgery," is both an attempt to incite guilt in the patient for driving the doctor south of the border and a raw threat that, if the patient does not acquiesce in the doctors' demands, the "state" system will collapse and American free style enterprise medicine will take over. The subliminal Marxist overtone in the word, "state", was to suggest that private enterprise medicine might be superior. In other words, the patient is caught between the Scylla and the Charybdis. The disadvantages of the completely subsidized British health care system in which doctors are slaves, i.e. they do not have the right to set their prices, were decried. Total government control in this country, it was implied, has lead to inefficiency: "Patients wait and wait." Guilt is again aroused in the old blame-the-patient argument: the system is free and, therefore, abused.

Pregnancy is a time when a woman must have the care of a doctor, midwifery not being legal in Canada, and, therefore the repetition of this image and these words at this vulnerable time could only be intended to arouse fear that care may not be available when needed if the patient does not comply with the doctors' demand to set their own prices. The choice of picture is intentional. The young, uninformed woman will immediately feel fear for what is dearest to her heart, her unborn child. The picture also has another typical powerful subliminal message: the elderly doctor is "daddy", the voice of authority, who can always be trusted to know best. Many women who have not yet shed the attitudes of their youth towards doctors still, unfortunately, relate to them, especially the older ones, as father figures. This little piece of public relations is predicated upon the medical profession's longstanding assumption that women are "weak, illogical, dependent and not fully rational" and thus doctors have the right to "pressure or coerce" them [69] openly or surreptitiously. Underlying all this invective is the distasteful equation that the higher the doctor's income the better the medical care. Whether Canada's health care system falls prey to U.S. style free enterprise medicine or the Marxist devils with more "state" control, the true message from this journalistic piece is that the patient is the hostage in the squabbles between the profession and the government.

The public must begin now to discard its traditional, highly emotional image of the TV medical hero. Patients must catch up, modernize, become more objective and independent. Doctors are human; they are neither machines nor gods, nor priests, whatever the metaphorical disguise. They offer a service that should not be held above that of any other service. The attitude that we get well because an authority figures tells us we will or gives us a pill should be discarded in favour of the belief that we get well because we are informed about our bodies which, translated means, we want to get well. And doctors are primarily businessmen for whom, like any other individual or company, it's the bottom line that counts. Doctors should not be regarded as "messiahs" or "good samaritans" as the dentist who replaced Slapek's "tin can" once called himself. This puts too much pressure on doctors or dentists to be perfect, but correspondingly the public should be allowed to see their imperfections. The doctor has modernized, adapted to technology; it is now time for the public to come of age. A report from Zurich, Switzerland, entitled *Sick and Therefore Defenceless*, which details experiences patients have had with doctors, suggests the Swiss have no trouble at all in viewing the doctor-patient contact as a "business relationship".[70] Canadians and Americans must do the same. "We believe Canada's new Health Act may be hazardous to your health!"[71] the OMA shrieked about a statute that guarantees the poor equal access to medical services. It would be preferable for the profession to channel its energy and time into rooting out incompetence or preventing doctors, like mine and Margo's, from practicing "hazardous" medicine.

Life is cheap to medi-businessmen who can joke, as Margo's doctor did, when she groggily awoke from surgery, "I bet you wish you had hair on your chest now!" What this doctor's reaction meant was that the most precious thing to a woman is her beauty, that appearance, in fact, is more important than health, that whether there is a scar on her chest is of more concern to her than valve replacement. The only message from this comment is that women are vain and shallow and, so, place more emphasis on appearance than reality. Imagine a doctor making a similar joke to a man who has just had open heart surgery. Women are, this doctor is saying, inferior to men; they are little girls whose only purpose in life is to look pretty to please men. In short, women must be protected by daddy-doctor from knowledge about the risks to their health, whether that be birth control pills or IE. Such medi-businessmen doctors place little importance on their patient's feelings and obviously give no thought to the quality of life the patient must face after open heart surgery and valve replacement. Why, therefore, should the public's response to doctors be primarily emotional? In fact, is it feeling, emotional support, that we want from the doctor-patient relationship? Rather than competence and knowledge and assurance that we will get this through parity that comes only with access to the medical record? Dr. Rosenberg, speaking at an OMA meeting, said "It's time to stop being nice" and it's time "to scare the hell out of the public."[72] For people who regard the doctor as daddy, priest, hero or god, this should be particularly offensive. What Rosenberg meant was that business was more important than patient health. At that time, the doctors were considering a strike in order to coerce the government and the public to comply with their demands to extra bill.

But it is certainly not the fault entirely of the medical profession that there is such inequity in the patient-doctor **contract**. If there is any genuine need to blame the patient, it is certainly for his or her attitude toward his business partner. The fact that we cannot look at doctors as businessmen is a dimension of our inability to accept reality, disease and death with rationality and objectivity. Instead, we dye our hair, undergo costly, dangerous cosmetic surgery, diet and exercise to the point of perhaps threatening our health, a real risk in the case of a **MVP** patient, hoard money, possessions, social and political power to delude ourselves that we are not fragile, are not mortal. And we anesthetize ourselves with the belief that medicine can accomplish miracles, that "daddy-doc" or "daddy-god", like the god in the basket, the deus ex machina, in Greek drama, will swoop down from the skies and extract us from peril. That we see doctors as miracle workers and medicine as miraculous is the reason that we remain incredibly uninformed about our bodies which then become damaged by that lack of knowledge. We prefer that medicine's activities remain mysterious because we believe blind faith, as in religion, works, and, when it doesn't, we are devastated and blame the medical profession.

What can we do to achieve a truly "balanced", equitable medical care system? We must look first to the political and legal systems because that is where injustice exists and, ultimately, that is where the power is to bring about change. In his paper delivered at the 1981 annual meeting of the Canadian Institute of Law and Medicine, Justice Linden reassured doctors that the "courts are not the enemies of physicians" and "our law is more favorable to doctors."[73] This reassurance was extended because of the doctors' exaggerated fear of a malpractice epidemic as is believed to exist in the US. "The chance," Justice Linden said, "of a doctor being successfully sued in Canada is extremely slight" because in court "the judiciary will approach the matter cautiously and reluctantly with the full knowledge that it is unqualified to do so."[74] The law recognizes unquestionably no other authority, no other source of medical information, than the doctor. It is because of this attitude of the legal profession towards the medical profession that we do not have access to our personal health information contained in the medical records held by all health care workers.

This imbalance must be redressed. What contract, other than that of patient-doctor, does an individual enter into with so little knowledge, so little understanding of risks, of what is being given and what is being taken away and so little protection? And, yet, this could be a contract on one's life. There can be no prevention of disease without patient knowledge, and there can be no knowledge without patient-doctor equality before the law. The sick, like any other minority group, must demand their rights. Doctors have tremendous legal and political influence in both Canada and the U.S. This was made abundantly clear in our country with the successful defeat of a very significant judicial proposal that would, literally, have catapulted the patient out of the dark ages.

On September 30, 1980, Honorable Justice H. Krever, a somewhat iconoclastic, provincial judge, a truly lone wolf, submitted his three volume *Report of the Commission of Inquiry into the Confidentiality of Health Information* to the then Health Minister for Ontario, Dennis Timbrell. A very brief section of that report contained Justice Krever's bold recommendation that a statute be introduced which grants patients direct right of access "to inspect and receive copies of any health information, of which he or she is the subject, kept by a health care provider."[75] At the time of his report, statutes existed only in Nova Scotia, Alberta and Quebec, granting patients direct access to hospital records though not to the doctors' office records. At the time of this writing, the situation remains the same. This same topic is being discussed in American legal circles, and the State of Massachusetts, in 1979, actually passed a law, The Patients' Bill of Rights,[76] which grants, among other things, the right of direct access to medical records which the Canadian judge had recommended. In Britain, there exists as of November, 1987, a Data Protection Act which gives patients the right to have copies of all personal health information held in a computer within 40 days of the request. While there is a section in that Act allowing doctors to censor certain information from the patient, a joint analysis by experts in medical information science, public health and medicine concluded that there is very little information, "only one percent of all problems" that would have to be censored from the patient.[77]

Krever's proposed statute would have protected patients, such as myself, from vanishing medical records, whether personal or hospital since I would have, as a matter of course, requested copies of everything as soon as they were available. Such a law, I venture to add, would also have caused a significant decline in the number of malpractice cases because it would have forced careless doctors, who now had someone to account to, to weed out errors. Rather than the courts, why can't the informed patient be the watchdog of his or her own care? Access would allow that. As Professor Westin stated for the Krever Report, access reflects "a growing citizens' movement to affirm individual self-determination and place limits on the power of institutions to determine important aspects of people's lives."[78]

The principle upon which Krever would base patient access was expressed thus:

> First, as an incident of human dignity a patient ought to have the right of access to the most personal information about himself or herself. No person, even though he or she may be a professional with much knowledge and experience, should be entitled to withhold that information. Second, the patient in his or her own interest, should be able to correct any misinformation which may appear on his record. Third, the patient will have a better understanding of his or her treatment and be in a better position to assist in future care. Fourth, access to the file will allow a patient to make an informed consent to the release of information from the file to a third party when necessary. Fifth, access creates a feeling of trust and openness between patient and health-care providers, and the quality of health care will thereby be enhanced.[79]

Human dignity, as Krever sees it, suffers without freedom of information, especially personal information kept by an institution, whether that be the court system or the health system. In oppressive regimes, prevention of access to information and deprival of education are the weapons that keep the poor powerless, in danger and victimized by an unjust, deceitful system. The right to correct errors in the medical record implies that the doctor is not infallible, is not all powerful. Krever envisions the patient as sharing in his treatment and this can only come about with access to knowledge. How can a patient, for example, sign a release of personal information for another party if he/she has never seen the information. In truth, in all such releases, the patient's signature is a mockery, a blow at human dignity because it is literally not worth the paper it's written upon. And, lastly, as Krever astutely saw, there can never be trust between the patient and the doctor when the doctor has all the information, all the power and the right to keep what he wishes hidden.

Krever's recommendation for a statute granting patient access to personal health information was defeated by the medical profession. In keeping with the law's view, that the doctor is the only authority in health care matters, the Ontario Health Minister, Dennis Timbrell, chose a doctor, J.D. Galloway, to prepare a report of the response of health care providers to Krever's proposal. Nowhere in this report are the opinions of users of the health care system represented. In Galloway's document, entitled, *The Review of The Report on The Confidentiality of Health Information*, the bulk of the opinion came from the medical profession, the most negative response being from physicians, psychiatrists, psychologists. In fact, discussion of this topic was the "most controversial and emotional."[80]

Doctors correctly saw Krever's statute as a challenge to their monopoly over medical information. Inevitably, opposition poured in from the medical profession as it flexed its defensive muscles. The OMA argued that "legislation allowing full disclosure of a physician's records may affect the completeness of the information placed in the record."[81] The College of Physicians and Surgeons of Ontario (CPSO) which is responsible for maintaining the standards of the profession and thus criticizing the care given by its physicians, unequivocally supported the OMA, claiming that such a statute would be "detrimental to the very quality of these records and thus to the quality of health care."[82] Such a statement implies that the skill and the knowledge of the doctor would deteriorate if the patient had access to personal medical information. This is, of course, absurd. An incomplete record would be one that would not contain the suggestion of error, likely the provisional or differential diagnosis.

The doctors' union and their governing body both found ways to claim that what was of benefit to patients would harm them, but few examples of such harm were offered by these medical groups in the Report. It is very difficult to understand how knowledge can harm except if the patient is presumed to be intellectually deficient or emotionally unbalanced and, therefore, cannot handle unpleasant facts about his or her health. And, even then, this is not a valid reason for obstructing access since patient responsibility must be encouraged. If patients were allowed access at all, both groups maintained, it must be through the attending physician or another appointed to care for the patient.[83] In other words, the patient must only be allowed to see the record at the discretion of the physician or his substitute and only in his presence. This amounts to no access at all.

The College of Family Physicians (CFPO), the GPs, likewise cried out vehemently against patient knowledge. The personal office record was "unquestionably and unequivocally"[84] sacrosanct, meant only for the eyes of the doctor. If there is nothing in there that shouldn't be in there, why is this so? The patient has entered a contract with a doctor to share a common object, a common resource of information, the patient's body. Why, therefore, does the patient not have the right to know to what use his or her body is made, what descriptions are given of it, what test findings, what observations are made and conclusions drawn about it? Does the client not have the right to know what descriptions of test findings or observations are made in regard to his or her automobile? I stress once again that, had my family physician not given me copies of the letters to him from the doctors I saw, I would have had no understanding of the change in my health. A sound physiological explanation, that intermittent, minimal regurgitation had become severe enough at the time of my illness, to cause my heart to enlarge, my murmur to change from late systolic to pansystolic, according to Dr. Austin, himself, my spleen to enlarge and my heart to be subject to excessive tachycardia, would have resolved the confusion and at least some of the anxiety, while attributing my lack of wellbeing to an obscure neurosis did not.

During the Commission's investigation, in endeavoring to defeat these arguments of the medical bodies, Justice Krever pointed out that the patient has the right, protected in law, to refuse an operation, even if such refusal is harmful, and, therefore, the patient should have the correlative right, even if it is harmful, to see information about his or her health. It is the patient's responsibility, as it is in any other contract, to accept the risk involved, in this case the risk of knowing. Krever argued convincingly that to refuse treatment could have far more dangerous consequences than seeing the medical records.[85] The doctors' argument that extending information is harmful and that withholding it is in the patient's best interests is no more valid than the argument that banning extra billing would result in deterioration in patient care, unless it can be construed that doctors perform sloppier work when they are paid less than when they are paid more.

The "dumb patient argument" or "the intellectual subordinate" of Geoff Issac, was another inadequate reason advanced for refusing access. A CPSO spokesman declared that the medical records contained information that patients could not possibly comprehend or might misinterpret. A ridiculous example was given. The patient might interpret a term like SOB as "son of a bitch".[86] Or perhaps BUN might indicate the doctor thinks the patient is an ass. This attitude is the fruit of a long history of elitism, exemplified in the views of doctors like Alvarez and the makers of the Minnesota Multiphasic Personality Test. When I examined Margo's medical records, my only difficulty was in reading the exceptionally poor copy. Pages of it were illegible with line after line of scribbles, stray marks and dots. Were they meant to be intelligible to anything other than a Morse code machine? It seems that giving the patient access would assure that the doctor's notes were legible, accurate and complete. If the patient does not understand a term such as SOB then the onus is upon him or her to find out from a doctor, medical dictionary or medical journal what that term means.

The word, "trust", was bandied about frequently during the Royal Commission's investigations. In the doctor's view, requests to see the medical records mean the patient mistrusts the doctor. "The request to review records indicates a degree of mistrust,"[87] the OMA representative stated, but its opposite, the denial of the records, or withholding of information, should not mean the doctor mistrusts the patient. The OMA claimed that doctors believe in "open, frank and honest communications between providers and consumers of health services"[88] and maintained that this already existed. The doctors argued unabashedly that patients must trust, must have blind faith, that their doctors are being frank and honest in transmitting information, without actually seeing that information, because good medicine is based on the fact that *"physicians are paternalistic"* and because *"paternalism"* is an approach *"that is expected by most patients."*[89] Direct access to health information conflicts, in the view of the doctors, with the patient's need to believe that the doctor knows best. If the public is, in fact, dependent upon such a primitive need, then it is time to change, time to realize that the doctor's service is not better because it is mysterious.

Deprived of knowledge and with no remedy in law to acquire such knowledge, the patient in desperate need of medical services is at the mercy of the institution, its doctors and its nurses. What patients feel is not trust but fear and begrudging submission. In Krever's opinion, access creates trust; to the doctors, mistrust. The "trust equals good medicine" argument is an irrational one based upon the monopolization of knowledge and information highly specific to the individual. In its efforts to resist challenges of that monopoly, the profession behaves not unlike the Church in the Middle Ages or any currently repressive regime which strives to keep people uneducated, uninformed and thus impotent.

In our age of explosion of knowledge, the refusal to grant direct access to personal medical records is an indefensible position which not only doctors but also hospitals believe is acceptable. A Toronto hospital administrator, who represented the Ontario Hospital Association (OHA), in a discussion with the Commissioner of the Inquiry, said that a hospital would provide personal health information about a patient to a third party, most often a physician or a lawyer, but not to the patient. The lawyer is not legally required to show this personal information to the patient who has no means of forcing him to do so. In reality then, the lawyer acts on behalf of the medical profession, not the client, as is commonly believed. The OHA representative alluded to that very strong bond between lawyers and doctors when he revealed, somewhat reluctantly, that the medical profession views lawyers as "wise persons" with "good judgement", and, therefore, qualified to decide whether the information contained in the medical record is "harmful" or not to the patient.[90] The converse is, of course, implied: the patient is neither "wise" nor has "good judgement" and is, thus,incapable of distinguishing what is or is not harmful to him or herself.

On behalf of the patient, the Commissioner of the investigation challenged the position of the administrator. The hospital, the Commissioner said, has elevated the lawyer to a status he does not merit, that of medical interpreter. In attempting to deny that the hospital accorded the lawyer a status higher than the patient, the hospital administrator resorted to the familiar "dumb patient" argument. The patient would not understand what was in the medical records while the lawyer would, and this misinterpreted information could be harmful to the patient. The only logical rebuttal to such an argument was that of the Commissioner who pointed out that the lawyer was no more capable of understanding medical terminology, for example, the meaning of an "elevated BUN", than the patient and might even be less capable since the matter is not of personal concern to him.[91] Certainly, a lawyer who refers to the mitral valve as "micro" valve and an enlarged spleen as an infected spleen, has no more facility than the patient in medical matters.

The hospital administrator's answers were evasive, and the arguments advanced for prevention of patient access were nothing more than attempts to disguise the real truth. The OHA administrator said "It is simply that if he (the lawyer) judges that there could be something in the information that would be worrisome for the patient, not just a legal matter, but that the lawyer would then perhaps consult with the physician and try to clarify this issue before he upsets the patient."[92] If, in fact, a medical matter were being referred to here, this would mean that the hospital administrator was, indeed, according the lawyer a status higher than that of the patient, the ability to interpret the "worrisome" detail and decide whether it was harmful and, therefore, should be withheld from the patient. The truth, however, is that the medical profession, out of fear, does not want the patient to know the meaning of the "worrisome" detail. This small phrase and the "legal matter", sandwiched casually in among these confused meanderings, has more importance than the administrator implied. What it means, ultimately, is that the lawyer is the unacknowledged watchdog, the spy, to put it bluntly, whose job is to screen out dangerous elements and prevent frivolous malpractice suits. This role he plays is established by long tradition; it represents the bond that exists between law and medicine. And since the legal system, in Canada, discourages malpractice and since the malpractice case is so difficult to win, the lawyer would not want, in any case, to proceed with a frustrating, profitless task.

That this was, indeed, the major concern of the hospital administrator and the entire medical profession became undeniable when the hospital administrator admitted that medical documents would not be forwarded to the lawyer if it were known that the patient were contemplating a malpractice suit. The patient would not, of course, seek a lawyer's opinion unless he or she were contemplating a malpractice suit. The decision to proceed can only come from the lawyer to whom the patient has turned for independent help. "To do so," the OHA administrator equivocated, "would not be in the patients' best interests because it would facilitate frivolous lawsuits."[93] This response echoed Alvarez's charge that "paranoic" patients undertake "foolish lawsuits". As I pointed out earlier, "frivolous" is a word favoured by the CMPA, the doctors' protective association in Canada.

Behind these specious arguments of "good medicine" and "the best interests of the patient" is the powerful motive of self-protection. It, in fact, is the major reason why patients do not have access to information about their own health and why doctors, without exception, discourage reading of the medical literature. According to one doctor represented in the report, "our surest and best protection against unfair litigation lies in full and complete written notes"[94] which, he said, doctors would be reluctant to prepare if the patient had direct access. If the doctor's process of thinking and his decisions were reasonable and justifiable, there should be no harm in including them in the record whether the patient sees them or not.

One must realize that **all litigation** is unfair to a doctor. This position is, of course, understandable. The highest stakes possible, the life of, the wellbeing of the patient, can rest upon the doctor's decisions. This suggests that the matter of compensation for injury should, somehow, be facilitated through other channels, especially in the U.S. where financial reimbursement can be significant. In Canada, malpractice, as a solution to the problem, is extremely ineffective because the physician's protective organization, the conspiracy of silence and the court system are stacked against the patient.

A few enlightened opinions of members of the medical profession, such as Professor Greenland, a psychiatrist from the Clarke Institute in Toronto, were included in the Galloway report. Greenland pointed out that there is evidence that the supposed harm that patient access to medical records would do to both the doctor and patient "is found in fact to be fantasy." The doctors' notes became, he said, "more objective" which is "all to the good."[95] And Professor Nahum Spinner of McMaster University's Psychiatry Department added that he could find no plausible reason why "information that is professionally sound and ought to be in the record ought not to be accessible to the patient."[96] It is noteworthy, however, that such opinions in favour of patient access, came from psychiatrists rather than practicing physicians, and it would seem that information from a psychiatrist about the patient's mind and personality, would be far more offensive and, therefore, harmful to the patient, than medical facts about the body. I am tempted to ask whether subjective comments, such as "labile mentality" and "pathological anxiety", were professionally sound in view of the clinical evidence found of a genuine cardiac malady, a significant enlargement of my heart over a period of a year? Such opinions can be dangerous if they prevent the doctor from properly investigating in order to arrive at a correct diagnosis. In my case, blood tests, not x-rays, are the means to diagnose IE along with clinical examination.

That the medical institutions view their rights as superseding all other rights is expressed in the Galloway Report through the opinions of two internists from London and St. Thomas, Ontario who spoke for the 16,000 doctors in Ontario. A Dr. Gunton commented that we live in an age of a more informed citizenry which now demands fairness, truth and the same rights formerly granted only to specialized groups, hence the burgeoning, he says, of "women's rights, civil liberty in all its forms, full disclosure, freedom of information."[97] Gunton, however, does not classify doctors with the civil libertarians nor the jurists who might support them through "the wish to remain contemporary".[98] Gunton chose to interpret the emphasis on civil rights as purely faddish, and advocated the preservation of the sanctity of the medical record which must remain absolutely untouched by the "freedom of information" movement. The individual's right to self-determination, expressed by Professor Westin, is secondary to the right of the institution to control. The CPSO had expressed the same attitude when it stated that "practices which relate to the freedom of information in other settings may not be compatible with the best interests of the patient, or society, when applied to health records."[99] There is no rational argument here; it is a matter of deferment to the unshakable status of the doctor as guardian of medical information, and, therefore, the entrenchment of power solely in the hands of the medical institution.

The views of the doctors' professional groups, the OMA and the governing colleges are also the views of the medical profession's most powerful institution, its protective body, the Canadian Medical Protective Association, the CMPA, which insures the doctors against malpractice litigation. At their annual meeting, Charles F. Scott, General Legal Counsel for the CMPA at the time of this writing, echoed Dr. Gunton. The new information society, Scott complained, has lead to the *Doctrine of Informed Consent* which allows the injured patient to recover damages in the courtroom on the grounds that the doctor did not fully disclose the nature of the risks of an investigative or surgical procedure. The *Doctrine of Informed Consent*, an American phenomenon, implies, at least, that there is some recognition by the courts that the patient is entitled to personal medical information, despite the fact that there is no statute granting access and that this doctrine is rarely invoked in Canadian courts. The doctors' legal representative complained that this ruling is a way for "making awards for bad results"[100] and that it encourages "the mistaken opinion . . . that those who perform services cannot be trusted."[101] An informed society is, in the opinion of the doctors and their legal advisor, a dangerous society because it signifies the end of the patient's blind trust in the doctor and the miracles of medicine and thus the termination of paternalistic control.

Attitudes such as these reflect a belief in class consciousness and inviolable privilege accorded only to the few who are entitled to knowledge, and patient access to personal health information is seen as a battle between the traditional rights of elitism and the evils of egalitarianism. "Theories of participatory democracy and egalitarianism . . .", Scott declared, "are used to push the assumed virtue of the citizenry beyond the limits of democracy."[102] What is at issue here is the patient's need and right to personal medical information. That right, this group is saying, is "beyond the limits of democracy".

The opinions expressed by Dr. Gunton are those of his legal counsel. "Those advocates of full disclosure"[103], the civil libertarians, do not, in his opinion, understand that patients must not have direct access because of the nature of the medical record, specifically the "provisional diagnosis" or the "differential diagnosis". Citizens, he said, are not "enlightened" enough to forgive "the theoretical errors" found in such diagnoses.[104] Among Gunton's examples of differential diagnosis are psychiatric illness, hysteria and malingering[105], labels that can easily be applied to MVP patients and were applied to myself and Margo as well as many of the MVP women who contacted me.

The provisional diagnosis in my case was that my knowledge of my MVP was causing "pathological anxiety" or cardiac neurosis. The provisional diagnosis, did not, of course, give way to the definitive diagnosis since tests for IE were never done, unless the missing x-rays and echocardiograms contained evidence of vegetations which would have altered the provisional diagnosis. However, they were not done as a diagnostic test for IE. The sudden chest pain, disruptive tachycardia, fever, changing murmur and cardiac enlargement in the presence of a highly suspicious source of infection, endodontal interventions and an aveolar abscess, did not obviously figure in Austin's "provisional diagnosis" or perhaps even a tricuspid murmur if, in fact, there had been vegetations on the tricuspid valve which subsequently showed up on echo as nodules. In Margo's case, her GP's preliminary opinions were clearly neurosis and hysteria, and, later in hospital, collagen vascular disease, lymphoma, lupus erythematosus and systemic infection. This term, "differential diagnosis", in reality, can cover a doctor's inability to identify the source of the trouble because he lacks the knowledge to know what to look for. Dr. Gunton was correct, of course, in predicting that an injured patient would not be able to see such provisional diagnoses "as an intellectual exercise designed to arrive at the correct diagnosis".[106]

The "differential diagnosis" argument exposes the doctor's real fear about patient access, the same fear expressed by Counsel Scott in his opposition to Informed Consent. If we consider some of the facts, that only one in six incidents of malpractice ever results in litigation,[107] according to a prominent provincial court judge, and that the number of cases the doctors lost in 1982 was virtually the same as in 1970, twelve years earlier, and that the number of patient's cases that the court dismissed rose from 35 in 1970 to 201 in 1982,[108] then opinions such as the following of Dr. Gunton seem tinged with paranoia, hysteria and exaggerated fear. "When one considers on a numerical basis the sheer size of the problem in respect to medical records and the vagaries of the human personality," he declared, "one would predict legal actions against physicians would increase beyond reason."[109] But, in fact, there is no evidence that access to one's own personal health information has produced an epidemic of malpractice suits. In Alberta, where access is enshrined in law, patients have not made more use of their right, which would precede the undertaking of any malpractice litigation, than in provinces which do not have legal access.[110]

With the successful defeat of Krever's recommendation, it became evident that legal and medical circles believed it perfectly justifiable for the doctor to fear the patient, but not for the patient to fear the doctor. And, likewise, for the doctor to mistrust the patient but not vice versa. An enemy lurks in the patient. This is the attitude of Alvarez and Lewis. Those patients with neurosis, almost anyone if the doctor lacks a defense, are bound to undertake a malpractice suit unjustly for greed or whatever base motive might be attributed to them. Given the power, the status, the political influence, and, most important of all, the precious bargaining tool, the threat of withdrawal of their salvation medicine in any form, by strike or emigration, it is not surprising that the OMA, the OHA, the CPSO, the CFPO and the CMPA, despite support for the public's right of direct access to their medical records from some psychiatrists, nurses and pharmacists, succeeded in persuading the law making bodies to crush a long overdue statutory recommendation that could have become the most just, civilized and enlightened piece of legislation since women were granted the vote.

Health care is a right, not a privilege. If the AIP can invoke the Charter of Rights, the patient ought to be able to do so as well. In the doctor-patient contract, the patient should have, in any country, "the right to life, liberty and security of person and the right not to be deprived thereof" as is stated in the *Canadian Charter of Rights and Freedoms* and in the *American*

Constitution. When one is sick, one does not have freedom and security if one must trust blindly and depend, out of fear and ignorance, on the institution, the hospital and the doctors. Margo and I were deprived of that security of health, mind and person. We were not told of the risks of the MVP condition nor how to protect ourselves from them. I was then deprived of a proper investigation and treatment which would have given me that "security of person". Further, the curious loss of my medical records prevented me irrevocably from ever knowing the exact nature of my illness which I was then forced to piece together laboriously, an effort that consumed six years of my life. My health changed suddenly and dramatically without any explanation and has since deteriorated much more quickly than that of other people with MVP. The anxiety alone that this lack of knowledge created was a threat to me.

Before patients and a supportive public can unite to demand right of access to all personal medical information, they must psychologically recondition themselves to adopt a different view of medicine, one with less emotionalism and subjectivity. Blind trust in authority figures is dangerous. And, before we can change the attitudes of the legal, political and medical establishments towards the defenceless patient, we must change our own attitude towards these venerated bodies. Malpractice litigation, whether in the U.S. or Canada, is not an ideal means of preventing disease or injury. Nor does it improve the health care system as a whole. It only serves to make the doctor more hostile just as lack of access to personal medical information makes the patient hostile. If the patient, who has been genuinely injured does not win — and this is usually the case — then there will be little compulsion within the profession to upgrade its standards. And an atmosphere in which the malpractice threat is always imminent does nothing to improve patient-doctor relationships. The cold, hard facts, however, are that someone must foot the bill for the lifelong care of patients who can no longer function as a result of their injury. Perhaps for these patients, or for injured patients in general whose pleasure in life has been diminished through the omissions or commissions of a doctor or dentist should have some kind of recourse to a compensation fund where it is not necessary to establish guilt. This would relieve the families of the injured person of the stressful and expensive burden of malpractice litigation.

Because what the public really wants is the best, up-to-date health care and not revenge on any doctor or dentist, the only answer lies in creating a fair system through public education and, therefore, pressure on governments to introduce legislation granting direct right of access with copies of all personal medical records including hospital records, all doctors' and nurses' notes, all laboratory test results and copies of x-rays, echocardiograms and electrocardiograms for which the patient would be required to pay. This would bring money into the system. Direct access to personal medical information is not universally assured in the U.S. any more than in Canada. To have access would, however, be of little value unless patients take responsibility for their health by learning everything they can about their illness and, in particular, how to prevent deterioration of a condition and unless the public, in general, educates itself about the human body. Facts — the truth — heal us mentally and physically. Ignorance — impotence — causes sickness or perpetuates ill health as the experiment involving the two groups of rats with and without levers to stop electric shocks so dramatically illustrated. Ignorance, lack of control, can kill.

If doctors were truly open with us, that is, for instance, everytime we visited our doctor, he provided us with a copy of his assessment of our health situation at that point in time, and, if we had legal power, in the form of a statute, to enforce him or her to do so, the relationship between the doctor and the patient could only improve and the standards of the profession would improve individually and as a whole because that doctor would make very certain that he employed everything that was known to assure his patients' continued health. And, if he lacked current knowledge, he would be encouraged to bring himself up to date. Armed with the same information as the doctor of the disease and how to treat it, patients could, where the doctor is remiss, suggest he reconsider his management approach. The patient would then truly become, as Norman Cousins suggested, a partner in his or her care. Mistakes are made not only through negligence or incompetence but also through human error and that is why the patient should be allowed to adopt this truly responsible role. If medical science is as inexact as doctors claim it is, then the patient must be familiar with the different treatment options and be able to decide, with the help of the doctor, which treatment might be most beneficial. Patients must read in order to know what doctors are supposed to know about their conditions. Surely a MVP patient would sooner opt for antibiotic protection, considering the minimal risk involved in taking this medication and the gravity of the risk in not. To have parity of knowledge in the doctor-patient contract is of far more value and, in fact, would reduce inevitably and dramatically the extent of malpractice litigation as well as improve medical care.

The media is largely responsible for promoting false, highly subjective views of the doctor's role in society and of elevating him to a status superior to all other people and of making of doctors heroes who accomplish miracles on a par with the heroes of the Greek myths. An educated public can transform the content of the media. Book stores, for example, reek of simple-minded, romantic fiction about noble, heroic doctors who struggle against dishonesty and corruption in their profession, doctors who are willing to put their careers on the line to chastize a colleague, doctors with a charismatic love for their patients equivalent to that of the Messiah. Such portraits of the doctors as are shown in Arthur Hailey's *Strong Medicine* or Neil Ravin's *MD*, with blurbs that read "medical school did little to prepare Bill Ryan for colleagues who are heavily into patients as whole human beings"[111] do not acknowledge the evidence of the conspiracy of silence nor the true nature of the doctor-patient relationship. The doctor in these books is always a superhuman in intellect, in human endowments, in morality. The public swallows these romantic, unrealistic sagas of the "messiahs" of medicine[112], as Gifford-Jones called them, with as little friction as junket or jello.

Non-fiction medical books manifest the same puerile fascination with these "great" medical people. In Martin O'Malley's book, *Doctors*, for example, the doctors are not businessmen but the same old mystical, god-like figures who inspire nothing but awe and reverence in the public. Doctors, in O'Malley's book, remain, unquestionably, the experts, and such authority is still equated, without rationality, with the best in humanity, courage, nobleness of soul and dazzling intelligence, and, beside such paragons, all other people are inferior.

Television perpetuates the same myth of the superhuman hero in series like St. Elsewhere or Trapper John, offspring of a long line of bigger than life Dr. Kildares and Ben Caseys who could never do harm. The public is constantly brainwashed with doctors who are "beyond reproach" in the words of media Professor George Gerbner who is studying how television programmes sell us a specific definition of reality. These television doctors are "fairer, more sociable and warmer than other characters and are rated as more intelligent, more rational and more stable and fair than the female nurses . . . and possess an uncanny ability to dominate and control the lives of others."[113] Since the ratings are excellent, the public is obviously comfortable with this superior image of the traditional authority figure and that control by this person is right and good.

What is needed on television is a balance, some realistic docu-dramas of cases of patients who have been maimed or killed by the "good samaritans" of medicine, an examination of what went wrong and what can be done to improve in the future on the part of the patient and the doctor. They should not be punitive but instructive. A steady diet of glamorous, brave and noble doctors who would sacrifice their own personal comfort or career to live up to their Apollo Creed distorts the facts and perpetuates the myths in an age when knowledge should replace legend. In these dramas, ordinary people should be chosen to expose the problems in the medical profession, not doctors, as in the cops and robbers medical fantasies where the conspiracy of silence is unheard of.

Of questionable value are the self-help books, written by doctors, which claim to give the public what it needs to know about medical issues. These books perpetuate the myth that only the moguls of medibusiness are qualified to write them, that they must first digest the medical information before feeding it to the public. Frequently these books are undisguised apologias for doctors, their primary goal being to restore decaying public confidence in the medical profession. Often, they are unabashed public relations documents. These doctor-authors give the reader the impression that they have set themselves apart from their more unenlightened colleagues, that they are the new breed of physician, courageous, forthright, more human than god-like and more caring, intelligent and noble. These books attempt to persuade the public that it should have faith in a dramatically changing medical profession. In his book, *Confessions of a Medical Heretic*, the guru of popular medical literature, Robert Mendelsohn, describes the "new doctor":

The education of the new Doctor will include not only medical and clinical sciences but ethics and literature as well. All students in the new medical school will be shown how human behaviour relates to health and disease. New Doctors will be trained to communicate by means of the written as well as the spoken word. They will also learn the basic techniques and social implications of other media such as television. New Doctors must not only be able to communiate effectively with the community, but they must be aware of the processes by which they and their patients are influenced. Since legal procedures are important not only to the doctor's protection of his practice but to the protection of his patients as well, New Doctors will learn to deal with lawyers and the law.[114]

Consumers must learn to read the hard-core selling between the lines of such manifestos. Mendelsohn wants the public to believe that the doctors of the future will be "whole human beings", into people, reminiscent of the heroes in the popular doctor novels. They possess not only scientific but cultural perfection and are familiar with the sublime humanitarian thoughts contained in the world's great literatures. The public is expected to trust, without doubt, such impressive specimens of humanity. But why is a knowledge of literature necessary to diagnose and treat illness or repair a diseased organ? Would one hire a roofer because he can quote Plato? That they have mastered the craft of writing might suggest to the public only that these doctors are able to make use of the power of print in selling their heroic image.

Doctors, like Rhodes, feel they have the right to quote the profound thoughts of Pope to their patients who are teachers of English literature, but why do patients not have the concomitant right to discuss the research of Yale, Stanford or Witwatersrand that is confined to the pages of the medical journals? How is it that a patient can be thrown out of a doctor's office for attempting to discuss her own personal information in her own medical record? We are decidedly not their equals; they are to be trusted, respected and feared; we are not. We are, as they have clearly told us repeatedly, "their intellectual subordinates".

In the matter of how human behaviour relates to health and disease, Mendelsohn is really talking about the curious twilight zone of psychosomatic medicine. This was the purpose of Alvarez's book, to assist the doctor in assessing the effect of human behaviour on the patient's disease. Does this mean that the doctor will learn how to convince the patient to accept blame for iatrogenic disease in order to protect the physician? It is neither possible nor even just for patients to accept any responsibility for illness without complete knowledge of that illness. That cannot be done without access to one's own medical records.

In the new ambiance of freedom of information, the word, "communicate", can be much abused. Doctor-authors know the public loves this word. Lack of communication is the chief complaint that patients make against doctors. But the word has two definitions, one for the doctor and one for the public. For the doctor it does not mean communicating complete medical information about the patient's disease. It means conveying only what the doctor wishes, what he thinks is in the patient's best interests to know, just as was proven in the case of the doctors who opposed Judge Krever's recommendation for an official Act to grant patients access to their medical information. And for Mendelsohn's new breed of doctor, it means playing chum, being more friendly, more familiar than in the past, using first names, talking down, either to build up a practice, as Alvarez said, or to avoid a malpractice suit as the legal-medical writers, the Rozovskys, advise in their article, "Avoid Malpractice Suits by Communicating with Your Patients". The Rozovskys say doctors should "discourage patients from suing in the first place regardless of whether or not they have legal grounds to do so."[115] The sweet talk, the backslapping puts the patient off guard so that he or she asks no questions. The patient equates the doctor's friendliness with honesty and the corollary that he has told the patient all and will do no harm.

When Mendelsohn says doctors must make use of "the basic techniques and social implications" of the media, he is talking about using the media to restore the patient's confidence and trust in the medical profession. These new doctors will become politicized, able to understand the "processes" in our society that influence in order to maintain their elitist position of power and authority as was expressed by their CMPA legal counsel. Doctors did not begin the movement for direct access to medical records in either Canada or the United States. This was the work of patients and patients rights' groups. Few, if any, authors of these self-help books would agree with Krever's recommendations that patients should have direct access to their own medical records. Secrecy is essential to a doctor's self-protection, and human beings are genetically programmed to protect themselves.

Mendelsohn owes much to Alvarez, Lewis and White when he speaks of the New Doctor being a "priest" who will "officiate or mediate at the absolution or cleansing of the patient's "sins".[116] Taking responsibility for one's health, according to Mendelsohn and many other doctors, means blaming the patient more often for his or her illness; he or she has in true Alvarez fashion, "sinned". It does not matter that the patient has "sinned" without knowledge; he or she has still, like Oedipus, sinned. There is nothing more powerful than self-blame to protect a doctor from criticism. Teaching that human behaviour relates to health and disease is a very valid argument but not when doctors use it for self-protection. With such a prescription for future medicine, one can envisage the disappearance of the word, "iatrogenic", from the vocabulary of doctor and public alike to be replaced with some newly coined word like "autogenic", in the way that the term "endogenous anxiety" has emerged. All this means, it seems, is that the New Doctor will have the "savvy" of the "master of ceremonies", the slickness of the television medivangelist, with all the persuasive techniques of that media at his command to manipulate human weakness into belief of self-guilt.

The last line of Mendelsohn's eulogy points to the bare truth, the real objective of many doctor self-help books, which is to stop the hemorrhage of public confidence in the medical profession and thus stem the tide of malpractice litigation. The doctors monopolize knowledge, as the Krever Commission demonstrated, for that very same reason. Doctors will become versed, Mendelsohn says, in the ways of the law and lawyers to protect the doctors' practice. But we know that no lawyer will ever say to a doctor, "a little learning is a dangerous thing" as Rhodes said to me. In Canada, doctors already have formidable legal back-up. It is difficult to imagine how much more perfected it could be. It is also difficult to understand how a doctor's knowledge of the law can protect the patient especially since doctors will not criticize a colleague when a patient has been injured.

Because these books are written quickly to serve the current popular market, they often smack of a certain carelessness that the public should not overlook because this may be a reflection of the all round lack of integrity in the work. After all, these books are written in a paternalistic style for the "dumb" patient. Robert Mendelsohn's elaborate extended metaphor comparing the medical profession to the Roman Catholic Church is an appalling example of what does not belong in a supposedly serious book purporting to give the public information, no more than do diagnoses such as "labile mentality" and "pathological anxiety" belong in the medical, as opposed to psychiatric, record of any patient, much less one who has suddenly shown evidence of a serious illness. Almost every page of *Confessions of a Medical Heretic* contains references to tabernacles, sacraments, priests, Church Laws, Holy Waters, rituals of the Church, sacramental benefits, sacred vestments and even the Inquisition of the Middle Ages. Such imagery should offend Catholics everywhere. One wonders just what Mendelsohn was excoriating, the medical profession or the Catholic Church. Cleverness dissipates into tedious, distasteful remarks that manifest an ominous prejudice against Catholicism, disguised as a criticism of the medical profession. "The Church is not about to give up any power, especially where its own temple is concerned. Would Catholics allow Jews to tell them how to run their churches and schools?"[117] And "Like priests who "blessed" the hot dogs to save parishioners from the moral bane of eating meat at a Friday night Church carnival, doctors gave their blessing to bottle feeding."[118] The reader who is not so "dumb", as Mendelsohn would conceive, must surely ask what eating hot dogs has to do with bottle feeding. Metaphors have the purpose of enlarging the imaginative perspective; certainly these do not, except to arouse distaste for the rituals of the Catholic church. Perhaps Mendelsohn's anecdote of the priest wanting to baptize dying, premature infants with, as he describes, "overwhelming compulsion" provoked a life-long anti-Catholic sentiment.[119]

Leonard Tushnet's *The Medicine Men*, curiously employs the same offensive metaphor with liberal references to Holy Church, high priests, acolytes, birettas, censers. But all the vocabulary and ritualistic elements of the Catholic Church do nothing to convince the reader that doctors are not to be regarded as infallible like "gods" but only that the "paraphernalia" of the Roman Catholic Church is a nasty, hollow ritual. Doctors do not retain their infallibility by words but by actions, by maintaining control over the patient's personal medical information, a point which is made neither by Mendelsohn nor Tushnet. In fact, I was as deeply mystified by these stylistic similarities as I was by the most curious appearance of an almost identical passage in each book. Mendelsohn says of the patient and his psychiatrist, "If you arrive for your appointment late, he'll say you're hostile. If you're early, you must be anxious. And if you're right on time your're compulsive."[120] And Tushnet mimicks him with "If the patient is late for his appointment, he's resisting treatment; if he's early he's overanxious; if he's right on time, he's compulsive."[121] It can only be concluded that these authors believe the "dumb" patient would no more appreciate sloppy writing than sloppy medicine.

Many of these books that claim to be informing the public are really defensive responses to what doctors conceive of as a "malpractice crisis" in the United States and Canada. These doctor-writers, who see themselves as mediators in the conflict between the public and the profession, blame the patient. Tushnet appeals directly to the public to stop "unfair" malpractice litigation because "doctors are human; they make mistakes. They should be forgiven. But they are not."[122] But what these authors refuse to accept is that the malpractice suit is, unfortunately, the patient's only means, no matter how imperfect, for criticizing, for urging certain doctors to upgrade themselves and, in particular, for just bringing information about their health that doctors have kept from them out into the open. In maintaining that lawsuits have increased "not because doctors are mistreating patients but because patients and their families demand a surety of cure,"[123] Tushnet is using the same argument that the Registrar of the Ontario College of Dentistry used when he said that patients expect the impossible and, therefore, most malpractice litigation is inspired by an exaggerated, erroneous notion of what dentistry or medicine can do. It was not "expecting the impossible" to assume that any cardiologist, especially one who is Chief of his speciality at a major hospital in a big city, should know that ABP had been recommended for MVP for over fifteen years in numerous medical journals and textbooks at the time that he diagnosed my MVP and that MVP had been known to carry a high risk of IE at the time of my hospitalization, and, to be perfectly accurate, ever since the introduction of antibiotics in 1944. But doctors still hadn't learned this in 1982 and 1989 when Margo and Doug developed their IE.

In *Second Opinion*, Isidore Rosenfeld bluntly tells the public why doctors oppose public education about medical matters. His opinions are those doctors advanced in the Galloway report to prevent patient access to personal medical information. Like Rhodes, Rosenfeld argues that a little knowledge is dangerous when it convinces the patient that his or her doctor is out of date or is employing treatment unacceptable to many of his colleagues.[124] Rosenfeld shares the opinion of Krever's opponents that medicine must keep its knowledge to itself and deplores the fact that the media is now allowed at conferences and conventions where medical topics, medical controversy, what he calls "family disputes"[125] are discussed. The danger, he warns, is that the lay press publishes these reports for the public "before we have heard about them or had an opportunity to evaluate and discuss them among ourselves."[126] But the doctors' problem is not that he hasn't had time to see the "new" information but that he hasn't bothered to digest the old or he has rejected it in spite of overwhelming evidence that his opinion is out of date. The knowledge that IE attacked incompetent rather than stenotic valves, that IE was common and that orthostatic hypotension is related to the LSM and, therefore, to MVP is not new; these are old subjects as I have pointed out.

In Rosenfeld's view "all hell breaks loose" when the patient gains knowledge from the lay publications that makes his doctor's treatment appear dangerous. The reader can only assume that one dimension of the ensuing "hell" might well be a "frivolous" lawsuit. Blaming the doctor is unfair, Rosenfeld preaches, because medicine is full of contradictory views; it is an inexact science. "Your doctor," Rosenfeld concludes in the last lines of his book, "is not to blame . . . he is buffeted by the changing winds of new scientific information."[127] All the cardiologists I saw in Toronto used this same argument, that medicine was subject to the "state of the art" fragility and that there was no hard and fast rule regarding the use of ABP to prevent IE in a MVP patient. This knowledge had been around for sixteen years and was hardly "new scientific information"!

Why is it that medicine, unlike most other sciences, cannot be more exact? Since medical practitioners have the rare opportunity to see the same problems repeated over and over again in thousands of patients, why do they not know everything there is to know about the body? After all, evolution has presumably stopped, and the human body is not changing before their very eyes. It is understandable that a geologist would not know everything there is to know about an earthquake or a volcano since, often, he must wait years to observe such "diseases" in nature. The rapidity with which our society learned about AIDS belies the claim of inexactitude in medical science. It is public pressure that determines how fast the researchers will come up with answers. It took doctors 100 years to accept that MVP was a disease and not a neurotic disorder. But the public does not demand scientific perfection though I'm sure this could be achieved if more money were spent on researching the causes of disease than on technology to replace diseased parts or if there were more application of existing knowledge, gained from years of research, in the clinical arena. What the public demands is adherence to proven preventative strategies or treatments known for many years.

Though their purpose is to shape public opinion of the profession, popular medical books may be more than just ineffective; they may be "hazardous to your health", to use the OMA's words. As well as dismissing MVP as having no more effect on longevity than "crooked legs" or a "deviated nasal septum", Gifford-Jones[128], like Mendelsohn,[129] counselled doctors not to tell patients about "harmless heart murmurs". Alternatively, if the doctor does tell the patient, he should explain, Gifford-Jones says, that the murmur is of no importance or a cardiac neurosis will be iatrogenically created. Once again, I stress, that research keeps showing consistently how great a risk IE is to the MVP patient.

In a 1988 letter to *The Journal of Family Practice*, it was said that MVP is present in 29 percent of the cases of IE and that "89 percent of the risk exists in the mitral valve prolapse patients with systolic murmurs."[130]

In his book, *The Doctor Game*, Jones speaks of an enlarged heart being as insignificant as a grey hair.[131] Although he is talking of an eighty year old man, one wonders if this is a general attitude of doctors to slight cardiac enlargement even in young people. An unusual enlargement of my heart did not alert Austin that there was something wrong, even though he regarded this as significant. Similarly, despite the fact that I have been given drugs used specifically to treat CHF and that there is improvement in my exercise tolerance, my symptoms are still said to be insignificant and I am not told, definitely, that I have heart failure though, on occasion, the suggestion has been made.

In his book, *Modern Medical Mistakes*, published in 1978, Edward Lambert makes no mention of MVP. However, he spends a lot of time rejecting the long held theory, still unchallenged today, that "localized pockets of bacterial infection around the teeth, tonsils, or other parts of the body produce or affect a wide variety of generalized diseases", including IE, and he claims that modern textbooks mention this theory only "to condemn it".[132] As this book demonstrates, the medical literature holds exactly the opposite opinion especially with regard to IE. But Lambert's objective is to show how this theory lead to too much surgery, specifically tonsillectomies or the extraction of teeth. Certain types of surgery go in and out of fashion, and, at the time of his writing, tonsillectomy was not popular. Lambert has set himself up as a medical critic whose aim is to protect the public from dangerous, inappropriate treatment and, in that role, the first thing a doctor does is attack unnecessary surgery as though a feud existed between diagnostician and surgeon over who should get the patient such as that which exists between general dentists and periodontist over the treatment of periodontitis. Lambert's criticism may be valid but not when he minimizes the dangers of bacteria associated with local infections in teeth and tonsils, particularly to susceptible patients with heart murmurs. My history and that of almost every person with diagnosed MVP who contacted me includes chronic tonsillitis recurring over many years, and Libman's studies as well as many after him have shown the riskiness of an "unclean" mouth.

Likewise, Gifford-Jones, riding high on the wave of public horror at too much surgery, says "children in North America are 12 times more likely to have their tonsils removed than are children in Sweden,"[133] and Tushnet even claims that 100-300 deaths occur annually from tonsillectomies.[134] A lot of questions arise in my mind about the circumstances and the actual cause of such deaths, including whether or not an unsuspected IE was present or whether antibiotics were used. Tushnet also claims that, after removal, these children were no better off and, in fact, were psychologically damaged though he gives no scientific proof of this. [135] Anyone who has suffered three to five bouts of tonsilitis annually well into adulthood knows this is not true and that life is immeasurably superior after the tonsils are removed, without even mentioning the cardiac risks that are thereby avoided.

But doctors like Tushnet who are so busy cashing in on popular topics like too much surgery rarely speak of the negligence in retaining diseased tonsils or in not testing for strep infection and prescribing antibiotics. Nor do they address the question of why some people's tonsils and not others are subject to chronic disease and whether poverty is a factor in chronic streptococcal infection of the tonsils. And when an author like Tushnet tells us that SBE has been conquered, his authority is suddenly shattered. Does he not know the statistics on IE, that the incidence is the same as in the the pre-antibiotic era? Mendelsohn states that in winter 20 percent of children harbour strep microorganisms in their throats.[136] This is misleading and creates a false conception about the process of disease, especially that of IE, since research has shown consistently for many years that microorganisms inhabit the mouth and throat or gastrointestinal tract at all times in everyone and that billions of staphylococci live on the skin[137]. When Mendelsohn says RHD "rarely appears except among the very poor",[138] we can only gasp in astonishment and ask does this doctor not know that 40 percent of people live below the poverty line in Canada and likely the same percentage in the U.S.? And does he not know that RHD still afflicts 1-3 percent of school-aged children? 12,930 people died from RHD in 1975.[139] RHD does not exist without many prior episodes of rheumatic fever which likely have been overlooked. But, then Mendelsohn's audience is not the poor, no more than Alvarez's was, nor that of any doctor who is the author of a self-help book.

The public must become very skeptical of these doctor-writers who claim to "communicate" better with the public than their colleagues or knowledgeable lay people might about a medical topic. This is not to say that these doctors I have referred to do not have valuable things to say. For instance, Robert Mendelsohn points out that the medical profession is reluctant to relinquish its power to any other health care groups such as the midwives, and everyone would likely concede that this is true. What I stress is that the public must no longer blindly accept medical information as accurate solely because it comes from a doctor. And they must stop passively allowing doctors to use their "tickerbelly-bum talk down" language. Lest we think the virulent snobbery of Alvarez is dead, consider Tushnet's remarks about patients, whom he calls, as Alvarez did, those "poor pathetic souls".[140] About one he says "maybe it's all in his mind. But he doesn't look or sound as though he had enough mind to have imagination."[141] This was said in 1971 and it is vintage Alvarez thinking of the 1950s. His influence is far from dead. Medical attitudes do not change; they are just better dressed, and they will not change until the public, through good, solid self-education, forces them to.

Very recently in June of 1988 in our House of Commons Debates, MP, Don Boudria, in a discussion about implementing the procedures to grant patients direct access and copies of their medical records, a matter which is once again being raised in our government, cited a case in which a doctor expressed an attitude toward his patient that was identical to that of Tushnet and Alvarez. It was a Workers' Compensation case, and a physician, who had not referred the patient to a psychiatrist for a complete examination but had come to his own conclusion, had recorded in his notes that the patient could not readjust to the workforce because he was suffering from "mental retardation".[142] Of course, the patient was not allowed to see his medical record which set out the reasons for the refusal of a disability pension. We have entered a period where it could be said, in the words of Shakespeare, that, for the doctors, "Robes and furr'd gowns hide all." But, for the patient, "through tattered clothes small vices do appear." If the public continues to "plate sin with gold", then surely "the strong lance of justice" will, indeed, break.

Ultimately these supposedly "freedom of information" books written by doctors drive us further from the real truth because they are in reality like a cow's second stomach. They break down the knowledge, chew it and regurgitate it so that the patient, the public, is able to digest it. The public should be content with nothing less than firsthand medical knowledge which can only be found at a university medical library or textbook store, in the journals and books from all over the world, written by doctors for doctors, not just doctors for the public, in the illustrated anatomical atlases and dictionaries, the tapes of heart murmurs, the medical equipment like blood pressure cuffs, stethoscopes and speculums, tools that were formerly sacred to the doctor but which must, like the thermometer, become part of the public domaine, just as the tools of the automechanic or the carpenter — the chisel, crowbar, wrench or sander — have become. Physiology courses should be mandatory or at least offered as electives in high school as they are in some schools in the United States. In talking to a seventeen year old niece of mine in the U.S., I was astonished to hear her use fluently the correct parts of the body, for example, such terms, as oral mucosa and brachial plexus. She is a third year high school student and is not intending to go into medicine. An editor once said to me that I must take such a word as oral mucosa out of my manuscript because readers wouldn't understand it. She had been brainwashed by the Tushnets and Alvarezes. To paraphrase Montaigne, "Know thy body as thou knowest thyself."

According to all research, MVP should remain stable unless the four major complications intervene, IE, thromboembolism, sudden death from an arrhythmnia or progression to severe regurgitation. There is a thread running through the medical literature indicating that MVP may be caused by IE, but no researcher has actually set out to prove this, although the majority of experts agree that progression to severe regurgitation does not happen quickly nor in the absence of IE. I began with an intermittent LSM. This means the murmur was not heard on every occasion and, therefore, there was likely no constant or chronic regurgitation. Perhaps there was only regurgitation when there were extra beats or episodes of tachycardia. This intermittent murmur became a pansystolic murmur within the short period of a year during a febrile illness. Dr. Barlow's observations, expressed in his book on the mitral valve, have convinced me, without a doubt, that I had IE in 1979-80 and that this has lead to my current health situation:

> We have observed patients with MVP reflected by a late systolic murmur advance to a pansystolic murmur during a 10-20 year period, but rapid progression is very unusual in the absence of infective endocarditis or Marfan's syndrome.[143]

However, because the continuity of my medical history was significantly disrupted with the disappearance of my documents during my 1979-80 illness, all my future contacts with the medical establishment will be shrouded in confusion, mystery and doubt. For instance, these records would have assisted doctors in dealing with my second unexplained febrile illness in September of 1989. If I had been able to present my medical history with the stamp of approval, I would likely have been given a more thorough investigation for IE and been treated for the full 4-6 weeks. Instead, I was only given a routine blood work-up done in the case of any disease, and, ultimately, the echocardiogram became the definitive diagnostic tool.

It is helpful to recall that the echocardiogram cannot distinguish accurately between "the lumps and bumps" of prolapse and the signs of IE, nor between old and fresh vegetations. For any doctor who has never seen an echocardiogram of mine, such as this cardiologist who reviewed my most recent one, he could not be anything but confused if he relies solely on this resource and especially if his experience has largely been in reviewing the echocardiograms of patients with uncomplicated MVP and a LSM who have never had IE. He would not expect to see "shaggy" or "fluffy" echoes of billowing leaflets in a person of my age group. My echocardiogram print-out would appear to him to be very atypical indeed.

My future remains clouded and uncertain. Were these "healed vegetations" of the past or fresh vegetations superimposed on old, fibrosed ones and "involuted" or shrunken by ten days of antimicrobial treatment? Needless to say, when I asked, I was refused a copy of this 1989 echocardiogram likely because the internist was protecting himself in the advent he had released me too early.

Dr. Jerry Yee of the Brooke Army Medical Center in Fort Sam Houston, Texas explains what happens to vegetations subjected to antimicrobial treatment:

> In infective endocarditis, it has long been observed that lesions can appear after the termination of antibiotic therapy, presumably after the patient has been 'cured'. The period between the appearance of the lesions and the end of therapy may be considerable, when vegetations have presumably healed or undergone spontaneous involution.[144]

This statement, once again, underlines the great confusion surrounding the use of "the machine" as a diagnostic tool for IE. It would also appear to strongly support the observations of Libman, Durack, Freedman and others that vegetations which would have, in the preantibiotic era, undergone "spontaneous involution", or, currently, regressed with antibacterial treatment, could become reinfected if not adequately treated. Repeated episodes of IE, when treatment is delayed or inadequate, cause increasingly severe regurgitation. This much at least is accepted by the medical community. And, therefore, the risk of sudden death from arrhythmia or from thromboembolism is greater.

In their 1977 Annual Report, the CMPA legal Counsel, Scott, compared doctors to "Pipers". He said, "The old cliché that he who pays the piper calls the tune is, in fact, not true of music. Piper-payers make occasional suggestions; by and large they let the pipers select the tunes and they cannot tell the pipers how to play."[145] Scott is of course talking about the doctors' demand to set their own prices during the war over extra billing in Canada. Like the pipers, Scott says, the doctors should be allowed to select the tunes since they alone know how to play them. We all know the story from our childhood of the Pied Piper of Hamelin and we all know how he rid Hamelin town of rats by playing music that lured them into the sea. And we know, too, that when the piper was not allowed to set his price in keeping with his conception of his worth, he piped the children to their deaths.

We, the patients, the public, pay the piper. We pay with our most precious possession, our health, our lives. But we cannot tell the pipers what tunes to play or how to play them because they have kept their art to themselves. We are without knowledge of how they play upon us, upon our bodies. We are not permitted to make suggestions for improvement in the way they play upon us. Will we, the sick, and those who are strong and healthy, continue to allow these pied pipers of medicine to fashion their mysterious instruments upon which they play their secretive tunes? Will we allow them to hoard their knowledge, their craft? And will we allow their inscrutable, insidious rhythms to lure us like helpless rats, or will we, as is our right, wrest from them their ancient arts and save ourselves from dancing blindly to our deaths?

APPENDIX

Terms Physicians Have Used Synonymously with the Term "Innocent Murmur"

The following list has been taken from Caceres, Cesar A. and Lowell W. Perry, The Innocent Murmur (London: J & A Churchill Ltd., 1967), pp. 63-66.

NB: Any individual who has been told by a physician that he or she has one of these murmurs should have an echocardiogram to rule out Mitral Valve Prolapse. The stethoscope is the best means of identification if the physician listens for the sounds of MVP in the different postures as described in this book. A second opinion may be necessary. The names marked with an asterisk have, at one time or another, been given to MVP.

Accessory murmur
Accidental murmur
Adventitious murmur
Anemic murmur
Anorganic murmur
Apical innocent murmur*
Atonic murmur

Basal ejection murmur*
Basal ejection vibrations
Basilar innocent murmur*
Benign murmur*
Benign murmur of no consequence*
Benign "physiologic" bruit
Benign precordial, systolic murmur of unknown origin*
Benign systolic ejection murmur*
Benign systolic murmur*

Completely benign murmur*

Dynamic murmur*

Ejection systolic murmur of innocent nature*
Ejection vibratory sound
Entirely insignificant murmur*

Fiddle-string murmur
Flow murmur*
Functional benign murmur*
Functional murmur*
Functional (innocent) murmur*
Functional (physiologic) murmur*
Functional systolic ejection murmur*
Functional systolic murmur*
Functional vibratory murmur

Groaning murmur

Harmless murmur*
Hemic murmur
Hemodynamically insignificant
    systolic murmur*

Incidental murmur
Innocent adventitious cardiac sound
Innocent apical systolic murmur*
Innocent early systolic ejection
    murmur*
Innocent ejection murmur*
Innocent functional ejection systolic
    murmur*
Innocent functional murmur*
Innocent (functional) murmur*
Innocent left parasternal murmur
Innocent mitral systolic murmur*
Innocent parasternal precordial
    murmur
Innocent parasternal systolic
    murmur
Innocent physiologic murmur*
Innocent precordial murmur, coarse
    variety, fine variety*
Innocent pulmonary systolic murmur
Innocent pulmonic ejection murmur
Innocent pulmonic murmur
Innocent systolic murmur*
Innocent systolic murmur over the
    pulmonary area
Innocent systolic parasternal
    precordial murmur
Innocent vibratory ejection murmur
Innocent vibratory murmur
Innocuous murmur
Inorganic murmur*
Insignificant murmur*
Isolated minor cardiac murmur*

Left sternal border vibratory murmur

Murmur of uncertain origin*
Murmur of unknown origin*
Musical apical systolic murmur*
Musical murmur*
Musical normal systolic murmur*

Musical precordial systolic murmur*
Myatonic murmur
Non-blowing (innocent) murmur
Non-blowing precordial and apical
    systolic murmur
Non-disease murmur of normal
    children
Non-musical apical systolic murmur
Nonorganic murmur*
Nonpathologic systolic murmur*
Nonpathologic vibratory murmur
Nonpathological murmur*
Nonsignificant murmur*
Normal ejection vibrations*
Normal heart murmur*
Normal pulmonary artery murmur
Normal systolic murmur*
Normal vascular hemodynamic
    noises*
Normally-occurring murmur*
Not significant murmur*

Occasional murmur*

Parasternal-precordial murmur*
Physiologic murmur*
Physiologic systolic murmur*
Physiological ejection murmur*
Physiological murmur*
Precordial systolic murmur*
Precordial vibratory murmur
Pulmonary blowing ejection murmur
Pulmonary ejection systolic murmur
Pulmonary innocent murmur
Pulmonic systolic murmur
Pulmonic systolic murmur of
    functional nature

"S" murmur
Simple-murmur
Sinus-shaped murmur
So-called functional murmur*
Still's murmur
Systolic murmur of no significance*
Systolic vibratory murmur

Temporary murmur*

Tinny murmur
Transient systolic murmur*
Truly innocent systolic murmur*
Twanging murmur*
Twanging string murmur*
"Twangy" murmur

Uncomplicated innocent systolic
    murmurs*

Unexplained murmur*
Unimportant murmur*
Universal systolic murmur
Unknown murmur*

Vibratory murmur
Vibratory non-blowing murmur
Vibratory parasternal-precordial
    murmur
"Vibratory" systolic murmur

Bibliography

Introduction: Flies to the Gods

1. West, G. L. "Sudden Death in a Case of Asymptomatic Endocarditis." (Oct 1, 1931) *The New England Journal of Medicine*: 675-78.
2. Weyman, J. "Antibiotics in General Dental Practice." (May 21, 1974) *British Dental Journal*: 404.
3. Clemens, J. et al. "A Controlled Evaluation of the Risk of Bacterial Endocarditis in Persons with Mitral Valve Prolapse." (1982) *The New England Journal of Medicine* 307: 776-781.
4. Roberts, W. C. "The 2 Most Common Congenital Heart Diseases." (1984) *The American Journal of Cardiology* 53 (8): 1198.
5. Barlow, J. B., et al. "MVP: Primary, secondary, both or neither?" (July, 1981) *American Heart Journal* 102 (1): 140-143.
6. *Medical Post*, February 23, 1982, p. 75.
7. Bor, D. H. et al. "Endocarditis Prophylaxis for Patients with MVP." (1984) *The American Journal of Medicine* 76: 711-717.
8. Markiewicz W., et al. "MVP in One Hundred Presumably Healthy Young Females." (March, 1976) *Circulation* 53 (3): 464-473.
9. Sbarbaro, J. A. et al. "A Prospective Study of Mitral Valvular Prolapse in Young men." (May 5, 1979) *Chest* 75: 555-59.
10. Cheitlin, M. D. and R. C. Byrd. "Prolapsed Mitral Valve: The Commonest Valve Disease?" (June, 1984) *Current Problems in Cardiology* 10: 1-54.
11. Greenwood, R. D. "Mitral Valve Prolapse: Incidence and Clinical Course in a Pediatric Population." (June, 1984) *Clinical Pediatrics* 23 (6): 318-20.
12. Chandraratna, P. A. N. et al. "Incidence of MVP in One Hundred Clinically Stable Newborn Baby Girls: An Echocardiographic Study." (1979) *American Heart Journal* 98: 312.
13. Cheitlin and Byrd, op. cit., p. 35.
14. MacMahon, S. W. et al. "Mitral Valve Prolapse and Infective Endocarditis." (1987) *American Heart Journal* 113 (5): 1291-1298.
15. *Statistics Canada*. (1986) Causes of Death: Vital Statistics Vol 4. Detailed categories of the "International Classification of Diseases" (ICD). Catalogue 84-203.
16. MacMahon et al., op. cit., p. 1294.
17. Bensman, M. et al. "Echocardiographic Follow-up of Patients with Late Systolic Murmur and/or Midsystolic Click." (October, 1975) *Circulation* 51 & 52 (II-159): 628.
18. *Statistics Canada*, 1986, op. cit.
19. Kligfield, P. et al. "Arrhythmias and Sudden Death in Mitral Valve Prolapse." (1987) *American Heart Journal* 113: 1298-1307.
20. Legge, W. "Callas Remembered: La Divina." (Nov 19, 1977) *Opera News* 42 (5): 11.

21. *Toronto Star*, January 23, 1982.
22. Krever, Hon. Justice H. *Report of the Commission of Inquiry into the Confidentiality of Health Information* Vol 2. (Toronto: J. C. Thatcher, Queen's Printer for Ontario, 1980), p. 468.
23. *Canadian Charter of Rights and Freedoms*, article 7.
24. Des Pres, T. "A Child of the State." (July 19, 1981) *The New York Times Book Review*."

Chapter Two

1. Krogh, C. M. E. et al. *Compendium of Pharmaceuticals and Specialties.* 21st ed. (Ottawa: Canadian Pharmaceutical Assoc., 1986), p. 635.
2. Nickerson, M. "Drugs Inhibiting Adrenergic Nerves and Structures Innervated by Them" in *The Pharmacological Basis of Therapeutics.* 4th ed., Goodman, L. S. and A. Gilman, eds. (New York: The MacMillan Co., 1970), p. 568.
3. Habib, A. and J. S. McCarthy. "Effects on the Neonate of Propranolol Administered During Pregnancy." (1977) *Journal of Pediatrics* 91: 808.

Chapter Three

1. Myall, R. W. T. and H. S. Gregory. "Current Trends in the Prevention of Bacterial Endocarditis in Susceptible Patients Receiving Dental Care." (December, 1969) *Oral Surgery, Oral Medicine & Oral Pathology*: 813-818.

Chapter Four

1. Dubin, D. *Rapid Interpretation of EKG's* (Tampa, Florida: Cover Pub. Co., 1970), pp. 107-19.
2. Shappell, S. D., et al. "Sudden Death and the Familial Occurrence of Mid-Systolic Click, Late Systolic Murmur Syndrome." (1973) *Circulation* 48: 1128-34.
3. Barlow, J. B., et al. "Late Systolic Murmurs and Non-Ejection ("Mid-Late") Systolic Clicks: An Analysis of 90 Patients." (1968) *British Heart Journal* 30: 203-18.
4. Devereux, R. B., et al. "Mitral Valve Prolapse." (July, 1976) *Circulation* 54 (1): 3-14.
5. Dorney, E. R. "Endocarditis" in *The Heart.* 3rd ed., Hurst, J. W. et al., eds. (New York: McGraw-Hill Book Co., 1974), pp. 1290-1305.
6. Cobbs, B. W. "Clinical Recognition and Medical Management of Rheumatic Heart Disease and Other Acquired Valvular Disease" in *The Heart*, ibid., pp. 881-889.

Chapter Five

1. American Heart Association Committee on Prevention of Rheumatic Fever: Prevention of Bacterial Endocarditis. (1977) *Circulation* 55 (1).
2. Goldstein, J. "Antibiotics as Related to Endodontic Therapy." (May, 1978) *Journal of Endodontics* 4 (5): 135-139.

Chapter Six

1. Dorney, E. R. "Endocarditis" in *The Heart.* 3rd. ed., Hurst, J. W. et al. eds. (New York: McGraw-Hill Book Co., 1974), p. 1296.
2. Weinstein, L. "Antibiotics IV. Miscellaneous Antimicrobial, Antifungal and Antiviral Agents" in *The Pharmacological Basis of Therapeutics.* 4th ed., Goodman, L. S. and A. Gilman, eds. (New York, The MacMillan Co., 1970) pp. 1292-93.
3. Berkow, R. et al. *The Merck Manual of Diagnosis and Therapy.* 14th ed., (Rahway, New Jersey: Merck, Sharp & Dohme Research Laboratories, 1982), p. 359.

4. Gazes, P. C. and R. B. Logue. "Common Mistakes Made in Practice" in *The Heart*, op. cit., p. 1750.

5. Weens, H. S. and B. B. Gay. "Routine Radiologic Examination of the Heart" in *The Heart*, ibid., p. 324.

6. Berkow, R. et al., op. cit., p. 369.

7. *Health Disciplines Act: Revised Statutes of Ontario 1980*, (Toronto: Queen's Printer for Ontario, June 1982), Chapter 196, pp. 10-28.

8. Weine, F.S. *Endodontic Therapy* (Saint Louis, MO: C. V. Mosby, 1976), p. 14.

9. Gerstein, H. *Techniques in Clinical Endodontics* (Philadelphia: W. B. Saunders Co., 1983), p. 348.

10. Ibid., p. 348.

11. Grossman, L. *Endodontic Practice* (Philadelphia: Lea Febiger, 1981), p. 28.

12. Weine, op. cit., p. 14.

13. Cameron, C.E. "The Cracked Tooth Syndrome." (November, 1976) *Journal of the American Dental Association* 93: 971-975.

14. Arens, D. et al. *Endodontic Surgery* (New York: Harper and Row, 1981), p. 222.

15. Wechsler, S. M. et al. "Iatrogenic Root Fractures: A Case Report." (August, 1978) *Journal of Endodontics* 4 (8): 251-253.

16. Meister, F. et al. "A Periodontal Abscess Associated with Vertical Root Fractures." (December, 1976) *Wisconsin Dental Association Journal* 52: 562-63.

17. Arens, op. cit., p. 223.

18. Levine, M. *Manual of Pre-Clinic Endodontic Technique*. (Toronto: University of Toronto, Dept. of Endodontics, Faculty of Dentistry, 1978), p. 76.

19. Grossman, op. cit., pp. 56-57.

20. Levine, op. cit., p. 50.

21. Kennedy, D. R., et al. "Effects on Monkeys of Introduction of Hemolytic Streptococci into Root Canals." (1957) *Journal of Dental Research* 36: 496.

22. Bender, I. B. et al. "The Incidence of Bacteremia in Endodontic Manipulations." (1960) *Oral Surgery, Oral Medicine & Oral Pathology* 13: 353.

23. Bence, R. et al. *Handbook of Clinical Endodontics* (Saint Louis, MO: C. V. Mosby Co., 1976), p. 130 ff.

24. *Royal College of Dental Surgeons of Ontario*, Dispatch, August, 1979.

25. Holroyd, S. V. *Clinical Pharmacology in Dental Practice* (Saint Louis, MO: C. V. Mosby Co., 1978), pp. 471-75.

26. Brown, A. A. "Prevention of Bacterial Endocarditis." (1977) *Ontario Dentist* 54 (4): 14-16.

27. Ellen, R. "The Dental Practitioner and Systemic Infections of Oral Origin." (1978) *International Dental Journal* 28 (3): 296-308.

28. Ibid., pp. 296-298.

29. Dewberry, J. A. "The Cracked Tooth Syndrome: Vertical Fractures of Posterior Teeth" in Weine, op. cit., p. 15.

Chapter Seven

1. Jeresaty, R. M. *Mitral Valve Prolapse*. (New York: Raven Press, 1979), p. 19.

2. Devereux, R. B. et al. "Mitral Valve Prolapse." (1976) *Circulation* 54 (1): 3-14.

3. Adolph, R. J. "Second Heart Sound: The Role of Altered Electromechanical Events" in *Physiological Principles of Heart Sounds and Murmurs*. Shaver, L. D. and J. H. Shaver, eds., Proceedings of a Symposium held April, 1974, Pittsburg, PA. (New York: American Heart Association, Inc., 1975), pp. 45-57.

4. Empson, H. E. *The Doctor and the Law*. (Toronto: MacMillan of Canada, 1979, p. 93.

5. Canadian Medical Protective Association. *Annual Report* (Ottawa: CMPA, August 26, 1981), p. 34.

6. Ibid., p. 37.
7. Ibid., p. 35.
8. Ibid., p. 36.
9. Ibid., p. 13.
10. Canadian Medical Protective Association. *Annual Report*. (Ottawa: CMPA June 9, 1971), p. 12.

Chapter Eight

1. Krotz, L. "A Little Learning."(April, 1981) *Canadian Lawyer*: 19-21.
2. Gibson, J. M. and R. L. Swartz. "Physicians and Lawyers: Science, Art and Conflict." (1980) *American Journal of Law and Medicine* 6 (2): 173-182.
3. Brown, B. B. *Stress and the Art of Biofeedback* (New York: Harper and Row, 1977), p. 35-36.
4. *The Globe and Mail*, Toronto, September 3, 1983.
5. Cousins, N. *Anatomy of an Illness* (Toronto: Bantam Books, 1979), p. 11.
6. Ibid., p. 48.
7. Ibid., p.22.

Chapter Nine

1. *The Globe and Mail*, Toronto, July 23, 1983.
2. Nickerson, M. "Drugs Inhibiting Adrenergic Nerves and Structures Innervated by Them" in *The Pharmacological Basis of Therapeutics*. 4th ed., Goodman. L. S. and A. Gilman, eds. (New York: The MacMillan Co., 1970), pp. 565-570.
3. Krogh, C.M.E. et al. *Compendium of Pharmaceuticals and Specialties*. 21st ed. (Ottawa: Canadian Pharmaceutical Assoc., 1986), pp. 635-637.
4. Perloff, J.K. and W. C. Roberts. "The Mitral Apparatus: Functional Anatomy of Mitral Regurgitation." (August, 1972) *Circulation* 46: 227-239.
5. Ibid., p. 228.
6. Pomerance, A. "Ballooning Deformity (Mucoid Degeneration) of Atrioventricular Valves." (1969) *British Heart Journal* 31: 343-351.
7. Hill, D. G. et al. "The Natural History and Surgical Management of the Redundant Cusp Syndrome (floppy mitral valve)." (April, 1974) *The Journal of Thoracic and Cardiovascular Surgery* 67 (4): 519-525.
8. Mills, P. et al. "Long-Term Prognosis of Mitral Valve Prolapse." (July 7, 1977) *The New England Journal of Medicine* 297 (1): 13-18.
9. Fontana, M. E. et al. "Functional Anatomy of Mitral Prolapse." (Proceedings of a Symposium held April, 1974) in *Physiological Principles of Heart Sounds and Murmurs*. Leon, D. and J. H. Shaver, eds. (Pittsburgh, PA: American Heart Association, Inc., 1975), pp. 126-132.
10. Pomerance, A. "Pathology and Valvular Heart Disease." (1972) *British Heart Journal* 34: 437-443.
11. Hill et al., op. cit., p. 520.
12. Leatham, A. and W. Brigden. "Mild Mitral Regurgitation and the Mitral Prolapse Fiasco." (1980) *American Heart Journal* 99 (5): 659-664.
13. Davies, M.J. et al. "The Floppy Mitral Valve: Study of Incidence, Pathology and Complications in Surgical, Necropsy and Forensic Material." (1978) *British Heart Journal* 40: 461-81.
14. Kern, W. H. and B. L. Tucker: "Myxoid Changes in Cardiac Valves: Pathologic, Clinical and Ultrastructural Studies." (September, 1972) *American Heart Journal* 84 (3): 294-301.
15. Bowers, D. "Pathogenesis of Primary Abnormalities of the Mitral Valve in Marfan's Syndrome." (1969) *British Heart Journal* 31: 679-83.
16. Cobbs, B. W. "Clinical Recognition and Medical Management of Rheumatic Heart Disease and Other Acquired Valvular Disease" in *The Heart*, 3rd. ed., Hurst, J. W. et al., eds. (New York: McGraw-Hill Book Co., 1974), pp. 956-57.

17. Berkow, R. et al. *The Merck Manual of Diagnosis and Therapy* 14th ed. (Rahway, New Jersey: Merck, Sharp & Dohme Research Laboratories, 1982), pp.360-62.

18. Jeresaty, R. M., *Mitral Valve Prolapse* (New York: Raven Press, 1979), p. 13.

19. Hurst, J. W. and J. F. Spann. "Etiology and Clinical Recognition of Heart Failure" in *The Heart*, op. cit., p. 447.

20. O'Rourke, R. A. and M. H. Crawford. "The Systolic Click-Murmur Syndrome: Clinical Recognition and Management." (1976) *Current Problems in Cardiology* 1: 1-60.

21. Cheitlin, M. D and R. C. Byrd. "Prolapsed Mitral Valve: The Commonest Valve Disease?" (June, 1984) *Current Problems in Cardiology* 10: 1-54.

22. Dillon, J. C. et al. "Use of Echocardiography in Patients with Prolapsed Mitral Valve." (April, 1971) *Circulation* 43: 503-507.

23. Jeresaty, R. "The Syndrome Associated with Mid-Systolic Click and/or Late Systolic Murmur: Analysis of 32 Cases." (June, 1971) *Chest* 59 (6): 643-647.

24. Tilkian, A. G. and M. Boudreau Conover. *Understanding Heart Sounds and Murmurs* (Philadelphia, PA: W. B. Saunders Co., 1984), pp. 92-96.

25. Ibid., p. 103.

26. Braunwald, E. "Idiopathic Hypertrophic Subaortic Stenosis (Obstructive Cardiomyopathy)" in *The Heart*, op. cit., p. 1346 ff.

27. Ibid., p. 1344.

28. Knowles, J. H. et al. "Clinical Test for Pulmonary Function with Use of Valsalva Maneuver." (January 7, 1956) *Journal of the American Medical Association* 160 (1): 44-48.

29. Tilkian, op. cit., p. 193.

Chapter Ten

1. Cobbs, B. W. "Clinical Recognition and Medical Management of Rheumatic Heart Disease and Other Acquired Valvular Disease" in *The Heart*, 3rd ed., Hurst, J. W. et al., eds. (New York: McGraw-Hill Book Co., 1974), p. 875.

2. Langman, J. and M. W. Woerdeman. *Atlas of Medical Anatomy* (Philadelphia: W. B. Saunders Co., 1978), p. 71.

3. MacPherson, A. *The Spleen* (Springfield, Ill: Charles C. Thomas, 1973), p.152.

4. Weinstein, A. J. "Infective Endocarditis: Changes in Etiology, Diagnosis and Management." (June 6, 1980) *Comprehensive Therapy* 6: 31-35.

5. Hayward, G. W. "Infective Endocarditis: A Changing Disease - I." (1973) *British Medical Journal* 2: 706-709.

6. Laws, P. *X-rays: More Harm Than Good?* (Emmaus, PA: Rodale Press, 1977), pp.141-42.

7. MacPherson, op. cit., p. 152.

8. Brunson, J. G. and E. A. Gall. *Concepts of Disease* (New York: The MacMillan Co., 1971), p. 749.

9. Carson, D. A. et al. "IgG Rheumatoid Factor in Subacute Bacterial Endocarditis: Relationship to IgM Rheumatoid Factor and Circulating Immune Complexes." (1978) *Clinical Experimental Immunology* 31: 100-103.

10. Langman, op. cit., p. 72.

11. MacPherson: op. cit., p. 167.

12. Hamman L. "Healed Bacterial Endocarditis." (1937) *Annals of Internal Medicine* XI: 175-194.

13. Libman, E. "A Consideration of the Prognosis in Subacute Bacterial Endocarditis." (1925) *American Heart Journal* 1: 25-40.

14. Libman, E. "A study of the Endocardial Lesions of Subacute Bacterial Endocarditis." (1912) *The American Journal of Medical Science* 140: 313-327, reprinted in (November, 1952) The American Journal of Medicine: 544-49.

15. Libman. "A Consideration of the Prognosis in Subacute Bacterial Endocarditis," op. cit., pp. 25, 39.

16. Ibid., p. 26.
17. Ibid., p. 31.
18. Ibid., p. 37.
19. Libman, E. "The Clinical Features of Subacute Bacterial Endocarditis That Have Spontaneously Become Bacteria-Free." (November, 1913) *The American Journal of Medical Science* 146 (5): 625-45.
20. Libman, "A Study of the Endocardial Lesions of Subacute Bacterial Endocarditis," op. cit., p. 32.
21. Ibid., p. 34.
22. Osler, W. "Chronic Infectious Endocarditis." (1909) *Quarterly Journal of Medicine*: pp. 219-230.
23. Horder, T. J. "Infective Endocarditis." (1909) *Quarterly Journal of Medicine*: 289-324.
24. Hamman, op. cit.
25. Ibid., p. 176.
26. Jeresaty, R. M. *Mitral Valve Prolapse* (New York: Raven Press, 1979), p. 207.
27. Shah, P. M. and R. Gramiak. (1970) "Echocardiographic Recognition of MVP." *Circulation* 42: III-45.
28. Dillon, J. C. et al: "Echocardiographic Manifestations of Valvular Vegetations." (November, 1973) *American Heart Journal* 86 (5): 698-704.
29. Gilbert, B. W. et al. "Two-Dimensional Echocardiographic Assessment of Vegetative Endocarditis." (February, 1977) *Circulation* 55 (2): 346-53.
30. Wann, L. S. et al. "Echocardiography in Bacterial Endocarditis." (1976) *The New England Journal of Medicine* 295: 135-39.
31. Stewart, J. A. et al. "Echocardiographic Documentation of Vegetative Lesions in Endocarditis: Clinical Implications." (February, 1980) *Circulation* 61 (2): 374-80.
32. Dillon et al., op. cit.
33. Wann et al., op. cit.
34. Chandraratna, P.A.N. et al. "Limitations of the Echocardiogram in Diagnosing Valvular Vegetations in Patients with Mitral Valve Prolapse." (1977) *Circulation* 56: 436-38.
35. Martin, R. P. et al. "Clinical Utility of Two-Dimensional Echocardiography in Infective Endocarditis." (September, 1980) *The American Journal of Cardiology* 46: 379-85.
36. Mintz, G. S. and M. N. Kotler. "Clinical Value and Limitations of Echocardiography." (August, 1980) *Archives of Internal Medicine* 140: 1022-27.
37. Dillon et al., op. cit.
38. Roy, P. et al. "Spectrum of Echocardiographic Findings in Bacterial Endocarditis." (March, 1976) *Circulation* 53 (3): 474-82.
39. Dillon et al., op. cit.
40. Hickey, A. J. et al. "Reliability and Clinical Relevance of Detection of Vegetations by Echocardiography in Bacterial Endocarditis." (1981) *British Heart Journal* 46: 624-28.
41. Mintz et al., op. cit.
42. Wann et al., op. cit.
43. Freedman, L. R. *Infective Endocarditis and Other Intravascular Infections* (New York: Plenum Medical Book Co., 1982), pp. 36-37.
44. Stewart et al., op. cit.
45. MacPherson, op. cit., p. 160.
46. Berkow, R. et al. *The Merck Manual of Diagnosis and Therapy.* 14th ed. (Rahway, New Jersey: Merck, Sharp & Dohme Research Laboratories, 1982), p. 1159.
47. Martin et al., op. cit.
48. Stewart et al., op. cit.

Chapter Eleven

1. Corrigall, D. et al. "Mitral Valve Prolapse and Infective Endocarditis." (August, 1977) *The American Journal of Medicine* 63: 215-22.
2. Clapesattle, H. *The Doctors Mayo* (Minneapolis, Minn: University of Minnesota Press, 1941), p. 352.
3. Welt, L. G. and W. B. Blythe. "Cations: Calcium, Magnesium, Barium, Lithium and Amonium" in *The Pharmacological Basis of Therapeutics.* 4th ed. Goodman, L. S. and A. Gilman, eds. (New York: The MacMillan Co., 1970), p. 814.
4. *The House on the Rock, Inc.*, (Madison, Wisconsin: Straus Printing Company, 1983).
5. The Olmsted County Historical Society, Box 6411, Rochester, Minnesota.

Chapter Twelve

1. Zion, M. M. et al. "Echocardiographic Criteria for Diagnosis of Mitral Valve Prolapse." (October 1, 1988) *The American Journal of Cardiology*: 841.
2. Hurst, J. W. and R. C. Schlant. "Auscultation of the Heart" in *The Heart.* 3rd ed., Hurst, J. W. et al., eds. (New York: McGraw-Hill Book Co., 1974), p. 218.
3. Ibid., p. 219.
4. Ibid.
5. Da Costa, J. M. "On Irritable Heart: A Clinical Study of a Form of Functional Cardiac Disorder and its Consequences." (January, 1871) *The American Journal of the Medical Sciences* CXXI: 2-52.
6. Ibid., p. 19
7. Ibid., pp. 26-27.
8. Ibid., pp. 26-27.
9. Fiddler, G. I. and O. Scott. "Heart Murmurs Audible Across the Room in Children with Mitral Valve Prolapse." (1980) *British Heart Journal* 44: 201-203.
10. DaCosta, op. cit., p. 26.
11. Ibid., p. 2.
12. Ibid., pp. 18-19.
13. Ibid., p. 2.
14. Ibid., p. 36.
15. Ibid., p. 35.
16. Cuffer and Barbillion: "Nouvelles Recherches sur le Bruit de Galop Cardiaque: Mémoires Originaux." (Fevrier, 1887) *Archives Générales de Médicine*: 129-149, 201-320.
17. Luisada, A. A. and M. M. Alimurung. "The Systolic Gallop Rhythm." (1949) *Acta Cardiologica* (Brux) 4: 309-323.
18. Thompson, W. P. and S. A. Levine. "Systolic Gallop Rhythm: A Clinical Study." (1935) *The New England Journal of Medicine* 213 (21): 1021-25.
19. Wolferth, C. C. and A. Margolies. " Gallop Rhythm." (1933) *International Clinics* 1 (16):16-30.
20. Cuffer, Barbillion, op. cit., p. 304.
21. Ibid., p.304.
22. Da Costa, op. cit., p. 26.
23. Cuffer and Barbillion, op. cit., p. 306.
24. Ibid., p. 312.
25. Ibid., p. 308.
26. Ibid., p. 319.
27. Wolferth and Margolies, op. cit., p. 19.
28. Harvey, W. P. and S. A. Levine. *Clinical Auscultation of the Heart* (Philadelphia: W. B. Saunders Co., 1949), p. 47.
29. Harvey, W. P. "Gallop Sounds, Clicks, Snaps and Other Sounds" in *The Heart*, op. cit., p. 247.

30. Cuffer and Barbillion, op. cit., p. 304.
31. Hancock, E. W. and K. Cohn, "The Syndrome Associated with Mid-Systolic Click and Late Systolic Murmur." (1966) *The American Journal of Medicine* 41: 184-196.
32. Thompson and Levine, op. cit., p. 1022.
33. Ibid.
34. Ibid.
35. Griffith, J. P. C. "Mid'Systolic and Late Systolic Mitral Murmurs." (1892) *The American Journal of the Medical Sciences* 104: 285-294.
36. Hall, J. N. "Late Systolic Mitral Murmurs." (1903) *The American Journal of the Medical Sciences* 125: 663-666.
37. Griffith, op. cit., p. 294.
38. Burch, G. E. et al. "The Syndrome of Papillary Muscle Dysfunction." (March, 1968) *American Heart Journal* 75 (3): 399-415.
39. Thayer, W. S. "Reflections on the Interpretation of Systolic Cardiac Murmurs." (March, 1925) *The American Journal of the Medical Sciences* 109 (3): 313-321.
40. Wolferth and Margolies, op. cit.
41. Thompson and Levine, op. cit.
42. Johnston, F. D. "Extra Sounds Occurring in Cardiac Systole." ((1938) *American Heart Journal* 15: 221-231.
43. Luisada and Alimurung, op. cit.
44. Johnston, op. cit., p. 229.
45. Thompson, op. cit., p. 1024.
46. Lewis, T. *The Soldier's Heart and The Effort Syndrome* (London: Shaw and Sons, 1940), p. B Introduction.
47. Ibid., p. B.
48. Lewis, T. *The Soldier's Heart and The Effort Syndrome* (London: Shaw and Sons, 1918), p. 61.
49. Caceres, C. A. and L. W. Perry. *The Innocent Murmur* (London: J & A Churchill, Ltd., 1967), pp. 177-180.
50. Lewis, T. *Diseases of the Heart* (London: MacMillan and Co., 1922), p. 137.
51. Ibid., p. 137.
52. Ibid., p. 137.
53. Ibid., pp. 138 ff.
54. Lewis, (1918 edition), op. cit., p. 64.
55. Davies, M. J. et al. "The Floppy Mitral Valve: Study of Incidence, Pathology and Complications in Surgical, Necropsy and Forensic Material. (1978) *British Heart Journal* 40: 468-81.
56. Lewis, (1918 edition), op. cit. p. 65.
57. Lewis, *Diseases of the Heart*, op. cit., p. 139.
58. Ibid., p. 139.
59. MacKenzie, J. *Diseases of the Heart* (London: Oxford University Press, 1913), p. 327.
60. Ibid., p. 327.
61. Evans, W. "Mitral Systolic Murmurs." (January 2, 1943) *British Medical Journal*: 8-9.
62. Ibid., p. 8.
63. Ibid.
64. Carmichael, C. H. R. " Mitral Systolic Murmurs." (February 6, 1943) British *Medical Journal*: 172.
65. Gaskell, H. S. "Mitral Systolic Murmurs." (March 13, 1943) *British Medical Journal*: 332.
66. Ibid.
67. Ibid.
68. White P. *Heart Disease* (New York: MacMillan and Co., 1931), p. 105.
69. Barlow, J. B. et al. "Late Systolic Murmurs and Non-Ejection (Mid-Late) Systolic Clicks." (1968) *British Heart Journal* 30: 203-217.

70. Leatham, A and W. Brigden. "Mild Mitral Regurgitation and the Mitral Prolapse Fiasco." (May, 1980) *American Heart Journal* 99 (5): 659-64.
71. Leatham, A. "Auscultation of the Heart." (1958) *The Lancet*: 703-708.
72. Reid, J. V. O. "Mid-Systolic Clicks." (April, 1961) South African Medical Journal: 353-55.
73. Ibid., p. 355.
74. Ibid.

Chapter Thirteen

1. Barlow, J. B. "Conjoint Clinic on the Clinical Significance of Late Systolic Murmurs and Non-Ejection Systolic Clicks. (1965) *Journal of Chronic Diseases* 18: 665-73.
2. Barlow, J. B. et al. "The Significance of Late Systolic Murmurs." (October, 1963) *American Heart Journal*: 443-52.
3. Ibid., p. 445.
4. Barlow, J. B. and W. A. Pocock. "The Mitral Prolapse Enigma — Two Decades Later." (March, 1984) *Journal of the American Medical Association* 53 (3): 13-17.
5. Barlow et al., "The Significance of Late Systolic Murmurs", op. cit.
6. Criley, J. M. et al. "Prolapse of the Mitral Valve: Clinical and Cine-Angiographic Findings." (1966) *British Heart Journal* 28: 488-96.
7. Humphries, J. O. and V. McKusick. "The Differentiation of Organic and "Innocent" Systolic Murmurs." (1962) *Progress in Cardiovascular Disease* 5 (2): 152-171.
8. Caceres, C. A. and Perry, L. W. *The Innocent Murmur* (London: J. A. Churchill, Ltd., 1967), pp. 63-66.
9. Humphries and McKusick, op. cit., p. 168.
10. Segal, B. L. and W. Likoff. "Late Systolic Murmur of Mitral Regurgitation." (June, 1964) *American Heart Journal*: 757-763.
11. Ibid., p. 761.
12. Thompson, W. P. and S. A. Levine. "Systolic Gallop Rhythm: A Clinical Study." (1935) *The New England Journal of Medicine* 213 (21): 1021-25.
13. Hancock, E. W. and K. Cohn. "The Syndrome Associated with Midsystolic Click and Late Systolic Murmur. (August, 1966) *The American Journal of Medicine* 41: 183-196.
14. Ibid., p. 191
15. Barlow, J. B. et al. "Late Systolic Murmurs and Non-Ejection ("Mid-Late") Systolic Clicks: An Analysis of 90 Patients." (1968) *British Heart Journal* 30: 203-217.
16. Davies, M. J. and M. V. Braimbridge. "The Floppy Mitral Valve: Study of Incidence, Pathology and Complications in Surgical, Necropsy and Forensic Material. " (1978) *British Heart Journal* 40: 468-81.
17. Ibid., p. 476.
18. Oka, M. and A. Angrist. "Fibrous Thickening with Billowing Sail Distortion of the Aging Heart Valve." (1961) *Proceedings of the New York State Association of Public Health Laboratories* 46: 21.
19. Barlow et al., "Late Systolic Murmurs and Non-Ejection (Mid-Late) Systolic Clicks", op. cit.
20. Bittar, N. and J. A. Sosa. "The Billowing Mitral Valve Leaflet." (October, 1968) *Circulation* 38: 763-770.
21. Pomerance, A. "Ballooning Deformity (Mucoid Degeneration) of Atrioventricular Valves. (1969) *British Heart Journal* 31: 343-51.
22. Read, R. C. et al. "Symptomatic Valvular Transformation (The Floppy Valve Syndrome) A Possible Forme Fruste of the Marfan's Syndrome." (1965) *Circulation* 32: 897-910.
23. Hill, D. G. et al. "The Natural History and Surgical Management of the Redundant Cusp Syndrome (Floppy Mitral Valve)." (April, 1974) *The Journal of Thoracic and Cardiovascular Surgery* 67 (4): 519-525.
24. Natarajan, G. et al. "Myocardial Metabolic Studies in Prolapsing Mitral Leaflet Syndrome." (December, 1975) *Circulation* 52: 1105-1110.

25. Cobbs, B. W. "Clinical Recognition and Medical Management of Rheumatic Heart Disease and Other Acquired Valvular Disease" in *The Heart*. 3rd ed., Hurst, J. W. et al., eds. (New York: McGraw-Hill Book Co., 1974), p. 881.

26. Criley et al., op. cit.

27. Humphries and McKusick, op. cit.

28. Segal and Likoff, op. cit.

29. Facquet J. et al. "Sur la Signification du Souffle Frequémment Associé au Claquement Télésystolique." (1964) *Acta Cardiologica* 19: 417-422.

30. LeBauer, E. J. et al. "The Isolated Click with Bacterial Endocarditis." (April, 1967) *American Heart Journal* 73 (4): 534-537.

31. Linhart, J. W. and W. J. Taylor. "The Late Apical Systolic Murmur, Clinical Hemodynamic and Angiographic Observations." (August, 1966) *The American Journal of Cardiology* 18: 164-168.

32. Shell, W. E. et al. "The Familial Occurrence of the Syndrome of Mid-Late Systolic Click and Late Systolic Murmur." (March, 1969) *Circulation* 39: 327-337.

33. Pomerance, op. cit.

34. Jeresaty, R. "The Syndrome Associated with Mid-Systolic Click and/or Late Systolic Murmur." ((June, 1971) *Chest* 59 (5): 643-647.

35. Littler, W. A. et al. "Acute Mitral Regurgitation Resulting from Ruptured or Elongated Chordae Tendinae: Auscultatory and Phonocardiographic Findings." (January, 1973) *Quarterly Journal of Medicine* 42(65): 87-110.

36. Perloff, J. K. and W. C. Roberts. "The Mitral Apparatus: Functional Anatomy of Mitral Regurgitation." (August, 1972) *Circulation* 46: 227-239.

37. Pomerance, A. "Pathology and Valvular Heart Disease." (1972) *British Heart Journal* 34: 437-443.

38. Kern, W. H. et al. "Myxoid Changes in Cardiac Valves: Pathologic, Clinical and Ultrastructural Studies." (1972) *American Heart Journal* 84 (3): 294-301.

39. Hill et al., op. cit.

40. Kincaid, D. T. and R. E. Botti. "Subacute Bacterial Endocarditis in a Patient with Isolated Nonejection Systolic Click but Without a Murmur." (July, 1974) *Chest* 66 (1): 88-89.

41. Lachman, A. S. et al. "Infective Endocarditis in the Billowing Mitral Leaflet Syndrome." (1975) *British Heart Journal* 37: 326-330.

42. Malcolm, A. D. et al. "Clinical Features and Investigative Findings in the Presence of Mitral Leaflet Prolapse." (1976) *British Heart Journal* 38:244-256.

43. Mills, P. et al. "Long Term Prognosis of Mitral Valve Prolapse." (1977) *The New England Journal of Medicine* 297: 13-18.

44. Hammond, G. N. et al. "Two Cases of Hemophilus Endocarditis of Prolapsed Mitral Valves — Hemophilus Paraphrophilus or Parainfluenzae?" (September, 1978) *The American Journal of Medicine* 65: 537-541.

45. Weinstein, A. J. et al. "Bacterial Endocarditis in a Patient with Mitral Valve Prolapse." (1979) *Archives of Internal Medicine* 139: 1191-1191.

46. Ringer, M. et al. "Mitral Valve Prolapse: Jet Stream Causing Mural Endocarditis." (February, 1980) *The American Journal of Cardiology* 45: 383-385.

47. Shah, G. M. and R. L. Winer. "Glomerulonephritis Association with Endocarditis Caused by Actinobacillus Actinomycetemcomitans." (1981) *American Journal of Kidney Diseases* 1 (2): 113-115.

48. Rajan, R. K. et al. "Bacterial Endocarditis in Mitral Leaflet Prolapse Syndrome." (April, 1982) *Postgraduate Medicine* 71: 203-205.

49. MacMahon, S. W. et al. "Mitral Valve Prolapse and Infective Endocarditis." (1987) *American Heart Journal* 113 (5): 1291-1298.

50. Levine, S. A. and Harvey, W. P. *Clinical Auscultation of the Heart* (Philadelphia: W. B. Saunders Co., 1949), p. 174.

51. Jeresaty, R. M. *Mitral Valve Prolapse* (New York: Raven Press, 1979), p. 10-13.

52. Allen, H. et al. "Significance and Prognosis of an Isolated Late Systolic Murmur: A 9-22 year follow-up." (1974) *British Heart Journal* 36: 525-532.

53. Bowers, D. "Pathogenesis of Primary Abnormalities of the Mitral Valve in Marfan's Syndrome." (1969) *British Heart Journal* 31: 679-683.

54. Lindsay, J. "Diseases of the Aorta and Venae Cavae" in *The Heart*, op. cit., pp. 1588 ff.

55. Read et al., op. cit.

56. Jeresaty, *Mitral Valve Prolapse*, op. cit., p. 35.

57. Cobbs, B. W., op. cit., p. 955.

58. Carpentier, A. et al. "Reconstructive Surgery of Mitral Valve Incompetence." (1980) *The Journal of Thoracic and Cardiovascular Surgery* 79: 338-348.

59. Allen et al., op. cit., p. 529.

60. Baddour, L. M. and A. L. Bisno. "Infective Endocarditis Complicating Mitral Valve Prolapse: Epidemiologic, Clinical and Microbiologic Aspects." (January-February, 1986) *Reviews of Infectious Diseases* 8 (1): 117-137.

61. Dorney, E. R. "Endocarditis in *The Heart*, op. cit., p. 1291.

62. Ringer, op. cit.

63. Popp, R. L. and R. A. Winkle. "Mitral Valve Prolapse Syndrome." (1976) *Journal of the American Medical Association* 236 (7): 867-870.

64. Jeresaty, *Mitral Valve Prolapse*, op. cit., p. 209.

65. Ibid., p. 206.

66. Ibid., p. 205.

67. Shulman, S. T. et al. "Prevention of Bacterial Endocarditis: A Statement for Health Professionals by the Committee on Rheumatic Fever and Infective Endocarditis of the Council on Cardiovascular Disease in the Young." (December, 1984) *Circulation* 70(6): 1123A-1127A.

68. McShane, Kathleen. "Preventing Bacterial Endocarditis." (June, 1978) *Circulation* 57 (6): 1232.

69. LeBauer et al., op. cit.

70. Kincaid, op. cit.

71. Lachman et al., op. cit.

72. Barlow and Pocock, op. cit.

73. Linhart and Taylor, op. cit., p. 207.

74. Jeresaty, *Mitral Valve Prolapse*, op. cit., p. 207.

75. Corrigall, D. et al. "Mitral Valve Prolapse and IE." (1977) *The American Journal of Medicine* 63: 215-222.

76. Rodbard, S. "Blood Velocity and Endocarditis." (January, 1963) *Circulation* 27: 18-28.

77. Leon, D. F. et al. "Late Systolic Murmurs, Clicks and Whoops Arising from the Mitral Valve." (September, 1966) *American Heart Journal* 72 (3): 325-336.

78. Pomerance, A., "Ballooning Deformity (Mucoid Degeneration) of Atrioventricular Valves", op. cit., p. 349.

79. Hayward, G. "Infective Endocarditis: A Changing Disease." (1973) *British Medical Journal* 2: 706-709.

80. Rodbard, op. cit., p. 23.

81. Buchbinder, W. C. and N. A. Roberts. "Healed Left-Sided Infective Endocarditis: A Clinico-pathological Study of 59 Patients." (December, 1977) *The American Journal of Cardiology* 40: 876-888.

82. Libman, E. and C. K. Friedberg. *Subacute Bacterial Endocarditis* (New York: Oxford University Press, 1948), p. 13.

83. Corrigall et al., op. cit., p. 221.

84. Libman and Friedberg, op. cit., p. 7.

85. Guy, F. C. et al. "Mitral Valve Prolapse as a Cause of Hemodynamically Important Mitral Regurgitation." (March, 1980) *The Canadian Journal of Surgery* 23 (2): 166-170.

86. Waller, B. F. et al. "Etiology of Clinically Isolated, Severe, Chronic, Pure Mitral Regurgitation:

Analysis of 97 Patients Over 30 Years of Age Having Mitral Valve Replacement." (1982) *American Heart Journal* 104: 276-288.

87. Clemens, J. D. et al. "A Controlled Evaluation of the Risk of Bacterial Endocarditis in Persons with Mitral Valve Prolapse." (September, 1982) *The New England Journal of Medicine*: 776-781.

88. Freedman, L. R. *Infective Endocarditis and Other Intravascular Infections* (New York: Plenum Medical Book Company, 1982), p. 39.

89. Ibid., p. 69.

90. Waller et al., op. cit.

Chapter Fourteen

1. Osler, W. "The Gulstonian Lectures on Malignant Endocarditis. (March, 7, 14, 21, 1885) *British Medical Journal*: 467-470, 522-526, 577-579.

2. Gross, L. and B. M. Fried. "The Role Played by Rheumatic Fever in the Implantation of Bacterial Endocarditis." (1937) *American Journal of Pathology* 13: 769-798.

3. Rahimtoola, S. H. *Infective Endocarditis* (New York: Grune & Stratton, 1978), p. 2.

4. Osler, op. cit., p. 467.

5. Libman, E. and C. K. Friedberg. *Subacute Bacterial Endocarditis* (New York: Oxford University Press, 1941), p. 16.

6. Glynn, T. R. "Infective Endocarditis Mainly in its Clinical Aspects." (April 11, 18, 25, 1903) *The Lancet*: 1007-1010, 1073-1077, 1148-1153.

7. Thayer, W. S. "Bacterial or Infective Endocarditis." (1931) *Edinburgh Medical Journal* 38: 307-334.

8. Gregoratos, G and J. S. Karliner. "Infective Endocarditis: Diagnosis and Management." (January, 1979) *Medical Clinics of North America* 63 (1): 173-199.

9. Hepper, N. G. G. et al. " Mitral Insufficiency in Healed Unrecognized Bacterial Endocarditis." (December, 1956) *Staff Meetings of the Mayo Clinic* 31 (25): 659-664.

10. Lichtmann, S. S. "Treatment of Subacute Bacterial Endocarditis: Current Results." (1943) *Annals of Internal Medicine* 19: 787-794.

11. Ibid.

12. Loewe, L. et al. "Combined Penicillin and Heparin Therapy of Subacute Bacterial Endocarditis." (January 15, 1944) *Journal of the American Medical Association*: 144-149.

13. Levine, W. G. "Heavy Metals and Heavy-Metal Antagonists" in *The Pharmacological Basis of Therapeutics*. 4th ed., Goodman, L. S. and A. Gilman, eds. (New York: The MacMillan Co., 1970), pp. 959-960.

14. Kelson, S. R. and P. D. White. "Notes on 250 Cases of Subacute Bacterial (Streptococcal) Endocarditis Studied and Treated Between 1927 and 1939. (1945) *Annals of Internal Medicine* 22: 40-60.

15. Ibid., p. 54.

16. Ibid., p. 56.

17. Ibid., p. 54.

18. Ibid., p. 55.

19. Puckett, T. F. "Infection and Infectious Diseases" in *Concepts of Disease*. Brunson, J. G. and E. A. Gall, eds., (New York: The MacMillan Co., 1971), p. 603.

20. Weinstein, A. J. et al. "Infective Endocarditis: Changes in Etiology, Diagnosis and Management." (June 6, 1980) *Comprehensive Therapy* 6: 31-35.

21. Baddour, L. M. and A. L. Bisno. "Infective Endocarditis Complicating Mitral Valve Prolapse: Epidemiologic, Clinical, Microbiologic Aspects." (Jan-Feb, 1986) *Reviews of Infectious Diseases*: 8 (1): 117-137.

22. Freedman, L. R. *Infective Endocarditis and Other Intravascular Infections* (New York, Plenum Medical Book Company, 1982), p. 33.

23. Ibid.

24. Everett, E. D. and J.V. Hirschmann. "Transient Bacteremia and Endocarditis Prophylaxis: A Review." (1977) *Medicine* 56 (1): 61-77.

25. Ward, R. L. "Endocarditis Complicating Ulcerative Colitis." (November, 1977) *Gastroenterology*: 1189-90.

26. Everett et al., op. cit., p. 66.

27. Ibid., p. 66.

28. Ibid.

29. Freedman, op. cit., pp. 33, 184.

30. Cobbs, C. G. "IUD and Endocarditis." (1973) *Annals of Internal Medicine* 78: 541.

31. de Swiet M. et al. "Bacterial Endocarditis After Insertion of Intrauterine Contraceptive Device." (Case Report) (1975) *British Medical Journal* 117: 76.

32. Freedman, op. cit., p. 33.

33. Everett, op. cit., p. 68.

34. Lachman, A. S. et al. "Infective Endocarditis in the Billowing Mitral Leaflet Syndrome." (1975) *British Heart Journal* 37: 326-330.

35. Osler, op. cit., p. 522.

36. Freedman, op. cit., p. 33.

37. Everett et al., op. cit., p. 64.

38. Glynn, op. cit., p. 1073.

39. Libman, E. "A Consideration of the Prognosis in Subacute Bacterial Endocarditis." (1925) *American Heart Journal* 1: 25-40.

40. Hamman, L. "Healed Bacterial Endocarditis." (1937) *Annals of Internal Medicine* XI: 175-194.

41. Hobson, F. G. and B. E. Juel-Jensen. "Teeth, Streptococcus Viridans and Subacute Bacterial Endocarditis." (December 27, 1956) *British Medical Journal*: 1501-1505.

42. Bieger, R. C. et al. "Haemophilus Aphrophilus: A Microbiologic and Clinical Review and Report of 42 Cases." (1978) *Medicine* 57 (4): 345-355.

43. Sims, W. "Oral Haemophili." (1970) *Journal of Medical Microbiology* 3: 615.

44. Righter, J. and J. Zwerver. "infections Caused by Group F Streptococci." (November 1, 1981) *Canadian Medical Association Journal* 125: 1008-1010

45. Von Scupin, E. and E. Scupin. "Das Tonsillitis-Endocarditis-Syndrom beim Hund." (August, 1978) *Deutsche Tierarztliche Wochenschrift* 85: 313-317.

46. Hayward, G. "Bacterial Endocarditis." (1960) *Proceedings of the Royal Society of Medicine* 53 (551): 13-24.

47. Everett, op. cit., p. 62.

48. Okell, C. C. et al. "Bacteremia and Oral Sepsis with special Reference to the Aetiology of Subacute Endocarditis." (October, 1935) *The Lancet*: 869-872.

49. Everett., op. cit., p. 63.

50. Ibid., p. 61.

51. Murray, M. and F. Moosnick. "Incidence of Bacteremia in Patients with Dental Disease. (1941) *Journal of Laboratory and Clinical Medicine* 26: 801.

52. Harvey, W. P. and M. A. Capone. "Bacterial Endocarditis Related to Cleaning and Filling Teeth with Particular Reference to the Inadequacy of Present Day Knowledge and Practice of Antibiotic Prophylaxis for all Dental Procedures. " (1961) *The American Journal of Cardiology*: 793-797.

53. Vose, J. M. et al. "Recurrent Streptococcus Mutans Endocarditis." (March 23, 1987) *The American Journal of Medicine* 82: 630-632.

54. Chunn, C. J. et al. "Haemophilus Parainfluenzae Infective Endocarditis." (1977) *Medicine* 56 (2): 99-113.

55. Hammond, G. W. et al. "Two Cases of Haemophilus Endocarditis of Prolapsed Mitral Valves: Haemophilus Paraprophilus or Parainfluenze?" (September, 1978) The American Journal of Medicine 65: 537-41.

56. Sims, W. "The Clinical Bacteriology of Purulent Oral Infections." (1974) *British Journal of Oral Surgery* 12: 1-12.

57. Okell, op. cit., p. 869.

58. Petersdorf, R. G. "Antimicrobial Prophylaxis of Bacterial Endocarditis: Prudent Caution or Bacterial Overkill?" (August, 1978) *The American Journal of Medicine* 65: 220-223.

59. Bender, I. B. et al. "Dental Procedures in Patients with Rheumatic Heart Disease. " (April, 1963) *Endodontics* 16 (4): 466-473.

60. Hobson and Juel-Jensen, op. cit., p. 1504.

61. Wilkinson, M. "Bacterial Endocarditis and Focal Infection." (February, 1967) *The Dental Practitioner* 17 (6): 201-204.

62. Monroe, C. O. and T. L. Lazarus. "Predisposing Conditions of Infective Endocarditis." (1976) *Journal of the Canadian Dental Association* 42 (10): 483-494.

63. Cohn, L. H. et al. "Bacterial Endocarditis Following Aortic Valve Replacement. (February, 1966) *Circulation* 33: 209-217.

64. Bender, op. cit., p. 471.

65. Tarsitano, J. J. "The Use of Antibiotics in Dental Practice." (October, 1970) *Dental Clinics of North America* 14 (4): 697-711.

66. Everett and Hirschman, op. cit., pp. 69-70.

67. Sims, "The Clinical Bacteriology of Purulent Oral Infections", op. cit., p. 2.

68. Gregoratos and Karliner, op. cit., 175.

69. Hollanders, G. et al. "A Six Years Review on 53 Cases of Infective Endocarditis: Clinical Microbiological and Therapeutical Features. (1988) *Acta Cardiologica* XLIII: 121-132.

70. Welton, D. E. et al. "Recurrent Infective Endocarditis." (June, 1979) *The American Journal of Medicine* 66: 932-938.

71. Grant, R. T. et al. "Heart Valve Irregularities in Relation to Subacute Bacterial Endocarditis." (1927) *Heart* 14: 247-255.

72. Ibid., p. 248.

73. Osler, Op. cit., p. 469.

74. Ibid.

75. Glynn, op. cit., p. 1009.

76. Ibid., p. 1009.

77. Grant, op. cit., p. 249.

78. Davies, M. J. et al. "The Floppy Mitral Valve: Study of Incidence, Pathology and Complications in Surgical, Necropsy and Forensic Material." (1978) *British Heart Journal* 40: 461-481.

79. Grant, op. cit., p. 250.

80. Berkow, R. et al. *The Merck Manual of Diagnosis and Therapy* (Rahway, New Jersey: Merck, Sharp & Dohme Research Laboratories, 1982), p. 526.

81. Davies et al., op. cit., p. 473.

82. Pomerance, A. "Ballooning Deformity (Mucoid Degeneration) of Atrioventricular Valves." (1969) *British Heart Journal* 31: 343-351.

83. Glynn, op. cit., p. 1075.

84. Osler, op. cit., p. 468.

85. Grant, op. cit., p. 251.

86. Da Costa, J. M. "On Irritable Heart: A Clinical Study of a Form of Functional Cardiac Disorder and its Consequences." (1871) *The American Journal of the Medical Sciences* CXXI: 2-52.

87. Ibid., p. 26.

88. Freedman, op. cit., p. 99.

89. Lewis, T. *The Soldier's Heart and The Effort Syndrome* (London: Shaw and Sons, 1940), p. 15.

90. Ibid., p. 17.

91. Ibid., p. 81.

92. Lewis, T. *The Soldier's Heart and The Effort Syndrome* (London: Shaw & Sons, 1918), p. 64.

93. Davies et al., op. cit., p. 473.
94. Gross, L. and B. M. Fried. "The Role Played by Rheumatic Fever in the Implantation of Bacterial Endocarditis." (1937) *American Journal of Pathology* XIII: 769-798.
95. Barlow, J. B. et al. "The Significance of Late Systolic Murmurs." (1963) *American Heart Journal* 66 (4): 443-452.
96. McLaren, M. J. et al. "Non-ejection Systolic Clicks and Mitral Systolic Murmurs in Black School Children of Soweto, Johannesburg." (1976) *British Heart Journal* 38: 718-724.
97. Davies et al., op. cit., p. 473.
98. Luxton, M. et al. "The Floppy Mitral Valve Syndrome: A Review of 14 Patients Requiring Valve Surgery." (1975) *Australia and New Zealand Journal of Medicine* 5: 112-116.
99. Tamer, D. et al. "Streptococcal Antibodies in MVP." (1980) *Clinical Research* 28: 14a.
100. Ibid.
101. Horder, T. J. "Infective Endocarditis: With an Analysis of 150 Cases and with Special Reference to the Chronic Form of the Disease." (April, 1909) *Quarterly Journal of Medicine* 289: 304.
102. Grant, op. cit., p. 252.
103. Freedman, op. cit., p. 46.
104. Ibid., pp. 9, 12.
105. Ibid., p. 53.
106. Durack, D. T. and P. B. Beeson. "Experimental Bacterial Endocarditis: II Survival of Bacteria in Endocardial Vegetations." (1972) *British Journal of Experimental Pathology* 53: 50-53.
107. Durack, D. T. et al. "Experimental Bacterial Endocarditis: III Production and Progress of the Disease in Rabbits. (1973) *British Journal of Experimental Pathology* 54: 142-151.
108. Ibid., p. 145.
109. Freedman, op. cit., p. 18.
110. Clawson, C. C. "The Role of Platelets in the Pathogenesis of Endocarditis" in *Infective Endocarditis: An American Heart Association Symposium.* Monograph #52, Kaplan, E. L and A. V. Taranta, eds. (Dallas: The American Heart Association, Inc., 1977), pp. 24-27.
111. Wannamaker, L. and M. T. Parker, "Microbiology of Bacteria Often Responsible for IE," ibid., p. 16.
112. Stein, P. D. et al. "Scanning Electron Microscopy of Operatively Excised Severely Regurgitant Floppy Mitral Valves." (August, 1989) *The American Journal of Cardiology* 64: 392-394.
113. Sandok, B. A. and E. R. Giuliani. "Cerebral Ischemic Events in Patients with MVP." (July-August, 1982) *Stroke* 13 (4): 448-450.

Chapter Fifteen

1. Freedman, L. R. *Infective Endocarditis and Other Intravascular Infections* (New York: Plenum Medical Book Co., 1982), p. 79.
2. Weinstein, A. J. "Infective Endocarditis: Changes in Etiology, Diagnosis and Management." (June 6, 1980) *Comprehensive Therapy* 6: 31-35.
3. Dorney, E. R. "Endocarditis" in *The Heart.* 3rd ed., Hurst, J. W. et al., eds. (New York: McGraw-Hill Book Co., 1974), p. 1295.
4. Gregoratos, G. and J. S. Karliner. "Infective Endocarditis: Diagnosis and Management." (January, 1979) *Medical Clinics of North America* 63 (1): 173-199.
5. Jacoby, G. A. and M. N. Swartz. "Fever of Undetermined Origin." (1971) *The New England Journal of Medicine* 289 (26): 1407-1409.
6. Berkow, R. et al. *The Merck Manual of Diagnosis and Therapy.* 14th ed. (Rahway, New Jersey: Merck Sharp & Dohme Research Laboratories, 1982), p. 5.
7. Puklin, J. E. "Culture of an Osler's Node." (February, 1971) *Archives of Internal Medicine* 127: 296-298.
8. Ellner, J. J. et al. "Infective Endocarditis Caused by Slow-Growing, Fastidious, Gram Negative Bacteria." (1979) *Medicine*: 145-158.

9. Mazansky, C. et al. "Aspects of Bacterial Endocarditis in the Johannesburg General Hospital: An Analysis of 30 Cases." (March 10, 1973) *South African Medical Journal*: 413-418.

10. Osler, W. "The Gulstonian Lectures on Malignant Endocarditis." (March 7, 1885) *British Medical Journal*: 467-470, 522-526, 577-579.

11. Williams, T. W. et al. "Management of Bacterial Endocarditis — 1970." (1970) *The American Journal of Cardiology* 26: 186-191.

12. Mazansky et al., op. cit., p. 416.

13. Gregoratos, op. cit., p. 179.

14. Ibid., p. 178.

15. Ibid., p. 179.

16. Danchin, N. et al. "Mitral Valve Prolapse as a Risk Factor for Infective Endocarditis." (April 8, 1989) *The Lancet*: 743-745.

17. Perloff, J. K. "Systolic, Diastolic and Continuous Murmurs" in *The Heart*, op. cit., p. 261.

18. Ibid.

19. Ibid.

20. Leon, D. F. et al. "Late Systolic Murmurs, Clicks and Whoops Arising from the Mitral Valve." (1966) *American Heart Journal* 72 (3): 325-336.

21. Cates, J. E. and R. V. Christie. "Subacute Bacterial Endocarditis." (April, 1951) *Quarterly Journal of Medicine* 20 (8): 95-130.

22. Gregoratos, op. cit., p. 178.

23. Pankey, G. A. "Acute Bacterial Endocarditis at the University of Minnesota Hospitals 1939-1959." (November, 1962) *American Heart Journal* 64 (5): 583-591.

24. Braunwald, E. and W. H. Resnik. "Palpitation" in *Harrison's Principles of Internal Medicine*. 7th ed., Wintrobe, M. M. et al., eds. (New York: McGraw-Hill Book Co., 1974), p. 182.

25. Dubin, D. *Rapid Interpretation of EKG's: A Programmed Course*. (Tampa, Florida: Cover Publishing Company, 1978), pp. 117-119.

26. Pillsbury, P. L. and M. J. Fiese. "Subacute Bacterial Endocarditis." (1950) *Archives of Internal Medicine* 85: 675-691.

27. Dubin, op. cit., p. 253.

28. Ringer M. et al. "Mitral Valve Prolapse: Jet Stream Causing Mural Endocarditis." (February, 1980) *American Journal of Cardiology* 45: 383-385.

29. Pankey, G. "Subacute Bacterial Endocarditis at the University of Minnesota Hospitals 1939-1959." (1961) *Annals of Internal Medicine* 55 (4): 550-561.

30. Pankey, G. "Acute Bacterial Endocarditis at the University of Minnesota Hospitals 1939-59," op. cit., 583-591.

31. Buchbinder, N. A. and W. C. Roberts. "Left-sided Valvular Active Infective Endocarditis: A Study of 45 Necropsy Patients." (July, 1972) *American Journal of Medicine* 53: 20-35.

32. Weinstein, L. and J. J. Schlesinger. "Pathoanatomic, Pathophysiologic and Clinical Correlations in Endocarditis." (1974) *The New England Journal of Medicine*: 1122-26.

33. Sheldon, W. H. and A. Golden. "Abscesses of the Valve Rings of the Heart, a Frequent but Not Well Recognized Complication of Acute Bacterial Endocarditis." (July, 1951) *Circulation* IV: 1-12.

34. Dorney, E. R., op. cit., p. 1294.

35. Libman, E. and C. K. Friedberg. *Subacute Bacterial Endocarditis* (New York: Oxford University Press, 1948) p. 33.

36. Pankey, (1961), op. cit., p. 553.

37. Libman and Friedberg, op. cit., p. 34.

38. Alpert, J. S. et al. "Pathogenesis of Osler's Nodes." (1976) *Annals of Internal Medicine* 85: 471-473.

39. Libman and Friedberg, op. cit., p. 36.

40. Wilson, W. R. et al. "Management of complications of Infective Endocarditis." (1982 *Mayo Clinic Proceedings* 57: 162-170.

41. Hayward, op. cit., p. 708.

42. Libman and Friedberg, op. cit., p. 37.
43. Hayward, op. cit., p. 708.
44. Gregoratos, op. cit., p. 180.
45. Rahimtoola, S. H. *Infective Endocarditis* (New York: Grune & Stratton, 1978), p. 134.
46. Mazansky et al., op. cit., p. 414.
47. Libman and Friedberg, op. cit., p. 40-41.
48. Ahmad, N. et al. "Potentially Fatal Splenic Involvement in Infective Endocarditis." (September 3, 1988) *The Lancet*: 576.
49. Horder, T. J. "Infective Endocarditis with an Analysis of 150 Cases and with Special Reference to the Chronic Form of the Disease." (April, 1909) *Quarterly Journal of Medicine*: 289-324.
50. Churchill, M. A. et al. "Musculoskeletal Manifestations of Bacterial Endocarditis." (1977) *Annals of Internal Medicine* 87: 754-759.
51. Good, A. E. et al. "Streptococcal Endocarditis Initially seen as Septic Arthritis." (May, 1978) *Archives of Internal Medicine* 138: 805-806.
52. Churchill et al, op. cit., p. 755.
53. Libman, E. "The Clinical Features of Subacute Bacterial Endocarditis That Have Spontaneously Become Bacteria-Free." (1913) *The American Journal of the Medical Sciences* 146 (5): 625-645.
54. Kincaid, D. T. and R. E. Botti. "Subacute Bacterial Endocarditis in a Patient with Isolated, Nonejection Systolic Click but Without a Murmur." (1974) *Chest* 66 (1): 88-89.
55. Churchill et al., op. cit., p. 755.
56. Freedman, op. cit., p. 110.
57. Mund, D. J. "Pyogenic Vertebral Osteomyelitis: Manifestation of Bacterial Endocarditis." (May, 1980) *New York State Journal of Medicine*: 980-982.
58. Musher, D. M. et al. "Vertebral Osteomyelitis." (January, 1976) *Archives of Internal Medicine* 136: 105-110.
59. Freedman, op. ci., p. 133.
60. Musher, D. M. et al. op. cit., p. 107.
61. Churchill, op. cit., p. 756.
62. McCord, M. C. and J. Moberly. "Acute Hypertrophic Osteo-Arthropathy Associated with Subacute Bacterial Endocarditis." (February, 1953) *Annals of Internal Medicine* 39: 640-644.
63. Scully, R. E. and B. U. McNeely. "Case Records of the Massachusetts General Hopsital Weekly Clinicopathological Exercises." (August, 1974) *The New England Journal of Medicine* 291 (5): 243-249.
64. Ziment, I. "Nervous System Complications in Bacterial Endocarditis." (October, 1969) *American Journal of Medicine* 47: 593-607.
65. Wilson, W. R. et al. "Management of Complications of Infective Endocarditis." (1982) *Mayo Clinic Proceedings* 57: 162-170.
66. Pruitt, A. A. et al. "Neurologic Complications of Bacterial Endocarditis." (1978) *Medicine* 57 (4): 329-343.
67. Ibid., p. 341.
68. Wilson et al. op. cit., p. 167.
69. Ziment, op. cit., p. 595.
70. Hayward, op. cit. p. 708.
71. Ziment, op. cit., p. 595.
72. Pruitt et al., op cit., p. 341.
73. Ziment, op. cit., 598.
74. Dubin, op. cit., p. 121.
75. Ziment, op. cit., p. 595.
76. Ibid., p. 599.
77. Pruitt et al., op. cit., p. 339.
78. Ibid.
79. Ziment, op. cit., p. 596.

80. Wilson et al., op. cit., p. 168.

81. Ziment, op. cit., p. 600-601.

82. Ibid., p. 598.

83. Ibid., p. 596.

84. Rabinovich, S. et al. "A Longterm View of Bacterial Endocarditis." (1965) *Annals of Internal Medicine* 63: 185.

85. Alajouanine, T. et al. "L'Artérite Cérébrale de la Maladie d'Osler: Ses Complications Tardives. (1959) *Seminars Hopital Paris* 35: 1160.

86. Ziment, op. cit., p. 601.

87. Valtin, H. *Renal Function: Mechanisms Preserving Fluid and Solute Balance in Health* (Boston: Little, Brown & Co., 1983), pp. 3-8.

88. Epstein, F. H. "Glomerulonephritis" in *Harrison's Principles of Internal Medicine*, op. cit., p. 1388ff.

89. Bell, E. T. "Glomberular Lesions Associated with Endocarditis." (1932) *American Journal of Pathology* VIII (6): 639-662.

90. Rowlands, D. T. "Immunity" in *Concepts of Disease*. Brunson, J. G. and E. A. Gall. eds. (New York: MacMillan Co., 1971), p. 563.

91. Waldenstrom, J. G. *Monoclonal and Polyclonal Hypergammaglobulinemia: Clinical and Biological Significance.* (Nashville, Tenn. Vanderbilt University Press, 1968), pp. 3-6.

92. Libman and Friedberg, op. cit., p. 23.

93. Valtin, op. cit., pp. 46-49.

94. Bayer, A. S. "Use of Circulating Immunge Complex Levels in the Serodifferentiation of Endocarditic and Nonendocarditic Septicemias." (January, 1979) *The American Journal of Medicine* 66: 58-62.

95. Freedman, op. cit., p. 95.

96. Rowland, D. T. "Immunity in *Concepts of Disease*, op. cit., p. 568.

97. Woodroffe, A. J. et al. "Detection of Circulating Immune Complexes in Patients with Glomerulonephritis." (1977) *Kidney International* 12: 268-278.

98. Kaufman, D. B. and R. McIntosh. "The Pathogenesis of the Renal Lesion in a Patient with Streptococcal Disease, Infected Ventriculoatrial Shunt, Cryoglobulinemia and Nephritis." (February, 1971) *The American Journal of Medicine* 50: 262-268.

99. Hurwitz, D. et al. "Cryoglobulinemia in Patients with Infective Endocarditis." (1975) *Clinical Experimental Immunology* 19: 131-141.

100. Cabane, J. et al. "Fate of Circulating Immune Complexes in Infective Endocarditis." (1979) *The American Journal of Medicine* 66: 277-282.

101. Wurman, R. J. *Medical Access* (Los Angeles: Access Press Ltd., 1985), p. 57.

102. Epstein, F. "Approach to the Patient with Renal Disease" in *Harrison's Principles of Internal Medicine*, op. cit., p. 1368.

103. Kyle, R. A. and E. D. Bayrd. "Benign" Monoclonal Gammopathy: A Potentially Malignant Condition?" (1966) *The American Journal of Medicine* 40: 426-430.

104. Brunner-Sholtis, L. and D. Suddarth-Smith. *The Lippincott Manual of Nursing* 3rd. ed. (Philadelphia: J. B. Lippincott, 1982), p. 478.

105. Bell, op. cit., p. 654.

106. Freedman, op. cit., p. 99.

107. Morel-Maroger, L. et al. "Kidney in Subacute Endocarditis: Pathological and Immunoflorescence Studies." (1972) *Archives of Pathology* 94: 205-213.

108. Epstein, F. H. "Glomerulonephritis" in Harrison's Principles of Internal Medicine, op. cit., p. 1390.

109. Raphael, S. S. *Lynch's Medical Laboratory Technology* (Philadelphia: W. B. Saunders Co., 1983), p. 211.

110. Epstein, F. H. op. cit., p. 1388ff.

111. Wallach, J. *Interpretation of Diagnostic Tests* (Boston: Little, Brown and Co., 1978), p. 9.

112. Brunner-Sholtis and Suddarth-Smith, "Diagnostic Studies and their Meanings." (Appendix I) in *The Lippincott Manual of Nursing*, op. cit., p. 1470.
113. Wallach, op. cit., p. 175.
114. Bayer, A. S. et al. "Circulating Immunge Complexes in Infective Endocarditis." (1976) *The New England Journal of Medicine* 295: 1500-1505.
115. Ibid., p. 1500.
116. Raphael, op. cit., p. 694.
117. Ibid., p. 694.
118. Sheagren, J. N. et al. "Rheumatoid Factor in Acute Bacterial Endocarditis." (1976) *Arthritis and Rheumatism* 19 (5): 887-890.
119. Milgrom, F. and E. Witebsky. "Studies on the Rheumatoid and Related Serum Factors. (September, 1960) *Journal of the American Medical Association* 174 (1): 138-145.
120. Williams, R. C. "Subacute Bacterial Endocarditis as an Immune Disease." (June, 1971) *Hospital Practice*: 113-122.
121. Sheagren et al. op. ci., p. 887.
122. Hurwitz et al. op. cit., p. 138.
123. Ibid., p. 138.
124. Das S. and J. T. Cassidy. "Importance of Heart Antibody in Infective Endocarditis." (1977) *Archives of Internal Medicine* 137: 591-593.
125. Lukes, B. J. and J. W. Parker. "Disorders of the Hematopoietic System" in *Concepts of Disease*, op. cit., p. 950.
126. Libman and Friedberg, op. cit., 1948, p. 59.
127. Cordeiro, A. et al. "Immunologic Phase of Subacute Bacterial Endocarditis: A New Concept and General Considerations. (1965) *The American Journal of Cardiology* 16 (4): 477-481.
128. Hallen, J. A. N. "Discrete Gammaglobulin (M-) Components in Serum: Clinical Study of 150 Subjects Without Myelomatosis. (1966) *Acta Medica Scandavica* Supplement 462: 8-115.

Chapter Sixteen

1. Simor, A. E. and I. E. Salit. "Endocarditis Caused by M6." (May, 1983) *Journal of Clinical Microbiology* 17: (5): 931-933.

Chapter Seventeen

1. Beaty, H. N. and R.G. Petersdorf. "Iatrogenic Factors in Infectious Disease." (October, 1966) *Annals of Internal Medicine* 65 (4): 641-656.
2. Ibid., p. 641.
3. Parker, D. J. "The Patient After Cardiac Valve Surgery -Risks and Complications. (1984) *European Heart Journal* 5 (Supplement A): 141-145.
4. "Clinical Signs Can Eliminate Routine Endocarditis Test." *The Journal*. (Toronto: Addiction Research Foundation of Ontario, May 1, 1985), p. 8.
5. Weinstein, L. "The Penicillins" in *The Pharmacological Basis of Therapeutics*. 4th ed., Goodman, L. S. and A. Gilman, eds. (New York: The MacMillan Co., 1970), p. 1210.
6. "Benzylpenicillin" in *The Pharmaceutical Codex* (London: The Pharmaceutical Press, 1979), p. 93.
7. Weinstein, L. "The Penicillins" in *The Pharmacological Basis of Therapeutics*, op. cit., p. 1209.
8. *The Pharmaceutical Codex*, op. cit., p. 93.
9. Weinstein, L. "Antimicrobial Agents: Streptomycin, Gentamycin and Other Aminoglycosides" in *The Pharmacological Basis of Therapeutics*. 5th ed., Goodman, L. S. and A. Gilman, eds. (New York: The MacMillan Co., 1975), p. 1175.
10. Weinstein, L. "The Penicillins" in *The Pharmacological Basis of Therapeutics* (1970), op. cit., 1970, p. 1208.

11. Weinstein, L. "Chemotherapy of Microbial Disease" in *The Pharmacological Basis of Therapeutics* (1970), op. cit., p. 1171.
12. Weinstein, "Antimicrobial Agents: Streptomycin, Gentamycin and Other Aminoglycosides" in *The Pharmacological Basis of Therapeutics* (1975), op. cit., p. 1175.
13. *The Pharmaceutical Codex*, op. cit., p. 93.
14. Goth, A. *Medical Pharmacology: Principles and Concepts* (St. Louis, MO: C. V. Mosby Company, 1981), p. 82-83.
15. Ibid., p. 82.
16. Weinstein, L. "Antibiotics IV: Miscellaneous Antimicrobial, Antifungal and Antiviral Agents" in *The Pharmacological Basis of Therapeutics* (1970), op. cit., p. 1298.
17. Weinstein, "The Penicillins", ibid., p. 1216.
18. *Drug Information for the Health Care Provider.* Vol I (Rockville, Maryland: United States Pharmacopeial Convention, Inc., 1983), p. 411.
19. Weinstein, L. "Antibiotics IV: Miscellaneous Antimicrobial, Antifungal and Antiviral Agents" in *The Pharmacological Basis of Therapeutics*, (1970), op. cit., p. 1298.
20. Ibid.
21. Weinstein, "The Penicillins", (1970), op. cit., p. 1207.
22. Ibid. p. 1218.
23. Chunn, C. J. et al. "Haemophilus Parainfluenzae Infective Endocarditis." (1977) *Medicine* 56 (2): 99-113.
24. Scully, R. E. and B. U. McNeely. "Case Records of the Massachusetts General Hospital: Weekly Clinicopathological Exercises. (1974) *The New England Journal of Medicine* 29 (5): 242-249.
25. Ibid., p. 242.
26. Jacoby, G. A. and M. N. Swartz. "Current Concepts: Fever of Undetermined Origin." (1971) *The New England Journal of Medicine* 289 (25): 1407-1409.
27. Scully and McNeely, op. cit., p. 243.
28. Krogh, M. E. et al. *Compendium of Pharmaceuticals and Specialties.* 21st ed. (Ottawa: Canadian Pharmaceutical Association, 1986), p. 764.
29. Scully and McNeely, op. cit., p. 248.
30. Ibid., p. 246.
31. Wallach, J. *Interpretation of Diagnostic Tests: A Handbook Synopsis of Laboratory Medicine* (Boston: Little, Brown and Co., 1978), p. 7.
32. Libman, E. and C. K. Friedberg. *Subacute Bacterial Endocarditis* (New York: Oxford University Press, 1948), p. 33.
33. Scully and McNeely, op. cit., p. 248.
34. Brunner-Sholtis, L. and D. Suddarth-Smith. *The Lippincott Manual of Nursing*, 3rd ed. (Philadelphia: J. B. Lippincott, 1982), p. 1468.
35. Wallach, op. cit., p. 19.
36. Ibid.
37. Scully and McNeely, op. cit., p. 249.

Chapter Eighteen

1. Weyman, J. "Antibiotics in General Dental Practice." (May 21, 1974) *British Dental Journal*: 404.
2. Hayward, G. W. "Infective Endocarditis: A Changing Disease — I." (1973) *British Medical Journal* 2: 706-709.
3. Ibid., p. 706.
4. Wilkinson, M. "Bacterial Endocarditis and Focal Infection." (February, 1967) *The Dental Practitioner* 17 (6): 201-204.
5. Bayliss, R. et al. "The Teeth and Infective Endocarditis." (1983) *British Heart Journal* 50: 506-512.

6. Cherubin, C. E. and H. C. Neu. "Infective Endocarditis at the Presbyterian Hospital in New York City from 1938-1967." (July, 1971) *The American Journal of Medicine* 51: 83-96.

7. Freedman, L. *Infective Endocarditis and Other Intravascular Infections* (New York: Plenum Medical Book Company, 1983), p. 38.

8. Bor, D. H. et al. "Endocarditis Prophylaxis for Patients with MVP." (1984) *The American Journal of Medicine* 76: 711-717.

9. *Statistics Canada.* (1986) Causes of Death: Vital Statistics Vol IV. Detailed Categories of the "International Classification of Diseases" — ICD.

10. Dorney, E. R. "Endocarditis" in *The Heart*, 3rd. ed. Hurst, J. W. et al., eds. (New York: McGraw-Hill Book Co., 1974), pp. 1292.

11. Hepper, N. G. G. et al. "Cardiac Clinics. CXLVI. Mitral Insufficiency in Healed Unrecognized Bacterial Endocarditis." (1956) *Staff Meetings of the Mayo Clinic* 31 (25): 659-664.

12. Landefeld, C. S. et al. "Diagnostic Yield of the Autopsy in a University Hospital and a Community Hospital." (May 12, 1988) *The New England Journal of Medicine* 318: 1249.

13. Freedman, op. cit., p. 38-39.

14. Boulton-Jones, J. M. et al. "Renal Lesions of Subacute Infective Endocarditis." (1974) *British Medical Journal* 2: 11-14.

15. Morel-Maroger, L. et al. "Kidney in Subacute Endocarditis: Pathological and Immunofluorescence Findings." (September, 1972) *Archives of Pathology* 94: 205-213.

16. *Statistics Canada*, 1986, op. cit.

17. Freedman, op. cit., p. 38.

18. Hayward, G. "Bacterial Endocarditis." (1960) *Proceedings of the Royal Society of Medicine* 53: 551-562.

19. Reimann, H. A. "Antibiotic Therapy." (June, 1966) *Archives of Environmental Health* 12: 683.

20. Uwaydah, M. M. and A. N. Weinberg. "Bacterial Endocarditis: A Changing Pattern." (December, 1965) *The New England Journal of Medicine* 273 (23): 1231-1234.

21. Chapman, I. "Prophylaxis of Bacterial Endocarditis: A General Practice Audit. (March, 1988) *Journal of the Royal College of Dental Practitioners*: 113-114.

22. Shinebourne, E. A. et al. "Bacterial Endocarditis 1956-1965: Analysis of Clinical Features and Treatment in Relation to Prognosis and Mortality." (1969) *British Heart Journal* 31: 536-542.

23. Kaplan, E. L. "Infective Endocarditis in the Pediatric Age Group: An Overview" in *Infective Endocarditis: An American Heart Association Symposium*. American Heart Association Monograph #52, Kaplan, E. L. and A. V. Taranta, eds., (Dallas: The American Heart Association, Inc., 1977), pp. 51-54.

24. Greenwood, R. D. "Mitral Valve Prolapse: Incidence and Clinical Course in a Pediatric Population." (1984) *Clinical Pediatrics* 23 (6): 318-320.

25. McNeill, K. M. et al. "Bacterial Endocarditis: An Analysis of Factors Affecting Long-Term Survival. (April, 1978) *American Heart Journal* 95(4): 448-453.

26. Garvey, G. J. and H. C. Neu. "Infective Endocarditis: An Evolving Disease. A Review of Endocarditis at The Columbian-Presbyterian Medical Center 1968-1973." (1978) *Medicine* 57 (2): 105-127.

27. Ormiston, J. A. et al. "Infective Endocarditis: A Lethal Disease." (1981) *Australian-New Zealand Journal of Medicine* 11: 620-629.

28. Boyd, A. D. et al. "Infective Endocarditis: An Analysis of 54 Surgically Treated Patients." (January, 1977) *The Journal of Thoracic and Cardiovascular Surgery* 73 #1: 23-30.

29. Sadowsky, D. and C. Kunzel. "Recommendations for Prevention of Bacterial Endocarditis: Compliance by Dental Practitioners." (1988) *Circulation* 77 (6): 1316-1318.

30. Bisno, A. L. et al. "Failure of Prophylaxis for Bacterial Endocarditis: American Heart Association Registry." (September, 1979) *Annals of Internal Medicine* 91 (3): 493.

31. Lerner, P. I. "Infective Endocarditis: A Review of Selected Topics." (May, 1974) *Medical Clinics of North America* 58 (3): 605-622.

32. Drake, T. A. and M. A. Sande, "Experimental Endocarditis" in *Experimental Models in Antimicrobial Chemotherapy*, Vol. I, Zak, O. and M. A. Sande, eds., (New York: Academic Press, Harcourt Brace Jovanovich, Publishers, 1986), pp. 257-277.

33. Durack, D. T. et al. "Apparent Failures of Endocarditis Prophylaxis: Analysis of 52 Cases Submitted to a National Registry." (November 4, 1983) *Journal of the American Medical Association* 250 (17): 2318-2322.

34. Levine, S. A. and W. P. Harvey. *Clinical Auscultation of the Heart* (Philadelphia: W. B. Saunders Co., 1949), p. 174.

35. Hobson, F. G. and B. E. Juel-Jenson. "Teeth, Streptococcus Viridans and Subacute Bacterial Endocarditis." (December, 1956) *British Medical Journal*: 1501-1505.

36. McGowan, D. A. and O. Tuohy. "Dental Treatment of Patients with Valvular Heart Disease." (June, 1968) *British Dental Journal*: 519-520.

37. Harvey, W. P. and M. A. Capone. "Bacterial Endocarditis Related to Cleaning and Filling of Teeth." (June, 1961) *The American Journal of Cardiology*: 793-797.

38. Croxson, M. S. et al. "Dental Status and Recurrence of Streptococcus Viridans Endocarditis." (June, 1971) *The Lancet*: 1205-1209.

39. Pelletier, L. L. and R. G. Petersdorf. " Infective Endocarditis: A Review of 125 Cases from the University of Washington Hospitals 1963-1972." (1977) *Medicine* 56 (4) 287-313.

40. Bayliss, R. et al. "Endocarditis Prophylaxis: Do Patients Remember Advice and Know What to Do?" (December, 1986) *British Medical Journal* 293: 1539-1540.

41. Munroe, C. O. and T. L. Lazarus. "Part I: Predisposing Conditions of Infective Endocarditis." (1976) *Journal of the Canadian Dental Association* 42 (10): 483-494.

42. Ibid., p. 492.

43. Kaplan, E. and D. T. Durack. "Committee for the Prevention of Rheumatic Fever and Bacterial Endocarditis of the American Heart Association." (January, 1978) *Journal of the American Dental Association* 96: 29.

44. Levine, S. A. "Some Unproved Impressions Concerning the Subject of Heart Disease." (1928) *The New England Journal of Medicine* 198 (17): 885-887.

45. Rodbard, S. "Blood Velocity and Endocarditis." (January, 1963) *Circulation* XXVII: 18-28.

46. Buchbinder, W. C. and N. A. Roberts. "Healed Left-Sided Endocarditis: A Clinicopathological Study of 59 Patients." (December, 1977) *The American Journal of Cardiology* 40: 876-888.

47. Kaplan, "Infective Endocarditis in the Pediatric Age Group: An Overview," op. cit., p. 51.

48. Rosenberg, C. A. et al. "Hypomastia and Mitral Valve Prolapse: Evidence of a Linked Embryologic and Mesenchymal Displasia." (1983) *The New England Journal of Medicine* 309 (20): 1230-32.

49. Cherubin and Neu, op. cit., p. 83.

50. Cawson, R. A. "Infective Endocarditis as a Complication of Dental Treatment." (1981) *British Dental Journal* 151: 409-413.

51. Sadowsky and Kunzel, op. cit.

52. Hepper, N. G. et al. "Cardiac Clinics CXLVI. Mitral Insufficiency in Healed, Unrecognized Bacterial Endocarditis." (1956) *Staff Meetings of the Mayo Clinic* 31 (25): 659-664.

53. Pini, R. et al. "Comparison of Mitral Valve Dimensions and Motion in Mitral Valve Prolapse With Severe Mitral Regurgitation to Uncomplicated Mitral Valve Prolapse and to Mitral Regurgitation Without Mitral Valve Prolapse." (1988) *The American Journal of Cardiology* 62: 257-263.

54. Guy, F. C. et al. "Mitral Valve Prolapse as a Cause of Hemodynamically Important Regurgitation." (March, 1980) *The Canadian Journal of Surgery* 23 (2): 166-170.

55. Waller, B. F. et al. "Etiology of Clinically Isolated, Severe, Chronic, Pure Mitral Regurgitation: Analysis of 97 Patients over 30 Years of Age Having Mitral Valve Replacement." (1982) *American Heart Journal* 104: 276-288.

56. *Statistics Canada*. (March 8, 1983) International Classification of Diseases 9: Acute Care Separations for Selected Diagnoses and Procedures, Ontario Hospitals 1981-82. Ontario Ministry of Health, Data Development and Evaluation Branch.

57. Reimann, op. cit.
58. Tarsitano, J. J. "The Use of Antibiotics in Dental Practice." (October, 1970) *Dental Clinics of North America* 14 (4): 697-711.
59. Pelletier and Petersdorf, op. cit., p. 303.
60. Kaplan and Durack, op. cit.
61. Weinstein, A. J. "Infective Endocarditis: Changes in Etiology, Diagnosis, and Management." (June 6, 1980) *Comprehensive Therapy* 6: 31-35.
62. Pesanti, E. L. and I. M. Smith: "Infective Endocarditis with Negative Blood Cultures." (January, 1979) *The American Journal of Medicine* 68: 43-50.
63. Pelletier and Petersdorf, op. cit., p. 294.
64. Ibid.
65. Van Scoy, R. "Culture Negative Endocarditis." (1982) *Mayo Clinic Proceedings* 57: 149-154.
66. Pelletier and Petersdorf, op. cit., p. 309.
67. Felner. J. M. and V. R. Dowell. "'Bacteroides' Bacteremia." (1971) *The American Journal of Medicine* 50: 787-796.
68. Petersdorf, R. G. "Antimicrobial Prophylaxis of Bacterial Endocarditis: Prudent Caution or Bacterial Overkill?". (August, 1978) *The American Journal of Medicine* 65: 220-223.
69. Weinstein, L. "Chemotherapy of Microbial Diseases." in *The Pharmacological Basis of Therapeutics.* 4th ed., Goodman, L. S. and A. Gilman, eds. (New York: The MacMillan Co., 1970), p. 1160.
70. McNeill et al., op. cit., p. 449.
71. Blount, J. G. "Bacterial Endocarditis." (1965) *The American Journal of Medicine* 38: 909-922.
72. Pelletier and Petersdorf, op. cit., p. 303.
73. Hayward, "Bacterial Endocarditis," op. cit.
74. Meyers, O. L. and D. J. Commerford. "Musculoskeletal Manifestations of Bacterial Endocarditis." (1977) *Annals of the Rheumatic Diseases* 36: 517-519.
75. Preston, P. B. et al. "Negative Blood Cultures in Infective Endocarditis: A Review." (1976) *Southern Medical Journal* 69 (11): 1420-1424.
76. Roberts, W. C. and N. A. Buchbinder. "Right-Sided Valvular Infective Endocarditis: A Clinicopathological Study of 12 Necropsy Patients." (July, 1972) *The American Journal of Medicine* 53: 7-19.
77. Preston et al., op. cit.
78. Friedberg, C. K. et al. "Study of Bacterial Endocarditis: Comparisons in 95 Cases." (January, 1961) *Archives of Internal Medicine* 107: 74-83.
79. Freedman, op. cit., p. 143.
80. Van Scoy, op. cit., p. 152.
81. Freedman, op. cit., p. 88.
82. Freedman, op. cit., p. 112.
83. Righter, J. and J. Zwerver. "Infections Caused by Group F Streptococci." (November, 1981) *Canadian Medical Association Journal* 125: 1008-1010.
84. Lerner, P. "Infective Endocarditis: A Review of Selected Topics." (1974) *Medical Clinics of North America* 58 (3): 605-619.
85. Ellner, J. J. et al. "Infective Endocarditis Caused by Slow-Growing, Fastidious Gram-Negative Bacteria." (1979) *Medicine* 58 (2): 145-158.
86. Felner and Dowell, op. cit., pp. 787, 794.
87. Lerner, op. cit., p. 607-608.
88. Washington, J. A. "Blood Culture Techniques in the Diagnosis of Infective Endocarditis" in *Infective Endocarditis: An American Heart Association Symposium*, American Heart Association Monograph #52, op. cit., pp. 44-45.
89. Freedman, op. cit., p. 208.
90. Ibid., p. 161.

91. DeSilva, M. et al. "Haemophilus Paraphrophilus Endocarditis in a Prolapsed Valve." ((November, 1976) *American Journal of Clinical Pathology* 66: 922-926.

92. Ellner, J. J. et al., op. cit., p. 151.

93. Wilson, W. R. et al. "Cardiac Valve Replacement in Congestive Heart Failure Due to Infective Endocarditis." (1979) *Mayo Clinic Proceedings* 54: 223-226.

94. Wilson W. R. et al. "Management of Complications of Infective Endocarditis." (1982) *Mayo Clinic Proceedings* 57: 162-170.

95. Freedman, op. cit., p. 216-217.

96. Zion, M. M. et al. "Echocardiographic Criteria for Diagnosis of Mitral Valve Prolapse." (October, 1988) *The American Journal of Cardiology*: 841.

97. Freedman, op. cit., p. 217.

98. Parker, D. J. "The Patient After Cardiac Valve Surgery -Risks and Complications." (1984) *European Heart Journal* 5 (Supplement A): 141-145.

99. Freedman, op. cit., p. 217.

100. Solomon, J. et al. "Surgical Treatment of Degenerative Mitral Regurgitation." (1975) *The American Journal of Cardiology* 36: 32-36.

101. Libman, E. and C. K. Friedberg. *Subacute Bacterial Endocarditis* (New York: Oxford University Press, 1948), p. 7.

102. Berkow, R. et al. *The Merck Manual of Diagnosis and Therapy* (Rahway, New Jersey: Merck, Sharp and Dohme Research Laboratories, 1982), p. 82.

103. *The Globe and Mail*, Toronto, June 15, 1984.

104. *The Globe and Mail*, Toronto, April 26, 1984.

105. Ibid.

106. *The Globe and Mail*, Toronto, November 18, 1983.

Chapter Nineteen

1. Wooley, C. F. "Where are the Diseases of Yesterday?" (May, 1976) *Circulation* 53 (5): 749-751.

2. Jones, W. G., *The Globe and Mail*, Toronto, April 21, 1983.

3. Caceres, C. A and L. W. Perry. *The Innocent Murmur* (London: J & A Churchill, Ltd., 1967), p. 66.

4. Rabelais, F., *Oeuvres Complètes: Pantagruel* Tome I (Paris: Garnier Frères, 1962), Le Tiers Livre, Chapitre XXXII, (author's translation) p. 539.

5. Alvarez, W. C. *The Neuroses: Diagnosis and Management of Functional Disorders and Minor Psychoses* (Philadelphia: W. B. Saunders Co., 1955), p. 39.

6. Ibid., p. 395.

7. Ibid., Preface, p. iv.

8. Ibid., p. 4.

9. Ibid., p. 49.

10. Ibid., p. 50.

11. Ibid., p. 52.

12. Ibid., p. 424.

13. Ibid., p. 148-149.

14. Ibid., p. 155.

15. Ibid., p. 411.

16. Ibid., p. 53.

17. Ibid., p. 40.

18. Ibid., pp. 41-42.

19. Ibid., p. 44.

20. Ibid., p. 108.

21. Ibid., p. 41, p. 85.

22. Ibid., p. 500.

23. Ibid., p. 40.
24. Ibid., p. 7.
25. Ibid., p. 43.
26. Quoted in *The Patient's Advocate* (newsletter of the Patients' Rights Association), Fall, 1986, p. 9.
27. McCallum P. "MDs Mistreat Women, Meeting Told." *The Globe and Mail*, Toronto, November 11, 1978.
28. Alvarez. op. cit., p. 39.
29. Ibid., p. 29.
30. Ibid., p. 217.
31. Wood, Paul, *Diseases of the Heart and Circulation*, 3rd ed. (London: Eyre and Spottiswoode, 1968), p. 1074.
32. Alvarez, op. cit., p. 395.
33. Ibid., p. 398.
34. Ibid.
35. Ibid.
36. Da Costa, J. M. "On Irritable Heart: A Clinical Study of a Form of Functional Cardiac Disorder and its Consequences." (1871) *The American Journal of the Medical Sciences*: 17-52.
37. Ibid., p. 18.
38. Ibid., p. 51.
39. Ibid., pp. 36-37.
40. Lewis, T. *The Soldier's Heart and The Effort Syndrome* (London: Shaw & Sons, 1940), pp. 2-3.
41. Lewis, T. *The Soldier's Heart and The Effort Syndrome* (London: Shaw & Sons, 1918), p. vi.
42. Ibid., p. vii.
43. Ibid., p. iv.
44. Lewis (1940), op. cit., p. 7.
45. Ibid., p. 11.
46. Ibid., p. 13.
47. Ibid.
48. Alvarez, op. cit., p. 398.
49. Da Costa, op. cit., p. 17.
50. Lewis (1918), op. cit., p. vi.
51. Wooley, C. F. "From Irritable Heart to Mitral Valve Prolapse — World War I, The British Experience and Thomas Lewis." (October, 1986) *The American Journal of Cardiology* 58: 844-849.
52. Ibid., p. 844.
53. Lewis (1918), op. cit., pp. vi-viii.
54. Wood, op. cit., pp. 1074-1075.
55. Cohen, M. E. et al. "Neurocirculatory Asthenia, Anxiety Neurosis or The Effort Syndrome." (1946) *Archives of Internal Medicine*: 260-281.
56. Craig, H. R and P. D. White. "Etiology and Symptoms of Neurocirculatory Asthenia." (May, 1934) *Archives of Internal Medicine* 53 (5): 633-648.
57. Wood, op. cit., p. 1079.
58. Craig and White, op. cit., p. 643.
59. Alvarez, op. cit., p. 398.
60. Craig and White, op. cit., p. 633.
61. White, P. D. *Heart Disease*. 3rd ed. (New York: The MacMillan Co., 1947), p. 515.
62. Craig and White, op. cit., p. 634.
63. White, *Heart Disease*, op. cit., p. 520.
64. Magarian, G. J. "Hyperventilation Syndromes: Infrequently Recognized Common Expressions of Anxiety and Stress." (1982) *Medicine* 61 (4):219-236.

65. Craig and White, op. cit., p. 637.

66. Ibid., pp. 637-639.

67. Ibid., p. 644.

68. Grant, R. T. "Observations on the After Histories of Men Suffering from the Effort Syndrome." (1925) *Heart* XII: 121-142.

69. Craig and White, op. cit., p. 637.

70. Ibid., p. 645.

71. Ibid., p. 646.

72. Ibid.

73. Crile, G. W. "Recurrent Hyperthyroidism, Neurocirculatory Asthenia and Peptic Ulcer: Treatment by Operations on the Suprarenal Sympathetic System." (November 28, 1931) *Journal of the American Medical Association* 97 (22): 1616-1618.

74. Johnston, F. D. "Extra Sounds Occurring in Cardiac Systole." (1938) *American Heart Journal* 15: 221-231.

75. Evans, W. "Mitral Systolic Murmurs." (1943) *British Medical Journal*: 8-9.

76. Grant, op. cit., p. 124.

77. Levine, S. A. *Clinical Heart Disease*, 5th ed. (Philadelphia: W. B. Saunders Co., 1958), p. 265.

78. Wooley, C. F. "Where are the Diseases of Yesterday?", op. cit., 745-751.

79. Ibid., p. 750.

80. Leatham, A. and W. Brigden. "Mild Mitral Regurgitation and the Mitral Prolapse Fiasco." (1980) *American Heart Journal*: 649-664.

81. Gorlin, R. "The Hyperkinetic Heart Syndrome." (November 24, 1962) *Journal of the American Medical Association* 182 (8): 84-91.

82. Barlow, J. B. and W. A. Pocock. "The Mitral Valve Prolapse Enigma — Two Decades Later." (March, 1984) *Modern Concepts of Cardiovascular Disease* 53 (3): 13-17.

83. Bryhn, M. and S. Persson. "The Prevalence of Mitral Valve Prolapse in Healthy Men and Women in Sweden." (1984) *Acta Medica Scandinavia* 215: 157-160.

84. Leatham, op. cit.

85. Barlow, J. B. *Perspectives on the Mitral Valve* (Philadelphia: F. D. Davis Co., 1987), p. 108.

Chapter Twenty

1. Johnson, Lt. Col. J.H. "Mitral Valve Prolapse: — The Facts." (1989) *Journal of the Royal Army Medical Corps* 135: 76-78

2. Carmichael, D. B. "Reflections on Medical Heroes and Mitral Prolapse." (September, 1987) *The Canadian Journal of Cardiology* 3(6): 261-262

3. Sheehan, D. V. et al. "Treatment of Endogenous Anxiety with Phobic Hysterical and Hypochondriacal Symptoms."(January 30, 1980) *Archives of General Psychiatry* 37: 51-59.

4. Ibid., p. 51.

5. Ibid.

6. Ibid., p. 59.

7. Magarian, G. J. "Hyperventilation Syndromes: Infrequently Recognized Common Expressions of Anxiety and Stress." (1982) *Medicine* 61 (4): 219-236.

8. Kantor, J. S. et al. "Mitral Valve Prolapse Syndrome in Agoraphobic Patients." (April 4, 1980) *American Journal of Psychiatry* 137: 467-469.

9. Ibid., p. 468.

10. Sheehan et al., op. cit., p. 51.

11. Pariser, S. F. et al. "Panic Attacks: Diagnostic Evaluations of 17 Patients." (January 1, 1979) *American Journal of Psychiatry* 136: 105-106.

12. Gorman, J. M. et al. "The Mitral Valve Prolapse - Panic Disorder Connection." (1988) *Psychosomatic Medicine* 50: 114-122.

13. Shapiro J. and R. J. McFerran. "Psychological Aspects of Mitral Valve Prolapse." (October, 1980) *American Family Physician* 24 (4): 100-102.

14. Sheehan et al., op. cit., p. 58.

15. Cohen, M. et al. "Neurocirculatory Asthenia, Anxiety Neurosis or The Effort Syndrome." (1946) *Archives of Internal Medicine*: 260-281.

16. Ibid., p. 266.

17. Pitts, F. N. and J. N. McClure. "Lactate Metabolism in Anxiety Neurosis." (December, 1967) *The New England Journal of Medicine* 277 (25): 1329-1336.

18. Brody, J. "Panic: Sudden Waves of Fear Linked to Physical Disorder." *The Globe and Mail,* Toronto, October 27, 1983.

19. *The Toronto Star,* July 20, 1985.

20. Raphael, S. S. et al: *Lynch's Medical Laboratory Technology* (Philadelphia: W. B. Saunders Co., 1983), p. 128.

21. Natarajan, G. et al. "Myocardial Metabolic Studies in Prolapsing Mitral Leaflet Syndrome." (1975) *Circulation* 52: 1105-1110.

22. Ibid., p. 1110.

23. Steelman, R. B. et al. "Midsystolic Clicks in Arteriosclerotic Heart Disease: A New Facet in The Syndrome of Papillary Muscle Dysfunction." (1971) *Circulation* XLVI: 503-514.

24. Aranda, J. M. et al. "Mitral Valve Prolapse and Coronary Artery Disease. Clinical, Hemodynamic and Angiographic Correlations." (August, 1975) *Circulation* 52: 245-252.

25. Raizada, V. et al. "Mitral Valve Prolapse Patients with Coronary Artery Disease: Echocardiographic and Angiographic Correlation." (1977) *British Heart Journal* 39: 53-60.

26. Chesler, E. et al. "Acute Myocardial Infarction with Normal Coronary Arteries." (August, 1976) *Circulation* 54 (2): 203-209.

27. Izumi, S. et al. "Mechanism of Mitral Regurgitation in Patients with Myocardial Infarction: A Study Using Real-time Two-dimensional Doppler Flow Imaging and Echocardiography." (1987) *Circulation* 76: 777-785.

28. Peller, O. G. et al. " Lack of Association Between Acute Myocardial Infarction and Mitral Valve Prolapse." (December 1, 1988) *The American Journal of Cardiology* 62 (17): 1297.

29. Przybojewski, J. Z. et al. "Mitral Valve Prolapse Complicated by Acute Cerebral Embolism, Arrhythmias and Painless Myocardial Infarction." (1984) *South African Medical Journal* 65: 390-396.

30. Freedman, L. *Infective Endocarditis and Other Intravascular Infections* (New York: Plenum Medical Book Co., 1983), p. 12.

31. Kannel, W. B. and R. D. Abbott. "Incidence and Prognosis of Unrecognized Myocardial Infarction; An Update on the Framingham Study." (1984) *The New England Journal of Medicine* 311: 1144-1147.

32. Boudoulas, H. et al. "Metabolic Studies in Mitral Valve Prolapse Syndrome: A Neuroendocrine Cardiovascular Process." (1980) *Circulation* 61: 1200-1205.

33. Ibid., p. 1204.

34. Alpert, J. S. *Physiopathology of the Cardiovascular System* (Boston: Little, Brown and Company, 1984), p. 83.

35. Hunter, A. *The Heart: What it Does. How it Can Go Wrong. How to Keep it Healthy* (Kingswood, Surrey, UK: Elliot Right Way Books, 1982), p. 59.

36. Boudoulas, H. et al. "Mitral Valve Prolapse: A Marker for Anxiety or Overlapping Phenomenon?" (1984) *Psychopathology* 17 (Supplement #1): 98-106.

37. Gonzalez, E. R. "Medical News: Pandora's Box of Autonomic Ills Found in Some Heart Patients." (January 9, 1981) *Journal of the American Medical Association* 245 (2): 107-108.

38. Alvarez, W. C. *The Neuroses: Diagnosis and Management of Functional Disorders and Minor Psychoses* (Philadelphia: W. B. Saunders Co., 1955), p. 26.

39. Gaffney, F. A. et al. "Autonomic Dysfunction in Women with Mitral Valve Prolapse Syndrome." (1979) *Circulation* 59 (5): 894-901.

40. Master, A. M. "Effort Syndrome or Neurocirculatory Asthenia in the Navy." (1943) *U. S. Navy Medical Bulletin* XLI (3): 666-669.

41. Starr, I. and L. Jonas. "Syndrome of Subnormal Circulation in Ambulatory Patients." (1940) *Archives of Internal Medicine* 66: 1095-1111.

42. Levine, S. A. *Clinical Heart Disease* 5th ed. (Philadelphia: W. B. Saunders Co., 1958), p. 263.

43. Alpert, op. cit., p. 1.

44. Deglin, J. M. and S. M. Deglin. "'Munchaüsen' Case." (May, 1975) *Annals of Internal Medicine* 82 (5): 721.

45. Fialk, M. A. and H. W. Murray. "Cardiac Munchaüsen Syndrome. " (1974) *Annals of Internal Medicine* 81: 562.

46. Deglin and Deglin, op. cit., p. 721.

47. Fialk and Murray, op. cit., p. 562.

48. Deglin and Deglin, op. cit., p. 721.

49. Fialk and Murray, op. cit., p. 562.

50. Deglin and Deglin, op. cit., p. 721.

51. Fialk and Murray, op. cit., p. 562.

52. Sparandero, F. "'Munchaüsen Syndrome' Cases." (1975) *Annals of Internal Medicine* 82: 123.

53. Fialk and Murray, op. cit., p. 562.

54. Sparandero, op. cit., p. 123.

55. Deglin and Deglin, op. cit., p. 721.

56. Sparendero, op. cit., p. 123.

57. Berkow, R. et al. *The Merck Manual of Diagnosis and Therapy*, 14th ed. (Rahway, New Jersey: Merck, Sharp & Dohme Research Laboratories, 1982), pp. 1406-1407.

58. Deglin and Deglin, op. cit., p. 721.

59. Jeresaty, R. *Mitral Valve Prolapse* (New York: Raven Press, 1979), p. 44.

60. Ibid.

61. McKinley, J. C. and S. R. Hathaway. "The Identification and Measurement of the Psychoneuroses in Medical Practice. The Minnesota Multiphasic Personality Inventory." (1943) *Journal of the American Medical Association* 122 (3): 161-167.

62. Ibid., p. 163.

63. Ibid., p. 164.

64. Cox, K. "Illness Not Diagnosed Until Autopsy, Jury Told". *The Globe and Mail*, Toronto, June 8, 1983.

65. Szmuiluwicz, J. and J. G. Flannery. "Mitral Valve Prolapse Syndrome and Psychological Disturbance." (May, 1980) *Psychosomatics* 21 (5): 419-421.

66. Ibid., p. 420.

67. Ibid. p. 421.

68. Ibid. p. 420.

69. Personal Communication from Jane McCulley, Doctoral Candidate in Psychology at McMaster University, Hamilton, Ontario, Canada. This project was announced on CBC Radio's "Classy Classified".

70. "They've Got 'Heart' at St. Joseph's." *West Hamilton Journal*, Hamilton, Ontario, April 20, 1983.

71. Gadd, J. "Doctors Open Panic Clinic". *The Globe and Mail*, Toronto, November 16, 1983.

72. Ibid.

73. Brody, J. "Panic: Sudden Waves of Fear Linked to Physical Disorder." *The Globe and Mail*, Toronto, October 27, 1983.

74. Gorman, J. M. et al. "Effect of Imipramine on Prolapsed Mitral Valves of Patients with Panic Disorder." (July, 1981) *American Journal of Psychiatry* 138 (7): 977-978.

75. Grunhaus, L. et al. "Mitral Valve Prolapse and Panic Attacks." (1982) *Israel Journal of Medical Science* 18: 221-223.

76. Krogh, C. M. E. et al. *Compendium of Pharmaceuticals and Specialties*. 21st ed. (Ottawa: Canadian Pharmaceutical Association, 1986), p. 485.

77. Nickerson, M. "Antihypertensive Agents and The Drug Therapy of Hypertension" in *The Pharmacological Basis of Therapeutics*. 4th ed. Goodman, L. S. and A. Gilman, eds. (New York: The MacMillan Co., 1970), p. 732.

78. Krogh et al., op. cit., p. 486.

79. Ibid., p. 346.

80. Marshall, C. E. et al. "Sudden Death and the Ballooning Posterior Leaflet Syndrome." (1974) *Archives of Pathology* 98: 134-138.

81. Grunhaus, L. et al., op. cit., p. 222.

82. Hart, R. G. and D. Easton. "Mitral Valve Prolapse and Cerebral Infarction." (1982) *Stroke* 13 (4): 429-430.

83. Barlow, J. B. and C. K. Bosman. "Aneurysmal Protrusion of the Posterior Leaflet of the Mitral Valve: An Auscultatory-electrocardiographic Syndrome." (1966) *American Heart Journal* 71: 166-178.

84. Barnett, H. J. M. "Transient Cerebral Ischemia: Pathogenesis, Prognosis and Management." (1974) *Annals of the Royal College of Physicians and Surgeons of Canada* 7: 153-173.

85. Ibid., p. 154.

86. Barnett, H. J. M. "Embolism in Mitral Valve Prolapse." (1982) *Annual Review of Medicine* 33: 489-507.

87. Barnett, H. J. M. "Cerebral Ischemic Events Associated with Prolapsing Mitral Valve." (1975) *Trans American Neurological Association* 100: 84-87.

88. Barnett, H. J. M. et al. "Cerebral Ischemic Events Associated with Prolapsing Mitral Valve." (1976) *Archives of Neurology* 33: 777-782.

89. Barnett, H. J. M. et al. "Mitral Valve Prolapse — A Modern Epidemic?" (1977) *Annals of the Royal College of Physicians and Surgeons of Ontario* 10: 286-289.

90. Barnett, H. J. M. et al. "Further Evidence Relating Mitral Valve Prolapse to Cerebral Ischemic Events. (1980) *The New England Journal of Medicine* 302: 139-144.

91. Barnett, H. J. M. "Embolism in Mitral Valve Prolapse." (1982), op. cit.

92. Barnett, H. J. M. et al. "Further Evidence Relating Mitral Valve Prolapse to Cerebral Ischemic Events." (1980), op. cit., p. 139.

93. Sandok, B. A. and E. R. Giuliani. "Cerebral Ischemic Events in Patients with Mitral Valve Prolapse." (1982) *Stroke* 13 (4): 448-450.

94. Wolf, P. A. and C. Sila. "Cerebral Ischemia with Mitral Valve Prolapse." (1987) *American Heart Journal* 113 (5): 1308-1315.

95. Nishimura, R. A. et al. "Echocardiographically Documented Mitral Valve Prolapse Long Term Follow Up of 237 Patients." (1985) *The New England Journal of Medicine* 313 (21): 1305-1309.

96. Wolf, op. cit., p. 1309.

97. Walsh, P. N. et al. "Platelets, Thromboembolism and Mitral Valve Prolapse." (March, 1981) *Circulation* 63 (3): 552-559.

98. Woldoff, H. S. et al. "Retinal Vascular Lesions in Two Patients with Prolapsed Mitral Valve Leaflets." (1975) *American Journal of Opthamology* 79 (3): 382-385.

99. Kimball, R. W. and T. R. Hedges. " Amaurosis Fugax Caused by a Prolapsed Mitral Valve Leaflet in the Mid-Systolic Click, Late Systolic Murmur Syndrome." (April, 1977) *American Journal of Opthamology*: 469-470.

100. Saffro, R. and J. V. Talano. "Transient Ischemic Attack Associated with Mitral Systolic Clicks." (1979) *Archives of Internal Medicine* 139: 693-694.

101. Caltrider, N. D. et al. "Retinal Emboli in Patients with Mitral Valve Prolapse." (1980) *American Journal of Opthamology* 90: 534-539.

102. Hart and Easton, op. cit.

103. Jones, H. R. et al. "Mitral Valve Prolapse and Cerebral Ischemic Events. (July-August, 1982) *Stroke* 13 (4): 452-453.

104. Scharf, R. E. et al. "Cerebral Ischemia in Young Patients: Is it Associated with Mitral Valve Prolapse and Abnormal Platelet Activity in Vivo?" (July-August, 1982) *Stroke* 13 (4): 454-458.

105. Kouvaras, G. and G. Bacoulas. "Association of Mitral Valve Leaflet Prolapse with Cerebral Ischaemic Events in the Young and Early Middle-aged Patient." (1985) *Quarterly Journal of Medicine* 55 (219): 387-392.

106. Kelley, R. E. et al. "Cerebral Ischemia and Mitral Valve Prolapse: Case-Control Study of Associated Factors." (April, 1988) *Stroke* 19 (4): 443-446.

107. Adams, R. D. and Griffith, J. F. "Migraine" in *Harrison's Principles of Internal Medicine.* 7th ed., Wintrobe, M. M. et al., eds. (New York: McGraw-Hill Book Co., 1974), p. 1864.

108. Litman, G. I. and H. M. Friedman. "Migraine and the Mitral Valve Prolapse Syndrome." (November, 1978) *American Heart Journal* 96 (5): 610-614.

109. Guest, M. A. and A. L. Woolf. "Fatal Infarction of Brain in Migraine." (1964) *British Medical Journal* 1: 225.

110. Wallis, D.E. and J. Godwin. "Mitral Valve Prolapse, Cerebral Ischemia and Protein S Deficiency." (May, 1988) *The American Journal of Medicine* 84: 974.

111. *The Globe and Mail,* Toronto, April 20, 1984.

112. McQuaig, Linda. "Warning on Birth Control Pills Pale Version of US Caution." *The Globe and Mail,* Toronto, April 4, 1984.

113. Makin, K. "Pill Makers Deceived Women, Trial Told." *The Globe and Mail,* Toronto, March 14, 1984.

114. "MD Says He'd Still Give the Pill." *The Globe and Mail,* Toronto, March 3, 1984.

115. Cox, R. "Hospital's Doctors Blamed by Father for Woman's Death." *The Globe and Mail,* Toronto, August 30, 1983.

116. Cox, R. "Consumer Information with Birth Control Pill Described as Adequate." *The Globe and Mail,* Toronto, August 31, 1983.

117. "Inquest Ordered on Pill-related Death." *The Globe and Mail,* Toronto, August 13, 1984.

118. From the letters of Maria Callas quoted in Stassinopoulas, A. *Maria Callas* (London: Weidenfeld and Nicholson, Ltd., 1980), p. 362.

119. Meneghini, G. B. with R. Allegri. (trans. Wisneski, H.) *My Wife, Maria Callas* (New York: Farrar, Straus, Giroux, 1982), p. 319-320.

120. Legge, W. "Callas Remembered: La Divina." (November, 1972) *Opera News* 42 (5): 11.

121. Meneghini, op. cit., p. 29.

122. Schutte, J. E. et al. "Distinctive Anthropomorphic Characteristics of Women with Mitral Valve Prolapse." (October, 1981) *The American Journal of Medicine* 71: 533-538.

123. Lieberfarb, R. M. et al. "Letter to the Editor." (April 19, 1984) *The New England Journal of Medicine* 310 (16): 1054.

124. Stassinopoulas, op. cit., p. 395.

125. Barlow, J. B. and W. A. Pocock. "The Mitral Valve Prolapse Enigma — Two Decades Later." (1984) *Modern Concepts of Cardiovascular Disease* 53: 13-17.

126. Meneghini, op. cit., p. 6.

127. *Healthsharing,* Vol. 2, #2, March, 1986, p. 5.

128. Meneghini, op. cit., pp. 87-97.

129. Ibid., p. 210.

130. Stassinopoulas, A. op. cit., p. 396.

131. Czarnecki, M. "Glenn Gould, 1932-1982." (October, 1982) *Maclean's*: 38-44.

132. Barnett, H. J. M. "Embolism in Mitral Valve Prolapse," op. cit., p. 492.

133. Berkow et al., op. cit., pp. 389-391, 558.

134. Friedrich, O. H. *Glenn Gould: A Life and Variations* (Toronto: Lester and Orpen Denys, 1989), p. 318.

135. Ibid., p. 78-80.

136. Epstein, F. H. "Glomerulonephritis" in *Harrison's Principles of Internal Medicine,* op. cit., p. 1389.

137. Schrier, R. W. *Renal and Electrolyte Disorders* (Boston: Little, Brown and Co., 1986), p. 402-403.

138. Friedrich, op. cit., p. 318-319.

139. Ibid.

140. Ibid.

141. Wyngaarden, J.B. "Gout and Other Disorders of Uric Acid Metabolism" in *Harrison's Principles of Internal Medicine*, op. cit., p. 615.

142. Ibid., p. 608.

143. Friedrich, op. cit., p. 318 ff.

144. Fisher, C. M. et al. "Cerebrovascular Disease" in *Harrison's Principles of Internal Medicine*, op. cit., p. 1768.

145. Friedrich, op. cit., p. 332.

146. Ruskin, J. N. et al. "Antiarrhythmic Drugs: A Possible Cause of Out of Hospital Cardiac Arrest. (November, 1983) *The New England Journal of Medicine* 309 (21): 1302-1305.

147. *Statistics Canada.* (1986), Causes of Death: Vital Statistics. Vol IV. Detailed Categories of the "International Classification of Diseases", (ICD), Catalogue 84-203.

148. Marshall and Shappell, op. cit., p. 135.

149. Winkle, R. A. et al. "Life Threatening Arrhythmias in the Mitral Valve Prolapse Syndrome." (June, 1976) *The American Journal of Medicine* 60: 961-968.

150. Dubin, D. *Rapid Interpretation of EKG's* (Tampa, Florida: Cover Publishing Co., 1970), pp. 8-20.

151. Shappell, S. D. et al. "Sudden Death and the Familial Occurrence of Mid-Systolic Click, Late Systolic Murmur Syndrome." (November, 1973) *Circulation* 48: 1128-1134.

152. Koch, F. H. and E. W. Hancock. "Ten-year Follow-up of Forty Patients with the Mid-Systolic Click/Late Systolic Murmur Syndrome." (1976) *American Journal of Cardiology* 37: 149.

153. Kligfield, P. et al. "Arrhythmias and Sudden Death in Mitral Valve Prolapse." (1987) *American Heart Journal* 113(5): 1298-1307.

154. Ibid., p. 1299.

155. Kligfield, P. et al. "Relation of Sudden Death in Pure Mitral Regurgitation, With and Without Mitral Valve Prolapse, to Repetitive Ventricular Arrhythmias and Right and Left Ventricular Ejection Fractions." (August, 1987) *The American Journal of Cardiology* 60: 397-399.

156. Hurst, J. W. "Cardiac Arrhythmias and Conduction Disturbances: Approach to the Problems of Cardiac Arrhythmias" in *The Heart.* 3rd ed., Hurst, J. W. et al., eds. (New York: McGraw-Hill Book Co., 1974), p. 529.

157. Nishimura, R. A. et al. *op. cit.*

158. Kligfield et al, "Arrhythmias and Sudden Death in Mitral Valve Prolapse," op. cit., p. 1300.

159. Cheitlin, M. D. and R. C. Byrd. "Prolapsed Mitral Valve: The Commonest Valve Disease?" (January 8, 1984) *Current Problems in Cardiology* 10: 1-54.

160. Kligfield et al. "Arrhythmias and Sudden Death in Mitral Valve Prolapse," op. cit., p. 1301.

161. Barlow, J. B. *Perspectives on the Mitral Valve* (Philadelphia: F. D. Davis Co., 1987), p. 101.

162. Rayburn, W. F. and M. E. Fontana. "Mitral Valve Prolapse and Pregnancy." (November, 1981) *American Journal of Obstetrics and Gynecology* 141 (1): 9-11.

163. Ibid., p. 10.

164. Artal, R. et al. "Transient Ischemic Attack: A Complication of Mitral Valve Prolapse in Pregnancy." (June, 1988) *Obstetrics and Gynecology* 71 (6): 1028-1029.

165. Gonzalez, E. R. "Pandora's Box of Autonomic Ills Found in Some Heart Patients." (January 9, 1981) *Journal of the American Medical Association* 245 (2): 107-108.

166. "Many Sleep Apnea Patients May be Improperly Treated." *The Medical Post*, November 30, 1982.

167. Carswell, H. "Scan Shows Obstruction in Sleep Apnea Patients." *The Medical Post*, October 19, 1982.

168. Berkow, R. et al. op. cit., p. 1856.

169. Ibid.

170. Kaplan, E. L. "Infective Endocarditis in the Pediatric Age Group: An Overview" in *Infective Endocarditis: An American Heart Association Symposium*, American Heart Association Monograph #52, Kaplan, E. L. and A. V. Taranta eds., (Dallas: The American Heart Association, Inc., 1977), pp. 51-54

171. Mazza, D. L. et al. "Prevalence of Anxiety Disorder in Patients with Mitral Valve Prolapse." (March, 1986) *American Journal of Psychiatry* 143 (3): 349-352.

172. Rosenberg, C. A. et al. "Hypomastia and Mitral Valve Prolapse. " (November, 1983) *The New England Journal of Medicine* 309 (20): 1230-1232.

173. Starr, I. and L. Jonas. "Syndrome of Subnormal Circulation in Ambulatory Patients." (November, 1940) *Archives of Internal Medicine* 66: 1095-1111.

174. Rosenberg et al., op. cit., p. 1231.

175. Schlant, R. C. et al. "Mitral Valve Prolapse" in *Disease-A-Month* Vol XXVI (10): Dowling, H. F., ed., (Chicago: Year Book Medical Publishers, Inc., 1980), pp. 11-51.

176. O'Rourke, R. A. and M. H. Crawford. "Systolic-Click Murmur Syndrome." (1976) *Current Problems in Cardiology* 1: 1-60.

177. Perloff, J. K. and J. S. Child. "Clinical and Epidemiological Issues in Mitral Valve Prolapse: Overview and Perspective." (May, 1987) *American Heart Journal* 113 (5): 1324-1332.

178. Ibid., p. 1324.

179. Wolferth, C. C. and A. Margolies. "Gallop Rhythm." (1933) *International Clinics* 1: 16-30.

180. Santos, A. D. et al. "Orthostatic Hypotension: A Commonly Unrecognized Cause of Symptoms in Mitral Valve Prolapse." (November, 1981) *The American Journal of Medicine* 71: 746-750.

181. Coghlan, H. C. et al. "Dysautonomia in MVP." (1979) *The American Journal of Medicine* 67: 894-901.

182. MacLean, A. R. and E. V. Allen. "Orthostatic Hypotension and Orthostatic Tachycardia." (December, 1940) *Journal of the American Medical Association* 115 (25): 2163-2167.

183. Gonzalez, op. cit., p. 107.

184. Hickey, A. J. et al. "Independence of Mitral Valve Prolapse and Neurosis." (1983) *British Heart Journal* 50: 333-336.

185. Ibid., p. 335.

186. Brody, J., op. cit.

187. Mazza et al. op. cit., p. 349.

188. Bor, D. and D. U. Himmelstein. "Endocarditis Prophylaxis for Patients with Mitral Valve Prolapse: A Quantitative Analysis." (April, 1984) *The American Journal of Medicine* 76: 711-717.

189. Freedman, op. cit., p. 1.

190. Retchin, S. M. et al. "Endocarditis Prophylaxis and Mitral Valve Prolapse: What is the "risk"?" (1984) *International Journal of Cardiology* 5: 653-659.

191. Baddour, L. M. and A. L. Bisno. "Infective Endocarditis Complicating Mitral Valve Prolapse: Epidemiologic, Clinical and Microbiologic Aspects." (January-February, 1986) *Reviews of Infectious Disease* 8 (1): 117-137.

192. Freedman, op. cit., p.88.

Chapter Twenty-one

1. Alvarez, W. *The Neuroses: Diagnosis and Management of Functional Disorders and Minor Psychoses* (Philadelphia: W. B. Saunders Co., 1955), p. 172.

2. Berkow, R. et al. *The Merck Manual of Diagnosis and Therapy.* 14th ed. (Rahway, New Jersey: Merck, Sharp & Dohme Research Laboratories, 1982), pp. 172-179.

3. Vose, J. M. et al. "Recurrent Streptoccus Mutans Endocarditis." (March 23, 1987) *The American Journal of Medicine* 82: 630-632.

4. Wasilkoff, P. C. and C. G. Maurice. "Role of Endodontics in Current Dental Practice." (October, 1976) *Journal of the American Dental Association* 93: 802.

5. "Gum Disease: The Later Problem." *Consumer Reports*, March 1984, pp. 133-137.

6. Viewpoint. *Dental Economics*, March 1977, p. 22.

7. Alvarez. op. cit., p. 46.

8. French, O. *The Globe and Mail*, Toronto, July 24, 1984.

9. Miller, M. Letter from a Dental Patient, *Dental Economics*, June 12, 1977, pp. 52-53.

10. Lewis, D. W. "Dental Health Services Research in Ontario." (May, 1977) *Ontario Dentist* 54 (5): 26-28.

11. Ibid., pp. 27-28.

12. "Tooth Decay: The Early Problem". (March, 1984) *Consumer Reports*: 130-132.

13. Elliott, R. H. and J. M. Dunbar. "Antibiotic Sensitivity of Oral Alpha-Hemolytic Streptococcus from Children with Congenital or Acquired Cardiac Disease: A Prolonged Survey." (May 3, 1977) *British Dental Journal* 142: 283-285.

14. Simon, D. S. and J. F. Goodwin. "Should Good Teeth Be Extracted to Prevent Streptococcus Viridans Endocarditis?" (June 12, 1971) *The Lancet*: 1207-1209.

15. Harris, A. H. "President-elect Speaks on Dental Care Plans." (April, 1977) *Ontario Dentist* 54 (4): 7-9.

16. Ibid., pp. 7-8.

17. Pownall, K. "Malpractice." (October, 1977) *Ontario Dentist* 54 (10): 29-30.

18. Gifford-Jones, W. "Surgeon alone Can't Work Miracles". *The Globe and Mail*, Toronto, April 28, 1983.

19. Brody, J. E. "Self-Blame Helps Victims Recover: Study." *The Globe and Mail*, Toronto, January 18, 1984.

20. Silversides, A. "Review of 200 Physicians Reveals Problems with 26." *The Globe and Mail*, Toronto, June 6, 1984.

21. Stephens, R. "Monitor Doctors Over 80, Health Board Report Urges." *The Globe and Mail*, Toronto, July 27, 1984.

22. "College of Physicians, Surgeons Sued: Halt Snooping in Files: Docs." *The Toronto Sun*, August 27, 1982.

23. Brunner, L. S. et al. "Diagnostic Studies and Their Meaning" (Appendix) in *Medical Surgical Nursing* (Philadelphia: J. B. Lippincott Company, 1970), p. 977.

24. Sholtis-Brunner, L. and D. Smith-Suddarth. "Diagnostic Studies and Their Meaning" (Appendix I) in *The Lippincott Manual of Nursing* (Philadelphia: J. B. Lippincott, 1982), p. 1480.

25. Wallach, J. *Interpretation of Diagnostic Tests: A Handbook Synopsis of Laboratory Medicine* (Boston: Little, Brown and Co., 1983), p. 18.

26. Boulton-Jones, J. M. et al. "Renal Lesions of Subacute Infective Endocarditis." (April, 1974) *British Medical Journal* 2: 11-14.

27. Wurman, R. S. *Medical Access* (Los Angeles: Access Press Ltd., 1985), p. 57.

28. Welt, L. G. "Edema" in *Harrison's Principles of Internal Medicine*. 7th ed., Wintrobe, M. M. et al., eds., (New York: McGraw-Hill Book Co., 1974), p. 181.

29. Galloway, A. C. et al. "Current Concepts of Mitral Valve Reconstruction for Mitral Insufficiency." (November, 1988) *Circulation* 78 (5): 1087-1098.

30. Sheppard, R. "Too Quick With the Knife." *The Globe and Mail*, Toronto, September 27, 1983.

31. Oury, J. H. et al. "Mitral Valve Replacement Versus Reconstruction." (June, 1977) *The Journal of Thoracic and Cardiovascular Surgery* 73 (6): 825-833.

32. Ibid., p. 825.

33. Carpentier, A. "Cardiac Valve Surgery — The 'French Connection'." (1983) *The Journal of Thoracic and Cardiovascular Surgery* 86: 323-337.

34. Williams, Tennessee. "A Streetcar Named Desire" in *Penguin Plays* (Middlesex, England: Penguin Books Ltd., 1962), p.194.

35. Barlow, J. B. *Perspectives on the Mitral Valve* (Philadelphia: F. A. Davis Co., 1987), p. 261-264.

36. Galloway et al., op. cit., p. 1087.

37. Carpentier, A. "Valve Surgery — the 'French connection'," op. cit., p.324.

38. Ibid., p. 327ff.

39. Bonchek, L. I. "Correction of Mitral Valve Disease without Valve Replacement." (October, 1982) *American Heart Journal* 104 (4): 865-868.

40. Ibid.

41. Galloway et al., op. cit., p. 1088.

42. Kay, J. H. et al. "Mitral Valve Repair for Significant Mitral Insufficiency." (August, 1978) *American Heart Journal* 96 (2): 253-262.

43. Bonchek, op. cit., p. 865.

44. Galloway et al., op. cit., p. 1089.

45. Ibid.

46. Carpentier, "Valve Surgery — the 'French Connection'," op. cit., pp. 335-336.

47. Carpentier, A. et al. "Reconstructive Surgery of Mitral Incompetence." (1980) *The Journal of Thoracic and Cardiovascular Surgery* 79: 338-348.

48. Galloway et al., op. cit., pp. 1093, 1096.

49. Caidahl, K. et al. "Conservative Surgery for Mitral Valve Prolapse with Regurgitation: Clinical Follow-up and Noninvasive Assessment." (1987) *European Heart Journal* 8: 384-394.

50. Galloway et al., op. cit., p. 1097.

51. Barwinsky, J. "Cardiac Valve Replacement: Canadian Review 1978-86." (November-December, 1988) *Journal of Cardiology* 4 (8): 422-424.

52. Kay, op. cit.

53. Carpentier, "Valve Surgery — the 'French Connection'," op. cit., p. 337.

54. Kay, op. cit., p. 257.

55. Guy, F. C. "Mitral Valve Prolapse as a Cause of Hemodynamically Important Mitral Regurgitation." (March, 1980) *The Canadian Journal of Surgery* 23 (2): 166-182.

56. Waller, B. F. et al. "Etiology of Clinically Isolated, Severe, Chronic, Pure Mitral Regurgitation: Analysis of 97 Patients over 30 Years of Age Having Mitral Valve Replacement." (1982) *American Heart Journal* 104: 276-288.

57. Galloway et al., op. cit., p. 1089.

58. Brown, E. R. *Rockefeller Medicine Men: Medicine and Capitalism in The Progressive Era* (Los Angeles: University of California Press, Berkeley, 1979), p. 232.

59. Slotnik, L. "Billing Clause Enrages MDs", *The Globe and Mail*, Toronto, June 7, 1983.

60. "So . . . how would you like your open heart surgery done by a civil servant?", *The Globe and Mail*, March 24, 1984.

61. Cruickshank, J. "Ontario has too many MDs: Minister", *The Globe and Mail*, Toronto, September 1, 1983.

62. Slotnik, L. "Right-wing Group Fights Health Act: Give to Coalition OMA Urges Doctors", *The Globe and Mail*, Toronto, March 24, 1984.

63. "A Fight Between Freedom and Slavery. OMA Calls Health Act a Federal Power Play", *The Globe and Mail*, March 1, 1984.

64. "Changes to Health Act a Fraud, CMA Charges", *The Globe and Mail*, Toronto, March 21, 1984.

65. Montgomery, C. "CMA Cries Rape, Offers to Back Medicare Strike", *The Globe and Mail*, Toronto, December 14, 1983.

66. Ibid.

67. Silversides, A. "Proposed Extra-billing Ban Slur on Doctors, MD Charges", *The Globe and Mail*, Toronto, December 21, 1985.

68. "Your Doctor: Who Knows More About Health Care", *The Globe and Mail*, Toronto, April 13, 1983.

69. "Most MDs Feel They Have the Right to Coerce Patients if Necessary", *The Globe and Mail*, Toronto, August 18, 1983.

70. *Sick — and Therefore Defenceless.* (March, 1979) The Patients' Centre (Corbusier Community Workshop): A Forum for Community Action of The Gottlieb Duttweiler Institute, Zurich, Switzerland. A Report of Experiences on the Patient in our Health Care System, p. 3.

71. "We Believe Canada's New Health Act May be Dangerous to Your Health", *The Globe and Mail,* Toronto, February 29, 1984.

72. McLaren, C. "OMA Bears the Brunt of the Anger: Doctors Sick of Obeying Rules", *The Globe and Mail,* Toronto, March 7, 1984.

73. Linden, A. M. "The Patient, the Doctor and Their Duty to Communicate with One Another." (Spring, 1981) *Health Law in Canada*: 57-65.

74. Ibid., p. 63.

75. Krever, Hon. Justice H. *Report of the Commission of Inquiry into the Confidentiality of Health Information* Vol 2. (Toronto: J. C. Thatcher, Queen's Printer for Ontario, 1980), p. 489.

76. Curran, W. J. "Law Medicine Notes: Massachusetts Patients' Bill of Rights: Cabbages, Kings, Sausages and Laws." (December 27, 1979) *The New England Journal of Medicine* 301 (26): 1433-1435.

77. Jones, R. B. et al. "Censoring of Patient-held Records by Doctors." (March, 1988) *Journal of the Royal College of General Practitioners*: 117-118.

78. Krever, op. cit., p. 455.

79. Ibid., p. 468.

80. Galloway, J. D. *The Review of the Report on the Confidentiality of Health Information,* Ontario Ministry of Health, October 31, 1981, p. 5.

81. Krever, op. cit., p. 462.

82. Ibid., p. 470.

83. Ibid., p. 469.

84. Galloway, *The Review of the Report on the Confidentiality of Health Information,* op. cit., p. 60.

85. Krever, op. cit., p. 471.

86. Ibid., p. 469.

87. Galloway, *The Review of the Report on the Confidentiality of Health Information,* op. cit., p. 59.

88. Ibid., p. 59.

89. Ibid.

90. Krever, op. cit., p. 473.

91. Ibid., p. 476.

92. Ibid., p. 475.

93. Ibid., p. 478.

94. Galloway, *The Review of the Report on the Confidentiality of Health Information,* op. cit., p. 63.

95. Krever, op. cit., p. 485.

96. Ibid.

97. Galloway, *The Review of the Report on the Confidentiality of Health Information,* op. cit., p. 62.

98. Ibid.

99. Ibid., p. 57.

100. Canadian Medical Protective Association. *Annual Report,* Report of the General Counsel for the year 1980 (Ottawa: CMPA, August 26, 1981), p. 40.

101. Canadian Medical Protective Association. *Annual Report,* Report of the General Counsel for the Year 1976 (Ottawa: CMPA, June 22, 1977), p. 25.

102. Ibid.

103. Galloway, *The Review of the Report on the Confidentiality of Health Information,* op. cit., p. 62.

104. Ibid.
105. Ibid.
106. Ibid.
107. Linden, A., op. cit., p. 64.
108. Canadian Medical Protective Association. *Annual Reports*, (Ottawa: Canadian Medical Protective Association, June 9, 1971, p. 21 and October 1, 1983, p. 21.
109. Galloway, op. cit., p. 63.
110. Krever, op. cit., p. 461-462.
111. *The New York Times Book Review*, April 5, 1981, p. 10.
112. Gifford-Jones, W. *The Doctor Game* (Toronto: McClelland and Stewart, 1975), p. 21.
113. Reed, C. "TV as a Shaper of Culture: Life Imitates Unreality." *The Globe and Mail*, Toronto, May 30, 1985.
114. Mendelsohn, R. S. *Confessions of a Medical Heretic* (New York: Warner Books, 1979), p. 289.
115. Rozovsky, L. E. and F. A. Rozovsky. "Avoid Malpractice Suits by Communicating with Your Patients." (November, 1982) *Canadian Doctor*: 71-72.
116. Mendelsohn, op. cit., p. 283.
117. Ibid., p. 134.
118. Ibid., p. 171.
119. Ibid., p. 72.
120. Ibid., p. 165.
121. Tushnet, L. *The Medicine Men: The Myth of Quality Medical Care in America Today* (New York: St. Martin's Press, 1971), p. 104.
122. Ibid., p. 153.
123. Ibid.
124. Rosenfeld, I. *Second Opinion* (New York: The Linden Press/Simon & Schuster, 1981), p. 363.
125. Ibid., p. 364.
126. Ibid.
127. Ibid., p. 365.
128. Gifford-Jones, W. "Doctors Who Distort the Facts", *The Globe and Mail*, Toronto, July 18, 1985.
129. Mendelsohn, op. cit., p. 43.
130. Johnson, M. Letter to the Editor. (1988) *Journal of Family Practice* 26 (1): 18.
131. Gifford-Jones, W. *The Doctor Game*, op. cit., p. 26.
132. Lambert, E. *Modern Medical Mistakes*. (Toronto: Fitzhenry and Whiteside, 1978), p. 27.
133. Gifford-Jones, W. "When Does Tonsillitis Call for Surgery?", *The Globe and Mail*, Toronto, November 22, 1984.
134. Tushnet, op. cit., p. 127.
135. Ibid., pp. 127-128.
136. Mendelsohn, R. S. *Malepractice: How Doctors Manipulate Women* (Chicago: Contemporary Books, Inc., 1981), p. 46.
137. Loesche, W. J. "Indigenous Human Flora and Bacteremia" in *Infective Endocarditis: An American Heart Association Symposium*, American Heart Association Monograph #52, Kaplan, E. L. and A. V. Taranta, eds. (Dallas: The American Heart Association, Inc., 1977), p. 40-43.
138. Mendelsohn, R. S. Malepractice, op. cit., p. 46.
139. Berkow, R. et al. *The Merck Manual of Diagnosis and Therapy* (Rahway, New Jersey: Merck, Sharp & Dohme Research Laboratories, 1982) p. 82.
140. Tushnet, op. cit., p. 7.

141. Ibid., p. 65.
142. *House of Commons Debates*. Official Report (Hansard), Vol. 129, #321, 2nd Session, 33rd Parliament, Thursday, June 2, 1988, p. 16088.
143. Barlow, J. B. *Perspectives on the Mitral Valve* (Philadelphia: F. A. Davis Co., 1987). p. 98.
144. Yee, J. Letter to the Editor (November, 1988) *Chest* 94 (5), p. 1110.
145. Canadian Medical Protective Association. *Annual Report*, Report of General Counsel for the Year 1976 (Ottawa: Canadian Medical Protective Association, June 22, 1977), p. 25.

Index